Neuro-
degenerative
Diseases

Alzheimer's and Parkinson's Diseases: Advances, Concepts and New Challenges

9th International Conference AD/PD
Prague, Czech Republic, March 11–15, 2009

PROCEEDINGS

Guest Editors
Manfred Windisch, Graz
Roger M. Nitsch, Zürich
Abraham Fisher, Ness Ziona
Israel Hanin, Tucson, Ariz.

75 figures, 4 in color, and 22 tables, 2010

KARGER Basel · Freiburg · Paris · London · New York · Bangalore · Bangkok · Shanghai · Singapore · Tokyo · Sydney

S. Karger
Medical and Scientific Publishers
Basel • Freiburg • Paris • London •
New York • Bangalore • Bangkok •
Shanghai • Singapore • Tokyo • Sydney

Disclaimer
The statements, opinions and data contained in this publication are solely those of the individual authors and contributors and not of the publisher and the editor(s). The appearance of advertisements in the journal is not a warranty, endorsement, or approval of the products or services advertised or of their effectiveness, quality or safety. The publisher and the editor(s) disclaim responsibility for any injury to persons or property resulting from any ideas, methods, instructions or products referred to in the content or advertisements.

Drug Dosage
The authors and the publisher have exerted every effort to ensure that drug selection and dosage set forth in this text are in accord with current recommendations and practice at the time of publication. However, in view of ongoing research, changes in government regulations, and the constant flow of information relating to drug therapy and drug reactions, the reader is urged to check the package insert for each drug for any change in indications and dosage and for added warnings and precautions. This is particularly important when the recommended agent is a new and/or infrequently employed drug.

Printed in Switzerland
on acid-free and non-aging paper (ISO 9706) by
Reinhardt Druck, Basel
ISBN 978–3–8055–9358–8
e-ISBN 978–3–8055–9359–5

KARGER

Fax +41 61 306 12 34
E-Mail karger@karger.ch
www.karger.com

Neuro-degenerative Diseases

www.karger.com/neurodis

KARGER

Printed in Switzerland on acid-free and non-aging paper (ISO 9706) by Reinhardt Druck, Basel

Appears bimonthly: 1 volume per year (6 issues)

Guidelines for Authors

Neuro-degenerative Diseases

'Neurodegenerative Diseases' is a bimonthly, multidisciplinary journal for the publication of advances in the understanding of 'Neurodegenerative Diseases', including Alzheimer disease, Parkinson's disease, amyotrophic lateral sclerosis, Huntington disease and related neurological and psychiatric disorders. 'Neurodegenerative Diseases' publishes results from basic and clinical scientific research programs designed to better understand the normal functions of genes and proteins involved in 'Neurodegenerative Diseases', to characterize their role in pathogenic disease mechanisms, to model their functions in animals and to explore their roles in the diagnosis, treatment and prevention of 'Neurodegenerative Diseases'. It is our firm belief that successful strategies for novel treatments of 'Neurodegenerative Diseases' will emerge from the intelligent integration of basic neurobiology with clinical sciences. Therefore, 'Neurodegenerative Diseases' will accept high-quality papers from a broad spectrum of scientific research areas ranging from molecular and cell biology to neuroscience, pharmacology, genetics and the clinical sciences.
'Neurodegenerative Diseases' is a peer-reviewed journal that publishes original research in the form of Articles and Brief Communications to 'Neurodegenerative Diseases' as well as Review Articles, Mini Reviews and Commentaries.

Submission

Only original papers written in English are considered and should be submitted online:

www.karger.com/ndd

Should you experience any problems with your submission, please contact:

ndd@karger.ch

Editorial Office 'Neurodegenerative Diseases'
S. Karger AG
P.O. Box
CH–4009 Basel (Switzerland)
Tel. +41 61 306 1358
Fax +41 61 306 1434

Names, postal and e-mail addresses of four experts in the appropriate area of research should accompany each manuscript. Selected scientist(s) will be invited to act as referee(s). Referees suggested should not be from the same institution as the author and should have expert knowledge of the subject.

Articles should be fully documented reports of original research. They must describe significant and original observations to be critically evaluated and, if necessary, repeated. They do not normally exceed 6 printed pages including all figures, tables and references.
Brief Communications to Neurodegenerative Diseases are short reports of original research and are intended to provide a rapid means of reporting new findings of sufficient importance. They do not normally exceed 2 printed pages including an abstract, essential references and not more than 3 tables or figures.
Review Articles, Mini Reviews and Commentaries are either invited by the Editors or may be submitted for consideration. Authors who wish to contribute a manuscript to one of these categories should contact the Editor-in-Chief.

Review Articles describe new developments of interdisciplinary significance and highlight unresolved questions and future directions. They do not generally occupy more than 9 printed pages. Mini Reviews should focus on topics of current interest and not exceed 5 printed pages.

Commentaries should offer a more personalized perspective on a topic that will be of interest to the general readership and fill an integral number of printed pages, generally one or two, including one or two small figures. All contributions to these categories will be subjected to editorial review.
Reports should comprise title page, Key Words, Abstract, Introduction, Results and Discussion, References, tables, figure legends, and figures – in this order.

Special Section: Modeling Neurodegenerative Diseases in vivo

Editorial policies and guidelines for submission to this section are as those given for the prime section of 'Neurodegenerative Diseases', except that the editorial responsibility falls within the province of the section editors Jean-Philippe Loeffler and José-Luis Gonzalez de Aguilar, Strasbourg. Contributions should be submitted online:

www.karger.com/ndd

Please mention in your convering letter that your article is submitted for publication in 'Modeling Neurodegenerative Diseases in vivo'.

Conditions

Only manuscripts that conform to the Guidelines for Authors will be considered and are subject to editorial review.

The manuscript must be accompanied by a cover letter stating that all authors have seen and given their approval for submission of the manuscript to be considered for publication in 'Neurodegenerative Diseases'. Manuscripts are accepted for review with the understanding that persons cited in unpublished work have approved such citations. Authors may provide the names and contact information for three or four suggested reviewers for their papers.

Manuscripts are received with the explicit understanding that they are not under simultaneous consideration by any other publication or have not already been published elsewhere. Submission of an article for publication implies transfer of the copyright from the author to the publisher upon acceptance. Accepted papers become the permanent property of 'Neurodegenerative Diseases' and may not be reproduced by any means, in whole or in part, without the written consent of the publisher. It is the author's responsibility to obtain permission to reproduce illustrations, tables, etc. from other publications.

The authors agree that their articles will be accompanied, if necessary, by a simplified version written by a scientific writer.

Manuscripts that do not comply with the ethical standards recommended by the Helsinki Declaration will not be accepted.

Arrangement

Title page: The first page of each paper should indicate the title, the authors' names, the institute where the work was conducted, and a short title for use as running head.
NB: Authors wishing to preserve the phonetic meaning of diacritics (PubMed reduces diacritics to their root characters) must spell their names accordingly when submitting manuscripts (e.g. Müller should be Mueller).

Full address: The exact postal address of the corresponding author complete with postal code must be given at the bottom of the title page. Please also supply phone/fax numbers and e-mail address.

Key words: For indexing purposes, a list of 3–10 key words (no abbreviations) in English is needed.

Abstract: Each paper needs an abstract of about 200 words, and should be structured as follows:

Background:	What prompted the study?
Objective:	What is the purpose of the study?
Methods:	How was the study carried out?
Results:	What are the most important findings?
Conclusion:	What is the most important conclusion?

The abstract should not exceed 250 words, and any abbreviations must be explained.

Footnotes: Avoid footnotes. When essential, they should be numbered consecutively and typed at the foot of the appropriate page.

Tables and illustrations: Tables and illustrations (both numbered in Arabic numerals) should be prepared on separate sheets. Tables require a heading and figure legends should be supplied on a separate sheet. For the reproduction of illustrations, only good drawings and original photographs will be accepted; negatives or photocopies cannot be used. Due to technical reasons, figures with a screen background should not be submitted. When possible, group several illustrations in one block for reproduction (max. size 180 × 223 mm) or provide crop marks. Electronically submitted b/w halftone and color illustrations must have a final resolution of 300 dpi after scaling, and line drawings one of 800–1,200 dpi.

Color illustrations
Online edition: Color illustrations are reproduced free of charge. In the print version, the illustrations are reproduced in black and white. Please avoid referring to the colors in the text and figure legends.
Print edition: Up to 6 color illustrations per page can be integrated within the text at CHF 760.– per page.

References: Identify references in the text with Arabic numerals [in square brackets]. Material submitted for publication but not yet accepted should be noted as 'unpublished data' and not be included in the reference list. The list of references should include only those publications cited in the text. Do not alphabetize; number references in the order in which they are first mentioned in the text. The surnames of the authors followed by their initials should be given. There should be no punctuation other than a comma to separate the authors. Preferably, please cite all authors. Abbreviate journal names according to the Index Medicus system. (Also see International Committee of Medical Journal Editors: Uniform requirements for manuscripts submitted to biomedical journals. N Engl J Med 1997;336:309–315.)

KARGER

Fax +41 61 306 12 34
E-Mail karger@karger.ch
www.karger.com

The Guidelines for Authors are available at:
www.karger.com/neurodis_Guidelines

Examples

(a) Papers published in periodicals: Desai MY, De la Peña-Almaguer E, Mannting F: Abnormal heart rate recovery after exercise: A comparison with known indicators of increased mortality. Cardiology 2001;96: 38–44.

(b) Papers published only with DOI numbers: Theoharides TC, Boucher W, Spear K: Serum interleukin-6 reflects disease severity and osteoporosis in mastocytosis patients. Int Arch Allergy Immunol DOI: 10.1159/000063858.

(c) Books: Matheis G, Moritz A, Scholz M (eds): Leukocyte Depletion in Cardiac Surgery and Cardiology. Basel, Karger, 2002.

(d) Edited books: Gladish GW, Haponik EF: Virtual Bronchoscopy; in Bolliger CT, Mathur PM (eds): Interventional Bronchoscopy. Prog Respir Res. Basel, Karger, 2000, vol 30, pp 253–266.

Papers that have been submitted but are not yet accepted should not be listed in the bibliography, but can be referred to in the text as unpublished observations. If details of methods are only available in papers that are 'in press', copies of the papers should be included with the manuscript submitted to 'Neurodegenerative Diseases' so that the editorial referees can have adequate information to judge the manuscript.

Reference Management Software: Use of EndNote is recommended for easy management and formatting of citations and reference lists.

Digital Object Identifier (DOI)

S. Karger Publishers supports DOIs as unique identifiers for articles. A DOI number will be printed on the title page of each article. DOIs can be useful in the future for identifying and citing articles published online without volume or issue information. More information can be found at www.doi.org.

Drugs

Generic names should be used in text, tables, and figures. Trade names in upper case may be mentioned in parentheses in the first text reference to the drug but should not appear in titles, figures or tables. The chemical nature of new drugs must be given when known.

Abbreviations

When an abbreviation is used in the manuscript, it should be defined in the text the first time it is used. Abbreviations for commonly used substances should be those recommended by the *Journal of Biological Chemistry.* Abbreviations for drugs/chemicals may be used if properly defined with the chemical or generic name when the abbreviation is first used. Excessive use of abbreviations in the text, however, is strongly discouraged. Most abbreviations are used without punctuation, with no distinction between singular and plural forms.

Author's Choice™

With this option the author can choose to make his article freely available online against a one-time fee of CHF 2750.–. This fee is independent of any standard charges for supplementary pages, color images etc. which may apply. More information can be found at www.karger.com/authors_choice.

Proofs

Unless otherwise indicated, proofs are sent to the first-named author and should be returned with the least possible delay. Alterations made in proofs, other than the correction of printer's errors, are charged to the author. No page proofs are supplied.

Reprints

Order forms and a price list will be sent with the proofs. Orders submitted after the issue is printed are subject to considerably higher prices.

KARGER

Fax +41 61 306 12 34
E-Mail karger@karger.ch
www.karger.com

The Guidelines for Authors are available at:
www.karger.com/neurodis_Guidelines

General Information

Neuro-degenerative Diseases

ISSN Print Edition: 1660–2854
ISSN Online Edition: 1660–2862

Journal Homepage: www.karger.com/neurodis

Publication Data: 'Neurodegenerative Diseases' is published 6 times a year. Volume 7 with 6 issues appears in 2010.

Disclaimer: The statements, opinions and data contained in this publication are solely those of the individual authors and contributors and not of the publisher and the editor(s). The appearance of advertisements in the journal is not a warranty, endorsement, or approval of the products or services advertised or of their effectiveness, quality or safety. The publisher and the editor(s) disclaim responsibility for any injury to persons or property resulting from any ideas, methods, instructions or products referred to in the content or advertisements.

Subscription Rates: Subscriptions run for a full calendar year. Prices are given per year.

Personal subscription:

Print or Online	**Print+Online combined**
CHF 417.90	CHF 462.90
EUR 298.50	EUR 330.50
USD 379.20	USD 422.20

postage and handling (added to print and print+online)
CHF 37.80 Europe, CHF 56.70 Overseas
EUR 27.–
USD 53.70

Institutional subscription:

Print or Online	**Print+Online combined**
CHF 1393.–	CHF 1532.–
EUR 995.–	EUR 1094.–
USD 1264.00	USD 1390.00

postage and handling (added to print and print+online)
CHF 47.40 Europe, CHF 70.80 Overseas
EUR 33.60
USD 67.20

Airmail surcharge: CHF 48.– / USD 45.60

Back Volumes and Single Issues: Information on availability and prices of single print issues and print or electronic back volumes can be obtained from Customer Service at *service@karger.ch.*

Bibliographic Indices: This journal is regularly listed in bibliographic services, including *Current Contents®* and PubMed/MEDLINE.

Photocopying: This journal has been registered with the Copyright Clearance Center (CCC), as indicated by the code appearing on the first page of each article. For readers in the US, this code signals consent for copying of articles for personal or internal use, or for the personal or internal use of specific clients, provided that the stated fee is paid per copy directly to
Copyright Clearance Center Inc.
222 Rosewood Drive
Danvers, MA 01923 (USA)
A copy of the first page of the article must accompany payment. Consent does not extend to copying for general distribution, for promotion, for creating new works, or for resale. In these cases, specific written permission must be obtained from the copyright owner,
S. Karger AG, P.O. Box
CH–4009 Basel (Switzerland).

Subscription Orders:
Orders can be placed at agencies, bookstores, directly with the Publisher

S. Karger AG
Medical and Scientific Publishers
P.O. Box
CH–4009 Basel
Switzerland
(for courier services only:
Allschwilerstrasse 10
CH–4055 Basel)
Tel. +41 61 306 11 11
Fax +41 61 306 12 34
E-Mail karger@karger.ch
www.karger.com

or further Karger offices or representatives:

France:
Librairie Medi-Sciences Sarl
36, bd de Latour-Maubourg
75007 Paris
France
Tél. +33 (0) 1 45 51 42 58
Fax +33 (0) 1 45 56 07 80
E-Mail librairie@medi-sciences.fr
www.medi-sciences.fr

Germany:
S. Karger GmbH
Postfach
79095 Freiburg
Deutschland
(Hausadresse: Lörracher Strasse 16A
79115 Freiburg)
Tel. +49 761 45 20 70
Fax +49 761 45 20 714
E-Post information@karger.de
www.karger.de

India, Bangladesh, Sri Lanka:
Panther Publishers Private Ltd.
33, First Main
Koramangala First Block
Bangalore 560 034
India
Tel. +91 80 25505 836
Tel. +91 80 25505 837
Fax +91 80 25505 981
E-Mail panther_publishers@vsnl.com
www.pantherpublishers.com

Japan:
Karger Japan, Inc.
Yushima S Bld. 3F
4-2-3, Yushima, Bunkyo-ku
Tokyo 113-0034
Japan
Tel. +81 3 3815 1800
Fax +81 3 3815 1802
E-Mail publisher@karger.jp

China, Taiwan and Malaysia:
Karger China
Suite 409, Apollo Building
1440 Central Yan An Road
Shanghai 200040
China
Tel. +86-21-6133 1861
Fax +86-21-6133 1862
E-Mail karger.ray@gmail.com

South America and Central America:
Cranbury International LLC
7 Clarendon Ave., Suite 2
Montpelier, VT 05602
USA
Tel. +1 802 223 6565
Fax +1 802 223 6824
E-Mail
eatkin@cranburyinternational.com
www.cranburyinternational.com

United Kingdom, Ireland:
S. Karger AG
c/o London Liaison Office
4 Rickett Street
London SW6 1RU
United Kingdom
Tel. +44 (0) 20 7386 0500
Fax +44 (0) 20 7610 3337
E-Mail uk@karger.ch

USA:
S. Karger Publishers, Inc.
26 West Avon Road
P.O. Box 529
Unionville, CT 06085
USA
Toll free: +1 800 828 5479
Tel. +1 860 675-7834
Fax +1 860 675-7302
E-Mail karger@snet.net

Change of Address:
Both old and new address should be sent to the subscription source.

KARGER

Fax +41 61 306 12 34
E-Mail karger@karger.ch
www.karger.com

The Journal Home Page is available at:
www.karger.com/neurodis

Vol. 7, No. 1–3, 2010

Neuro-
degenerative
Diseases

Contents

5 **Preface**
Windisch, M. (Graz); Nitsch, R.M. (Zürich); Fisher, A. (Ness Ziona); Hanin, I. (Tucson, Ariz.)

History of Dementia Research

6 **History of Dementia Research in Bohemia and Middle Europe**
Kalvach, P.; Kalvach, Z. (Prague)

Biology of Neurodegeneration

10 **Dissecting Toxicity of Tau and β-Amyloid**
Götz, J.; Lim, Y.-A.; Ke, Y.D. (Camperdown, N.S.W.); Eckert, A. (Basel); Ittner, L.M. (Camperdown, N.S.W.)

13 **Tau Kinase I Overexpression Induces Dentate Gyrus Degeneration**
Avila, J.; Gómez de Barreda, E. (Madrid); Engel, T. (Dublin); Pérez, M.; Martín-Maestro, P.; Fuster-Matanzo, A.; Goñi-Oliver, P.; Lucas, J.J.; Hernández, F. (Madrid)

16 **Possible Role of Tau in Mediating Pathological Effects of apoE4 in vivo prior to and following Activation of the Amyloid Cascade**
Inbar, D.; Belinson, H. (Tel Aviv); Rosenman, H. (Jerusalem); Michaelson, D.M. (Tel Aviv)

24 **Transition of Tau Protein from Disordered to Misordered in Alzheimer's Disease**
Kovacech, B.; Skrabana, R. (Bratislava/Vienna); Novak, M. (Bratislava)

28 **'Prion-Like' Propagation of Mouse and Human Tau Aggregates in an Inducible Mouse Model of Tauopathy**
Sydow, A.; Mandelkow, E.-M. (Hamburg)

32 **Are Aβ and Its Derivatives Causative Agents or Innocent Bystanders in AD?**
Robakis, N.K. (New York, N.Y.)

38 **Neuroinflammation – An Early Event in Both the History and Pathogenesis of Alzheimer's Disease**
Eikelenboom, P.; van Exel, E.; Hoozemans, J.J.M.; Veerhuis, R.; Rozemuller, A.J.M.; van Gool, W.A. (Amsterdam)

42 **Analysis of APL1β28, a Surrogate Marker for Alzheimer Aβ42, Indicates Altered Precision of γ-Cleavage in the Brains of Alzheimer Disease Patients**
Okochi, M.; Tagami, S.; Takeda, M. (Osaka)

46 **Expression of Familial Alzheimer's Disease-Linked Human Presenilin 1 Variants Impair Enrichment-Induced Adult Hippocampal Neurogenesis**
Veeraraghavalu, K.; Choi, S.H.; Sisodia, S.S. (Chicago, Ill.)

50 **p53 Is Regulated by and Regulates Members of the γ-Secretase Complex**
Checler, F.; Dunys, J.; Pardossi-Piquard, R.; Alves da Costa, C. (Valbonne)

56 **Amyloid-β-Derived Diffusible Ligands Cause Impaired Axonal Transport of Mitochondria in Neurons**
Wang, X. (Cleveland, Ohio); Perry, G. (Cleveland, Ohio/San Antonio, Tex.); Smith, M.A.; Zhu, X. (Cleveland, Ohio)

60 **Acetylcholinesterase Variants in Alzheimer's Disease: From Neuroprotection to Programmed Cell Death**
Greenberg, D.S.; Toiber, D.; Berson, A.; Soreq, H. (Jerusalem)

64 **Neuroprotective and Neurotoxic Phenotypes of Activated Microglia in Neonatal Mice with Respective MPTP- and Ethanol-Induced Brain Injury**
Sawada, H. (Kobe/Toyoake); Suzuki, H. (Nagoya); Nagatsu, T. (Toyoake/Nagoya); Sawada, M. (Nagoya)

68 **LRRK2 and the Stress Response: Interaction with MKKs and JNK-Interacting Proteins**
Hsu, C.H.; Chan, D.; Wolozin, B. (Boston, Mass.)

76 **Misframed Proteins and Neurodegeneration: A Novel View on Alzheimer's and Parkinson's Diseases**
Dennissen, F.J.A.; Kholod, N.; Steinbusch, H.W.M.; Van Leeuwen, F.W. (Maastricht)

80 **Impaired Neurotransmitter Release in Alzheimer's and Parkinson's Diseases**
Shen, J. (Boston, Mass.)

84 **Stem Cell Biology in the Study of Pathological Conditions**
Sugaya, K. (Orlando, Fla.)

Disease Models

88 **Possible Involvement of Transthyretin in Hippocampal β-Amyloid Burden and Learning Behaviors in a Mouse Model of Alzheimer's Disease (TgCRND8)**
Doggui, S.; Brouillette, J.; Chabot, J.-G.; Farso, M.; Quirion, R. (Montreal, Que.)

96 **Early-Stage Inflammation and Experimental Therapy in Transgenic Models of the Alzheimer-Like Amyloid Pathology**
Cuello, A.C.; Ferretti, M.T.; Leon, W.C.; Iulita, M.F.; Melis, T.; Ducatenzeiler, A.; Bruno, M.A.; Canneva, F. (Montreal, Que.)

99 **Transgenic Zebrafish as a Novel Animal Model to Study Tauopathies and Other Neurodegenerative Disorders in vivo**
Paquet, D.; Schmid, B.; Haass, C. (Munich)

KARGER

Fax +41 61 306 12 34
E-Mail karger@karger.ch
www.karger.com

Access to full text and tables of contents, including tentative ones for forthcoming issues: www.karger.com/ndd_issues

103 **Generation of Tau Aggregates and Clearance by Autophagy in an Inducible Cell Model of Tauopathy**
Wang, Y.; Krüger, U.; Mandelkow, E.; Mandelkow, E.-M. (Hamburg)

108 **Silencing/Overexpressing Selected Genes as a Model of Sporadic Parkinson's Disease**
Fishman-Jacob, T.; Youdim, M.B.H.; Mandel, S.A. (Haifa)

Relationship Between Cerebrovascular Lesions and Primary Neurodegenerative Diseases

112 **Prevalence and Impact of Cerebrovascular Lesions in Alzheimer and Lewy Body Diseases**
Jellinger, K.A. (Vienna)

116 **The Vascular Hypothesis of Alzheimer's Disease: Bench to Bedside and Beyond**
de la Torre, J.C. (Sun City, Ariz.)

122 **Vascular Dementia and Alzheimer's Disease – Are We in a Dead-End Road?**
Cavalieri, M. (Graz/Ferrara); Enzinger, C.; Petrovic, K.; Pluta-Fuerst, A.; Homayoon, N.; Schmidt, H.; Fazekas, F.; Schmidt, R. (Graz)

127 **Vascular Contribution to Dementia in Parkinson's Disease**
Korczyn, A.D. (Ramat Aviv)

Imaging, Biomarkers, Genetics and Diagnostic Markers

131 **Early Detection of Alzheimer's Disease with PET Imaging**
Berti, V. (New York, N.Y./Florence); Osorio, R.S.; Mosconi, L.; Li, Y.; De Santi, S. (New York, N.Y.); de Leon, M.J. (New York, N.Y./Orangeburg, N.Y.)

136 **Amyloid Imaging in Early Detection of Alzheimer's Disease**
Nordberg, A. (Stockholm)

139 **Inability of Plasma and Urine F2A-Isoprostane Levels to Differentiate Mild Cognitive Impairment from Alzheimer's Disease**
Mufson, E.J.; Leurgans, S. (Chicago, Ill.)

143 **Increased CD44 Gene Expression in Lymphocytes Derived from Alzheimer Disease Patients**
Uberti, D.; Cenini, G.; Bonini, S.A. (Brescia); Barcikowska, M.; Styczynska, M.; Szybinska, A. (Warsaw); Memo, M. (Brescia)

148 **Human Analogue of the Morris Water Maze for Testing Subjects at Risk of Alzheimer's Disease**
Laczó, J. (Prague); Andel, R. (Tampa, Fla.); Vyhnalek, M.; Vlcek, K.; Magerova, H.; Varjassyova, A. (Prague); Tolar, M. (New Haven, Conn.); Hort, J. (Prague)

153 **Social Odor Recognition: A Novel Behavioral Model for Cognitive Dysfunction in Parkinson's Disease**
Monaghan, M.M.; Leddy, L.; Sung, M.-L.A.; Albinson, K.; Kubek, K.; Pangalos, M.N.; Reinhart, P.H.; Zaleska, M.M.; Comery, T.A. (Princeton, N.J.)

160 **Cognitive Event-Related Potentials and Oscillations in the Subthalamic Nucleus**
Rektor, I.; Baláž, M.; Bočková, M. (Brno)

163 **Oophorectomy, Menopause, Estrogen, and Cognitive Aging: The Timing Hypothesis**
Rocca, W.A.; Grossardt, B.R.; Shuster, L.T. (Rochester, Minn.)

167 **Pharmacogenomic Protocols in CNS Disorders and Dementia**
Cacabelos, R. (Coruña)

170 **Common Variant in *GRN* Is a Genetic Risk Factor for Hippocampal Sclerosis in the Elderly**
Dickson, D.W.; Baker, M.; Rademakers, R. (Jacksonville, Fla.)

175 **Leucine-Rich Repeat Kinase 2 Gene-Associated Disease: Redefining Genotype-Phenotype Correlation**
Wider, C.; Dickson, D.W.; Wszolek, Z.K. (Jacksonville, Fla.)

Treatment and Prevention

180 **Lipid-Lowering Treatment Is Related to Decreased Risk of Dementia: A Population-Based Study (FINRISK)**
Solomon, A. (Kuopio); Sippola, R. (Helsinki); Soininen, H. (Kuopio); Wolozin, B. (Boston, Mass.); Tuomilehto, J.; Laatikainen, T. (Helsinki); Kivipelto, M. (Kuopio/Stockholm)

183 **Cholesterol and Cognitive Performance in Normal Controls and the Influence of Elective Statin Use after Conversion to Mild Cognitive Impairment: Results in a Clinical Trial Cohort**
Sparks, D.L. (Sun City, Ariz.); Kryscio, R.J. (Lexington, Ky.); Connor, D.J.; Sabbagh, M.N.; Sparks, L.M. (Sun City, Ariz.); Lin, Y. (Lexington, Ky.); Liebsack, C. (Sun City, Ariz.)

187 **Effect of Heparin on APP Metabolism and Aβ Production in Cortical Neurons**
Klaver, D. (Hobart, Tas./Clayton, Vic.); Hung, A.C.; Gasperini, R.; Foa, L. (Hobart, Tas.); Aguilar, M.-I. (Clayton, Vic.); Small, D.H. (Hobart, Tas./Clayton, Vic.)

190 **Retinoids as a Perspective in Treatment of Alzheimer's Disease**
Fahrenholz, F.; Tippmann, F.; Endres, K. (Mainz)

193 **Treatment of Alzheimer's Disease with a Cholinesterase Inhibitor Combined with Antioxidants**
Cornelli, U. (Maywood, Ill.)

203 **Filamentous Phages Reduce α-Synuclein Oligomerization in the Membrane Fraction of SH-SY5Y Cells**
Dimant, H.; Solomon, B. (Tel-Aviv)

206 **Effects of Dopamine Agonists on Neuropsychiatric Symptoms of Parkinson's Disease**
Rektorová, I. (Brno)

210 **Future Strategies for Neuroprotection in Parkinson's Disease**
Schapira, A.H.V. (London)

213 **The Concept of Continuous Dopaminergic Stimulation: What We Should Consider when Starting Parkinson's Disease Treatment**
Stocchi, F. (Rome)

216 **Author Index**
217 **Subject Index**

Neurodegenerative Diseases

Neurodegenerative Dis 2010;7:5
DOI: 10.1159/000283473

Published online: February 13, 2010

Preface

The 9th International Conference on Alzheimer's and Parkinson's Diseases took place in Prague, Czech Republic, from March 11th to 15th, 2009. The unique composition of gothic and baroque buildings was a stimulating environment for a unique conference, now the biggest scientific meeting, where most recent research on Alzheimer's disease (AD), Parkinson's disease (PD) and related neurodegenerative disorders is presented and discussed. We are convinced that the comparison of underlying pathogenetic processes like protein misfolding, which characterizes practically all of these diseases, may lead to a better understanding of these disorders and allow the development of improved therapeutic strategies.

More than 2,500 participants took part in the conference in Prague, underlining the huge interest in this area of research. The constant growth in numbers of students, researchers, clinicians and people from pharmaceutical as well as biotechnological industry participating in the AD/PD conferences is certainly due to an outstanding scientific program, presenting newest findings about AD, PD and related disorders. The setting of the meeting stimulates interactive discussion among all the participants. The newly introduced 'Meet the Expert' sessions are an excellent opportunity for young scientists and students to meet with famous scientists in the field, and to openly interact with them. The Organizers have continually succeeded in attracting more young people at each meeting, by providing an aggressively increased number of travel supports, including the possibility for each senior invited speaker to bring one of his/her students free of charge to the meeting. The special character of the AD/PD conferences is also based on a balance between basic and applied science. This provides an excellent opportunity for scientists in basic and clinical research to learn from one another, and to appreciate progress in the different disciplines that might help to fight these devastating disorders.

The Local Scientific Advisory Board consisting of Prof. Irena Rektorova and Prof. Jacob Hort was invaluable to us in facilitating many local aspects of the conference, and in working with us to construct a well-balanced and strong scientific program. Their contribution of time, insight, and effort was definitely an important factor contributing to the success of the conference.

Of course, the organization of these international events depends, to a large extent, on generous financial support from industry. We are very grateful to the following companies for their support of the conference in Prague:

Gold sponsors: Elan, Medivation, Pfizer, Wyeth

Silver sponsors: Probiodrug

Bronze sponsors: Affiris, Cognitive Drug Research, Noscira

Other sponsors: ABCAM, BTG, Cornelli Foundation, JSW Life Sciences, LipiDiDiet, Lundbeck, MEMOSAD, MEMOLOAD, MemStick, Proteo Tech, Siena Biotech, Teva, Wako.

It would be impossible to run such a large international conference without the backing of an experienced, professional organizational company. The team of Kenes handled everything in a perfect, completely professional and efficient manner.

Last but not least, we also would like to acknowledge the professionalism of the S. Karger AG editorial personnel, who worked with us to bring this publication to fruition. Their collaboration has ensured a timely publication of these selected presentations from the 9th International Conference on Alzheimer's and Parkinson's Diseases.

We are looking forward to welcoming you at the 10th AD/PD Conference that will take place on March 9–13, 2011, in Barcelona.

Manfred Windisch
Roger Nitsch
Abraham Fisher
Israel Hanin

KARGER

Fax +41 61 306 12 34
E-Mail karger@karger.ch
www.karger.com

1660–2854/10/0073–0005$26.00/0

Accessible online at:
www.karger.com/ndd

Neurodegenerative Diseases

Neurodegenerative Dis 2010;7:6–9
DOI: 10.1159/000283474

Published online: February 13, 2010

History of Dementia Research in Bohemia and Middle Europe

Pavel Kalvach[a] Zdeněk Kalvach[b]

[a]Department of Neurology, 3rd Faculty of Medicine, Charles University, and
[b]Medistar, Private Outpatient Office for Gynecology and Psychiatry, Prague, Czech Republic

Key Words
Dementia research · St. Catherine asylum · Prague · Czech psychiatry · Senile plaques

Abstract
The clinical aspects and histopathology of dementia are best understood when based on knowledge of the historical milestones associated with its development. We studied archive materials and visited some of the psychiatric asylums that were active in Prague during the 19th century. ***Results:*** The gradual recognition of dementia and its histological correlates on the territory of the actual Czech Republic from the 1830s are described, together with its links to Austrian, German, and other foreign psychiatry and neurology. A stepwise differentiation between inborn mental incapacity and the acquired forms occurred between 1830 and 1890. This was followed by contributions from Emil Redlich, Arnold Pick, Karel Kuffner, Oskar Fischer and others between 1890 and 1930, elucidating features of senile plaques, and shedding light on behavioral-morphological correlations and on the role of inflammatory tissue changes. These discoveries allowed the distinction between neurodegenerative causes of dementia and other etiological categories. ***Conclusion:*** One hundred years ago, Prague was one of the cradles from which our modern understanding of neurodegenerative dementia emerged.

The roots of care for mental insanity in Bohemia reach as far back as 1458, when 'Hospitale hominum rationem non habentium' was established in Znojmo, Moravia. The period of reliably documented psychiatric care starts in the 19th century. At that time, the territory of today's Czech Republic was part of the Austro-Hungarian monarchy and existed as the Kingdom of Bohemia and Moravia. Although the majority of the population was Czech, the dominant intellectual influence on society was mostly German. German was also the language of the first written reports from this time period. The intellectual dominance of the German, mainly Jewish, community continued even after the imperial edict of Franz Joseph I in 1882, which divided Charles-Ferdinand University in Prague into two separate universities – one Czech, and one German.

With the erection of the Imperial-Royal General Hospital in Prague by Joseph II and Leopold II at the end of the 18th century, an official 'Tollhaus' (i.e. lunatic asylum) with 56 beds for the mentally insane became one of its wards. In 1822, this asylum was moved to the readapted monastery of St. Catherine (fig. 1) and psychiatry students were first allowed to go there twice weekly. Local care for 'Irrenwesen' (the mentally ill) in the first half of the 19th century already distinguished some twenty etiological units (fig. 2). In the report of 1827–1829, dementia was not yet recognized [1]. The word 'psychiatry', intro-

Prof. Pavel Kalvach, MD
Department of Neurology, Charles University
3rd Medical Faculty, Ruská 87
CZ–100 00 Praha 10 (Czech Republic)
Tel. +420 2 6716 3657, Fax +420 2 6716 2377, E-Mail kalvach@fnkv.cz

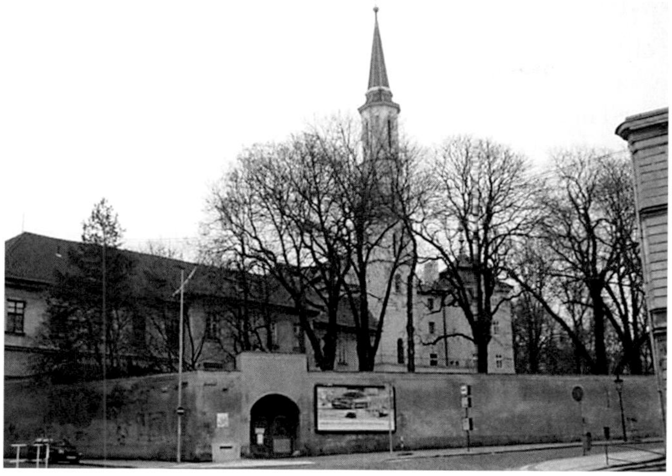

Fig. 1. St. Catherine asylum in Prague, readapted from its previous use as a monastery in 1822.

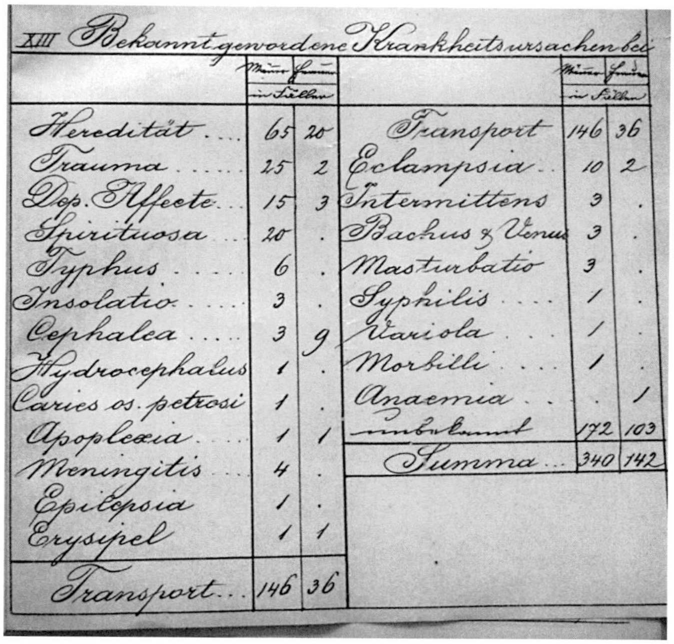

XIII Bekanntgewordene Krankheitsursachen bei

	Männer	Frauen		Männer	Frauen
	in Fällen			in Fällen	
Heredität	65	20	Transport	146	36
Trauma	25	2	Eclampsia	10	2
Dep. Affecte	15	3	Intermittens	3	.
Spirituosa	20	.	Bachus & Venus	3	.
Typhus	6	.	Masturbatio	3	.
Insolatio	3	.	Syphilis	1	.
Cephalea	3	9	Variola	1	.
Hydrocephalus	1	.	Morbilli	1	.
Caries os. petrosi	1	.	Anaemia	.	1
Apoplexia	1	1	unbekannt	172	103
Meningitis	4	.	Summa	340	142
Epilepsia	1	.			
Erysipel	1	1			
Transport	146	36			

Fig. 2. Etiological diagnoses used in Prague's 'Irrenanstalt' in 1828 [1].

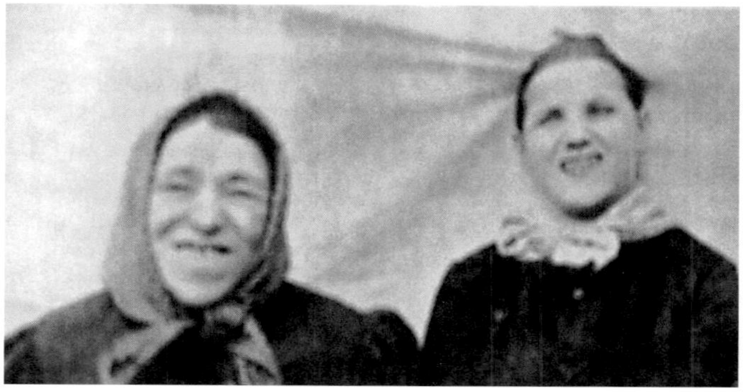

Fig. 3. 'Physiognomy of a person stupefied (left) compared with a girl stupid from birth (right)'. We can distinguish also acromegalic features, which at that time were not yet properly understood. From Karl Kuffner's *Psychiatry for Study and Practice* [10].

duced by Johann Christian Reil in 1811, was not used until the second half of the century. In the possession of Prague's asylum was a German translation of J.E.D. Esquirol's *Des Maladies Mentales*, dating from 1838; this would have allowed eventual knowledge of Esquirol's 'demence aigüé' (acute dementia) or 'idiotie acquise' (acquired idiocy). Nevertheless, not even the next important treatise regarding another of Prague's institutes – 'Die Idiotenanstalt in 1871–1883' – distinguished between inborn mental insufficiencies and acquired ones. Differential diagnostic attempts were aimed at a description of idiocy, epilepsy (both diseases understood as one and the same, with only different dynamics) and cretinism. The principle of cretinism was felt to be in embryogenesis: 'The cretin has vitia primae formationis already at conception and fetus creation' [2]. Traumatic, infectious, postapoplectic and nutritional reasons for an intellectual deterioration gradually started to be properly perceived, but not until the 1880s and 1890s. However, even at the end of the 19th century, differential diagnoses of congenital and the acquired mental incapacities were attempted only superficially, using e.g. physiognomy (fig. 3).

The years between 1880 and 1920 were an extremely fruitful period in Bohemian and Moravian neurosciences. Emil Redlich (1866–1930), born in Moravia and working in Vienna, described 'miliäre Sklerose' in two cases of senile dementia in 1898. These miliary sclerotic lesions were analogous to those previously described in 1892 by Paul Blocq and Georges Marinesco and named by them as 'amas ronds'. Redlich's paper was, however, the first to use the designation 'plaques' [quoted in 3].

Arnold Pick (1851–1924), a well-known member of the German psychiatry community, came from a Moravian Jewish family. After his studies in Vienna and a short working period at the Theodor Meynert (1833–1898) Institute, Pick followed his colleague Karl Wernicke (1848–

1905) to Berlin and began to work under Prof. Karl Westphal (1833–1890). Both of these famous scientists also gave their names to eponyms: the first one to Wernicke's temporal aphasia and to alcoholic encephalopathy, the latter together with Edinger to the mesencephalic nucleus. After several years as the director of a psychiatric asylum in Dobřany, Arnold Pick came to Prague, and in 1887 he was awarded the chair of the German Department of Psychiatry. Among his 280 publications, we find an unprecedented diversity of topics, including hysterical psychoses, spinal cord and brain histopathology, visual systems in dogs, psychological phenomena such as reduplicative paramnesia, and stress-related impact (I World War) on neuroses. All these topics provided considerable enrichment to the world psychiatry. In his review of the Bohemian 'Irrenwesen' in 1885, Pick estimated the need for one psychiatric bed per 1,000 inhabitants and reported about '7,794 mentally handicapped persons living in Bohemia, of whom 1,115 were institutionalized in Prague's asylums, 399 in the Kosmonosy asylum, and 117 in the Dobřany asylum; 6,980 idiots were at home'. Pick's classic paper on the relationship between senile brain atrophy and aphasia describes the case of August H., autopsied by Prof. Chiari in 1892 [4]. The main merit of this paper was in clarifying the role of the frontal lobe in the ideational component of language production.

There were two obstacles to properly deciphering the principles of neurodegenerative deterioration: first was the relatively short average life span, and second was the widespread nature of dementia paralytica of inflammatory origin. The fact that progressive paralysis was due to the 'syphilitic virus', as it was called by Friedel Pick in 1892, was generally not acknowledged even 12 years later. Histopathological changes in meningeal gummata, in luetic endarteritis (Heubner, 1874) and in tabic myelopathies were well studied in Prague in the early 1890s as is evident from autopsies done by Chiari and F. Pick [5]. While still admirable work, it was not as detailed as that described 14 years later in the remarkable 'Habilitationsschrift' (postdoctoral thesis) 'Histological studies on the differential diagnosis of progressive paralysis' by Alois Alzheimer in 1904.

The clinical views of dementias were represented best by Karl Kuffner in his *Psychiatry for Study and Practice* in 1900. Kuffner was head of the Czech Department of Psychiatry in Prague in 1895–1929, in fact during 25 years parallel to the German Department of Psychiatry with Arnold Pick. In this work, he clearly distinguished between inborn stupidity and acquired stupefaction. For dementias as the final stage of other primary psychoses 'after prior states of melancholy, maniac stupidity, etc.' he coined the term dementia simplex consecutiva, which is close to one of the historical meanings of dementia praecox. Those dementias, which developed without any psychotic overtures (equivalent to our contemporary neurodegenerative development), he called dementia simplex primitiva.

The admirably detailed studies of senile plaques by Oskar Fischer (1876–1942) deserve special attention. Fischer worked under A. Pick in Prague at the beginning of the 20th century. He graduated in 1900 and became associate professor in 1917 after defending his thesis 'Causes and relevance of CSF pleocytosis'. His main scientific merit lies in three large articles on 'granular necroses' or 'Sphaerotrichia multiplex cerebri', i.e. on inclusions of 10–120 μm corresponding to plaques. In 1907, he observed and reported on this phenomenon in 12 out of 16 demented brains, and by 1910 he had published observations on plaques in 58 demented persons found among 275 autopsies including also normal individuals and people with different psychoses and paralyses [6–8]. Due to his meticulous histological analyses, combined with his prior clinical observations, Oskar Fischer was able to arrive at the opinion that these tissue alterations are the principle cause of presbyophrenic dementia. He described maturation of presbyophrenic plaques in eight stages, similar to Bielschowsky's staging described 4 years later. He also speculated on the inflammatory character of the plaques, a theory which 100 years later was further elaborated using the sophisticated instruments of modern histochemistry [9].

A century ago, the city of Prague and the surrounding area of Bohemia and Moravia represented one of the important cradles of our modern understanding of the neurodegenerative principles of dementia.

In later years of the 20th century, a number of neuroscientists and neuroclinicians of Czech origin achieved international fame. These were, e.g., Jan Janský, who in 1907, while working in Prague's Department of Psychiatry, completed Landsteiner's discovery of three blood groups (1901) to the final number of four. Kamil Henner and Jiří Vítek brought neurology and Jan Jirout neuroradiology to flourishment after the II World War. Similarly, Zdeněk Mysliveček and Vladimír Vondráček fostered development in psychiatry. The basic research in neurosciences was most successfully pursued by Zdeněk Servít in epilepsy during the 1950s and 1960s and by Jan Bureš in the field of memory. The latter one's animal experiments performed at the Academy of Sciences achieved international reputation, as did the physiological studies by Vilém Laufberger. Very successful were also publications by Stanislav Grof in the field of transpersonal psychology and by his brother Pavel in research of affective disorders – especially after their immigration to the USA and Canada.

Acknowledgement

This article was supported by grant MSM CR VZ 0021620816.

References

1 Riedel J: Prag's Irrenanstalt und ihre Leistungen in den Jahren 1827–1829. Prague, Sommersche Buchdruckerei, 1830.
2 Amerling K: Die Idiotenanstalt des Sct. Anna-Frauen-Vereines in Prag 1871–1883. Prague, Selbstverlag, 1883.
3 Goedert M: Oskar Fischer and the study of dementia. Brain DOI 10.1093/brain/awn256.
4 Pick A: Über die Beziehungen der senilen Hirnatrophie zur Aphasie. Prager Med Wochenschr 1892;16:165–167.
5 Pick F: Über cerebrospinale Syphilis. Prager Med Wochenschr 1892;24:261–264.
6 Fischer O: Miliäre Nekrosen mit drusigen Wucherungen der Neurofibrillen, eine regelmässige Veränderung der Hirnrinde bei seniler Demenz. Monatsschr Psychiatr Neurol 1907;22:361–372.
7 Fischer O: Die presbyophrene Demenz, deren anatomische Grundlage und klinische Abgrenzung. Zeitschr Ges Neurol Psychiatr 1910;18:371–471.
8 Fischer O: Ein weiterer Beitrag zur Klinik und Pathologie der presbyophrenen Demenz. Zeitschr Ges Neurol Psychiatr 1912;12:99–135.
9 Eikelenboom P, Veerhuis R, Scheper W, Rozemuller AJM, van Gool WA, Hoozemens JJM: The significance of neuroinflammation in understanding Alzheimer's disease. J Neural Transm 2006;113:1685–1695.
10 Kuffner K: Psychiatrie pro studium i praktickou potřebu Lékaře. Vol. II. Prague, Bursík a Kohout, 1900.

Biology of Neurodegeneration

Neuro-degenerative Diseases

Neurodegenerative Dis 2010;7:10–12
DOI: 10.1159/000283475

Published online: February 13, 2010

Dissecting Toxicity of Tau and β-Amyloid

Jürgen Götz[a] Yun-An Lim[a] Yazi D. Ke[a] Anne Eckert[b] Lars M. Ittner[a]

[a]Alzheimer's and Parkinson's Disease Laboratory, Brain and Mind Research Institute, University of Sydney, Camperdown, N.S.W., Australia; [b]Neurobiology Laboratory for Brain Aging and Mental Health, Psychiatric University Clinics, University of Basel, Basel, Switzerland

Key Words
Alzheimer's disease · Axonal transport · Frontotemporal dementia · Kinesin · Oligomer · Tau · Transgenic mice · Type 2 diabetes

Abstract
Background: How β-amyloid (Aβ) and tau exert toxicity in Alzheimer's disease is only partly understood. Major questions include (1) which aggregation state of Aβ confers toxicity, (2) do amyloidogenic proteins have similar mechanisms of toxicity, and (3) does soluble tau interfere with cellular functions? ***Methods:*** To determine Aβ toxicity in P301L mutant tau transgenic mice, mitochondrial function was assessed after insult with monomeric, oligomeric and fibrillar Aβ. Amylin and Aβ toxicity were compared in cortical and hippocampal long-term cultures. To determine tau toxicity, K369I mutant tau mice were established as a model of frontotemporal dementia, analyzed biochemically and compared with human diseased brain. ***Results:*** Oligomeric and fibrillar Aβ42 were both toxic, although to different degrees. Human amylin shared toxicity with Aβ42, an effect not observed for nonamyloidogenic rat amylin. Clinical features of K369I tau mice were caused by aberrant interaction of phosphorylated tau with JIP1, a component of the kinesin transport machinery. ***Conclusion:*** Our data support the notion of a synergistic action of tau and Aβ pathology on mitochondria. A specific conformation of Aβ42 and human amylin determines toxicity. Finally, trapping of JIP1 by phosphorylated tau in the neuronal soma emerges as a fundamental pathomechanism in neurodegeneration.

A central question in Alzheimer's disease (AD) research is how β-amyloid (Aβ) and tau, principal components of amyloid plaques and neurofibrillary tangles, exert toxicity. Recent findings highlight the role of distinct Aβ species including Aβ*56, a dodecameric form of Aβ [1]. Others demarcate differences between oligomeric and fibrillar forms [2]. For tau, inducible transgenic mice reveal a toxicity independent of neurofibrillary tangles [3], a notion supported by studies in transgenic flies [4]. Irrespective of the form of toxic species, Aβ and tau seem to confer toxicity synergistically, as Aβ exacerbates a preexisting tau pathology [5], while Aβ toxicity is tau dependent [6].

An excellent read-out for functional impairment is mitochondrial respiration [7]. A sophisticated set of functional assays is available determining activities of all mitochondrial complexes separately, as well as different forms of respiration. Mitochondrial function is vital for any type of cell, in particular neurons; however, mitochondria are also the major source of reactive oxygen spe-

KARGER

Fax +41 61 306 12 34
E-Mail karger@karger.ch
www.karger.com

1660–2854/10/0073–0010$26.00/0

Accessible online at:
www.karger.com/ndd

Jürgen Götz
Alzheimer's and Parkinson's Disease Laboratory
Brain and Mind Research Institute, University of Sydney
Camperdown, N.S.W. 2050 (Australia)
Tel. +61 2 9351 0789, Fax +61 2 9351 0731, E-Mail jgoetz@med.usyd.edu.au

cies. Microtubules are needed to properly distribute mitochondria, establishing a link to tau as microtubule-stabilizing protein. To determine how mitochondrial function is impaired by Aβ, we isolated mitochondria from P301L tau transgenic mice [5] and incubated them with different forms of Aβ [8]. Both oligomeric and fibrillar, but not disaggregated (mainly monomeric) Aβ42 caused a decreased mitochondrial membrane potential in cortical brain cells obtained from the transgenic mice. This was not observed with cerebellar preparations (an area where the transgene is not expressed), indicating a role for tau in mediating Aβ42 toxicity. Furthermore, we found reductions in state 3 respiration, the respiratory control ratio and uncoupled respiration when incubating transgenic mitochondria either with oligomeric or fibrillar preparations of Aβ42. Finally, aging of the peptides specifically increased the sensitivity of mitochondria to oligomeric Aβ42. We found that oligomeric and fibrillar Aβ42 are both toxic, but to a different degree. Furthermore, we found that aging of the mice increased sensitivity of mitochondria to Aβ damage, in agreement with studies in Aβ plaque-forming amyloid precursor protein transgenic mice [9].

Epidemiological, clinical and biochemical studies establish a link between AD and type 2 diabetes, another leading cause of morbidity and mortality in the elderly [10]. Both diseases are characterized by amyloidosis in their target tissue; amylin aggregation in type 2 diabetes is associated with β-cell loss while Aβ aggregation in AD brain is associated with neuronal loss. Aβ and human amylin are similar in size; however, while sharing little similarities in their primary sequence, they fold into similar secondary structures. Given these similarities, we asked whether human amylin would exert neurotoxic effects similar to Aβ [11]. Cell type specificity of toxicity was explored by comparing cortical to hippocampal long-term cultures, and aged peptide preparations were compared with nonaged preparations. We found that, different from nonamyloidogenic rat amylin, Aβ42 and human amylin both caused a dose-, time- and cell type-specific neurotoxicity, supporting the notion of a similar toxic mechanism [11]. Depending on the cell type, this finding is also supported by coincubation of amylin and Aβ. We observed that in general, hippocampal neurons were more sensitive than cortical neurons to toxicity exerted by either human amylin or Aβ42. We also found that rat amylin, which does not form fibrils, is virtually not toxic to hippocampal neurons but surprisingly, toxic to cortical neurons under some conditions. Coincubation of Aβ42 and human amylin suggests the possibility of a shared pathway in hippocampal neurons, whereas more than one pathway may be activated in cortical neurons. Our results imply that specific conformational changes in peptides are important determinants of toxicity. In support, conformational antibodies can be generated that recognize a generic amyloid fibril epitope found on amyloid-like aggregates derived from proteins such as transthyretin, amylin or β_2-microglobulin [12].

Not only is the toxicity of Aβ42 not fully understood, the same holds true for tau, where soluble species more so than the fibrillar forms seem to be a culprit in disease initiation. To determine tau toxicity, we generated a novel transgenic mouse strain, K3, which expresses human tau carrying the mutation K369I found in a familial case of frontotemporal dementia (FTD). The mice develop a progressive histopathology reminiscent of the human patient. Furthermore, they show early onset memory impairment and amyotrophy, that precedes neurodegeneration as the mice age. Different from our previously generated tau transgenic strains, K3 mice express the transgene in the substantia nigra, associated with an early onset motor phenotype that reproduces parkinsonism with tremor, bradykinesia, abnormal gait and postural instability. Interestingly, motor performance of young, but not old K3 mice could be improved upon L-dopa treatment, which bears similarities to parkinsonism in FTD. The early onset symptoms in the mice are mechanistically related to selectively impaired anterograde transport of distinct cargos, which precedes loss of dopaminergic neurons in aged mice. The impaired axonal transport affects, among others, vesicles containing the dopamine-synthesizing enzyme tyrosine hydroxylase. Distinct modes of transport are also impaired in sciatic nerve, which may explain amyotrophy [13]. We found that impaired axonal transport in the K3 mice is due to a cargo-selective impairment of kinesin-driven anterograde transport by tau. Specifically, formation of the kinesin motor complex formation is disturbed in K3 mice, as hyperphosphorylated tau interacts with JIP1, a protein associated with the kinesin motor protein complex. Consequently, JIP1 transport into the axon is impaired causing accumulation in the soma. Since we found trapping of JIP1 in the soma and a pathological tau/JIP1 interaction also in AD brain, this has pathomechanistic implications for tauopathies. We also found JIP1 sequestration in the soma of tau-transfected primary neuronal cultures. The pathological tau/JIP1 interaction depends on tau phosphorylation, with tau competing with the physiological binding of JIP1 to kinesin light chain. Since JIP1 is involved in regulating cargo binding to kinesin motors, our findings may, at least in part, explain how hyperphosphorylated tau, independent of effects mediated by amyloid precursor protein/Aβ42, mediates impaired axonal transport in both AD and FTD [14].

Together, this highlights the validity of transgenic animal models [15] and underscores the role of impaired axonal transport in human neurodegenerative disease [16].

Acknowledgments

J.G. and L.I. have been supported by the ARC and NHMRC and A.E. by the Swiss National Science Foundation (No. 310000-108223).

References

1 Lesne S, Koh MT, Kotilinek L, Kayed R, Glabe CG, Yang A, Gallagher M, Ashe KH: A specific amyloid-beta protein assembly in the brain impairs memory. Nature 2006;440: 352–357.

2 Necula M, Kayed R, Milton S, Glabe CG: Small molecule inhibitors of aggregation indicate that amyloid beta oligomerization and fibrillization pathways are independent and distinct. J Biol Chem 2007;282:10311–10324.

3 Santacruz K, Lewis J, Spires T, Paulson J, Kotilinek L, Ingelsson M, Guimaraes A, DeTure M, Ramsden M, McGowan E, Forster C, Yue M, Orne J, Janus C, Mariash A, Kuskowski M, Hyman B, Hutton M, Ashe KH: Tau suppression in a neurodegenerative mouse model improves memory function. Science 2005; 309:476–481.

4 Wittmann CW, Wszolek MF, Shulman JM, Salvaterra PM, Lewis J, Hutton M, Feany MB: Tauopathy in drosophila: neurodegeneration without neurofibrillary tangles. Science 2001;293:711–714.

5 Gotz J, Chen F, van Dorpe J, Nitsch RM: Formation of neurofibrillary tangles in p301l tau transgenic mice induced by abeta 42 fibrils. Science 2001;293:1491–1495.

6 Roberson ED, Scearce-Levie K, Palop JJ, Yan F, Cheng IH, Wu T, Gerstein H, Yu GQ, Mucke L: Reducing endogenous tau ameliorates amyloid beta-induced deficits in an Alzheimer's disease mouse model. Science 2007;316:750–754.

7 Rhein V, Baysang G, Rao S, Meier F, Bonert A, Muller-Spahn F, Eckert A: Amyloid-beta leads to impaired cellular respiration, energy production and mitochondrial electron chain complex activities in human neuroblastoma cells. Cell Mol Neurobiol 2009;29: 1063–1071.

8 Eckert A, Hauptmann S, Scherping I, Meinhardt J, Rhein V, Drose S, Brandt U, Fandrich M, Muller WE, Gotz J: Oligomeric and fibrillar species of β-amyloid (aβ42) both impair mitochondrial function in p301l tau transgenic mice. J Mol Med 2008;86:1255–1267.

9 Hauptmann S, Scherping I, Drose S, Brandt U, Schulz KL, Jendrach M, Leuner K, Eckert A, Muller WE: Mitochondrial dysfunction: an early event in Alzheimer pathology accumulates with age in ad transgenic mice. Neurobiol Aging 2009;30:1574–1586.

10 Gotz J, Ittner LM, Lim YA: Common features between diabetes mellitus and Alzheimer's disease. Cell Mol Life Sci 2009;66: 1321–1325.

11 Lim YA, Ittner LM, Lim YL, Gotz J: Human but not rat amylin shares neurotoxic properties with abeta42 in long-term hippocampal and cortical cultures. FEBS Lett 2008;582: 2188–2194.

12 O'Nuallain B, Wetzel R: Conformational abs recognizing a generic amyloid fibril epitope. Proc Natl Acad Sci USA 2002;99:1485–1490.

13 Ittner LM, Fath T, Ke YD, Bi M, van Eersel J, Li KM, Gunning P, Gotz J: Parkinsonism and impaired axonal transport in a mouse model of frontotemporal dementia. Proc Natl Acad Sci USA 2008;105:15997–16002.

14 Ittner LM, Ke YD, Gotz J: Phosphorylated tau interacts with c-jun n-terminal kinase-interacting protein 1 (jip1) in Alzheimer disease. J Biol Chem 2009;284:20909–20916.

15 Gotz J, Ittner LM: Animal models of Alzheimer's disease and frontotemporal dementia. Nat Rev Neurosci 2008;9:532–544.

16 Gotz J, Ittner LM, Kins S: Do axonal defects in tau and amyloid precursor protein transgenic animals model axonopathy in Alzheimer's disease? J Neurochem 2006;98: 993–1006.

Biology of Neurodegeneration

Neuro-degenerative Diseases

Neurodegenerative Dis 2010;7:13–15
DOI: 10.1159/000283476

Published online: February 13, 2010

Tau Kinase I Overexpression Induces Dentate Gyrus Degeneration

Jesús Avila[a, b] Elena Gómez de Barreda[a] Tobias Engel[d] Mar Pérez[a, c] Patricia Martín-Maestro[a] Almudena Fuster-Matanzo[a] Paloma Goñi-Oliver[a, b] José J. Lucas[a, b] Félix Hernández[a]

[a]Centro de Biología Molecular Severo Ochoa (CSIC-UAM), [b]Departamento de Neurociencias y Centro de Investigación Biomédica en Red sobre Enfermedades Neurodegenerativas (CIBERNED), [c]Departamento de Anatomía, Histología y Neurociencia, Facultad de Medicina, Universidad Autónoma de Madrid, Madrid, Spain; [d]Department of Physiology and Medical Physics, Royal College of Surgeons in Ireland, Dublin, Ireland

Key Words
Alzheimer disease · Tau · Tau kinase I · GSK3 activity · Dentate gyrus

Abstract
Familial Alzheimer gene mutations result in a signaling mechanism that converges, downstream, in the activation of GSK3 activity. We have generated a GSK3 transgenic mouse model to study the consequences of GSK3 activation. In this model, dentate gyrus is degenerated in a process in which phosphorylated tau can be involved.

Introduction

Familial Alzheimer disease (AD) is a consequence of mutations in three genes: app, ps-1 and ps-2. The mutated proteins resulting from the expression of these genes may interfere with signal transduction cascades that will result, in all cases, in an increase in tau kinase I (GSK3) activity [1–4]. In sporadic AD, there are examples showing that GSK3β overactivation may also take place [5]. It is known that the expression of specific ApoE isoforms could be a risk factor for the disease [6]. One of ApoE cell receptors, LRP6, is a coreceptor of the Wnt/GSK3 pathway [7, 8]. Recently, a common genetic variation within LRP6 has been reported to be associated with late-onset AD [9]. Thus, the presence of this LRP6 variant could result in a decrease in Wnt signaling and an increase in GSK3 activity. More recently, an association between a single nucleotide polymorphism in the GSK3β gene and increased risk of AD has been reported [10].

GSK3β is a proline directed serine-threonine kinase [11], implicated in insulin-mediated signal transduction and, also, in the Wnt signaling pathway [12]. Thus, GSK3β activation could be a convergent point in AD pathology. To study the effects on brain of an increased GSK3β activity, a conditional transgenic GSK3β mouse was raised [13]. In this mouse, a decrease in dentate gyrus (DG) volume was observed [14].

GSK3 Activation Results in DG Degeneration

DG size decrease (degeneration) by GSK3 activation could be the consequence of an increase in the number of death neurons promoted by the activation of the kinase, followed by the modification of some substrates involved in cell death or cell survival. In addition, DG size decrease could be due to an effect of GSK3 activation on

KARGER

Fax +41 61 306 12 34
E-Mail karger@karger.ch
www.karger.com

1660–2854/10/0073–0013$26.00/0

Accessible online at:
www.karger.com/ndd

Jesús Avila
Centro de Biología Molecular Severo Ochoa (CSIC-UAM)
C/ Nicolás Cabrera 1, Universidad Autónoma de Madrid, Campus Cantoblanco
ES–28049 Madrid (Spain)
Tel. +34 91 196 44 20, Fax +34 91 196 45 64, E-Mail javila@cbm.uam.es

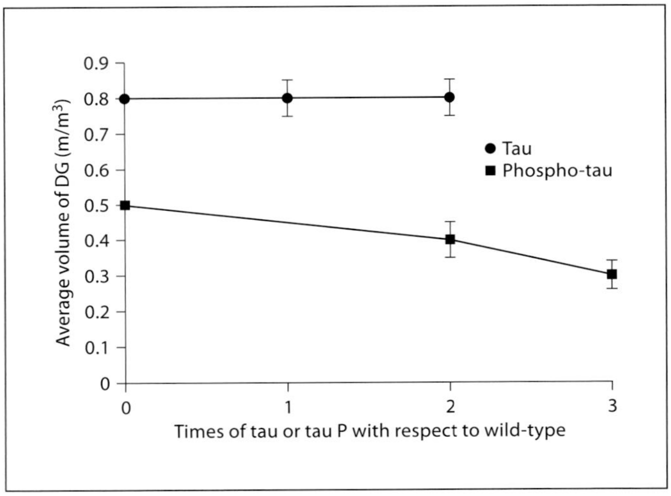

Fig. 1. Average size of DG in different mice. The volumes of DG from k.o. tau mice (0), wild-type mice (1), or mice overexpressing human tau [bearing three FTDP-17 mutations and with a total amount of expressed tau double (2) that of wild type] are shown. No changes in the average DG size were observed. In addition, DG volume was measured in some mice lines overexpressing GSK3 (those transgenic lines were obtained by crossing k.o. tau mice and FTDP-17 transgenic line with a mouse line overexpressing GSK3β [14]). Mice overexpressing GSK3β but lacking tau have no phospho-tau (0), while mice overexpressing GSK3β and with basal levels of tau present twofold (2) phospho-tau levels compared to those found in wild-type mice. Mice overexpressing GSK3β and human tau with FTDP-17 mutations have threefold levels (3) of phospho-tau compared to those of wild-type mice. It can be observed that an increase in tau phosphorylation correlates with a decrease in DG size. The volume of DG corresponds to 3-month-old animals. An average of three experiments per sample is shown.

neurogenesis, since DG is one of the few places in the central nervous system where neurogenesis occurs. It has been indicated [13] that GSK3 overexpression results in neuron death, perhaps by modification of the proapoptotic protein Bax-1. Also, an increase in β-catenin phosphorylation by GSK3 could be the cause of neuron-impaired survival [13]. However, little is known about the possibility that tau protein, phosphorylated by GSK3 [15], could also be a toxic agent for the cell. Our preliminary results, working with a transgenic mouse overexpressing GSK3 but lacking tau suggest that, indeed, the presence of an increased amount of phospho-tau could be toxic for neurons [Gómez de Barreda et al., unpubl. data]. These results agree with some previous data indicating that in double-transgenic mice overexpressing GSK3 and human tau (bearing some mutations that facilitate its phosphorylation by the kinase), DG degeneration is accelerated compared to the single transgenic mouse only overexpressing GSK3 [14].

Figure 1 shows the average size of the DG of a mouse lacking tau and a wild-type mouse, and the volume of a transgenic line expressing not only endogenous tau but also a similar amount of human tau bearing some FTDP-17 mutations [16]. The DG of these mice lines is similar. In addition, in figure 1 it is indicated how an increase in tau phosphorylation induced by GSK3β overexpression correlates with a decrease in the size of DG.

The decrease in DG size could be the consequence of a failure in neurogenesis promoted by GSK3 overexpression. Preliminary experiments performed in collaboration with Drs. Sirerol and García-Verdugo from the Universidad de Valencia, Spain, have suggested that an increase in GSK3 activity in the DG results in an impaired neurogenesis that could yield a decrease in the size of DG in those transgenic mice overexpressing GSK3.

References

1 Avila J: Tau phosphorylation and aggregation in Alzheimer's disease pathology. FEBS Lett 2006;580:2922–2927.
2 Baki L, Shioi J, Wen P, Shao Z, Schwarzman A, Gama-Sosa M, Neve R, Robakis NK: PS1 activates PI3K thus inhibiting GSK-3 activity and tau overphosphorylation: effects of FAD mutations. EMBO J 2004;23:2586–2596.
3 Kimura T, Yamashita S, Fukuda T, Park JM, Murayama M, Mizoroki T, Yoshiike Y, Sahara N, Takashima A: Hyperphosphorylated tau in parahippocampal cortex impairs place learning in aged mice expressing wild-type human tau. EMBO J 2007;26:5143–5152.
4 Townsend M, Mehta T, Selkoe DJ: Soluble Abeta inhibits specific signal transduction cascades common to the insulin receptor pathway. J Biol Chem 2007;282:33305–33312.
5 Pei JJ, Braak E, Braak H, Grundke-Iqbal I, Iqbal K, Winblad B, Cowburn RF: Distribution of active glycogen synthase kinase 3beta (GSK-3beta) in brains staged for Alzheimer disease neurofibrillary changes. J Neuropathol Exp Neurol 1999;58:1010–1019.

6 Strittmatter WJ, Saunders AM, Schmechel D, Pericak-Vance M, Enghild J, Salvesen GS, Roses AD: Apolipoprotein E: high-avidity binding to beta-amyloid and increased frequency of type 4 allele in late-onset familial Alzheimer disease. Proc Natl Acad Sci USA 1993;90:1977–1981.

7 Tamai K, Semenov M, Kato Y, Spokony R, Liu C, Katsuyama Y, Hess F, Saint-Jeannet JP, He X: Ldl-receptor-related proteins in Wnt signal transduction. Nature 2000;407:530–535.

8 Cselenyi CS, Jernigan KK, Tahinci E, Thorne CA, Lee LA, Lee E: LRP6 transduces a canonical Wnt signal independently of Axin degradation by inhibiting GSK3's phosphorylation of beta-catenin. Proc Natl Acad Sci USA 2008;105:8032–8037.

9 De Ferrari GV, Papassotiropoulos A, Biechele T, Wavrant De-Vrieze F, Avila ME, Major MB, Myers A, Saez K, Henriquez JP, Zhao A, Wollmer MA, Nitsch RM, Hock C, Morris CM, Hardy J, Moon RT: Common genetic variation within the low-density lipoprotein receptor-related protein 6 and late-onset Alzheimer's disease. Proc Natl Acad Sci USA 2007;104:9434–9439.

10 Schaffer BA, Bertram L, Miller BL, Mullin K, Weintraub S, Johnson N, Bigio EH, Mesulam M, Wiedau-Pazos M, Jackson GR, Cummings JL, Cantor RM, Levey AI, Tanzi RE, Geschwind DH: Association of GSK3B with Alzheimer disease and frontotemporal dementia. Arch Neurol 2008;65:1368–1374.

11 Woodgett JR: Molecular cloning and expression of glycogen synthase kinase-3/factor A. EMBO J 1990;9:2431–2438.

12 Barth AI, Nathke IS, Nelson WJ: Cadherins, catenins and APC protein: interplay between cytoskeletal complexes and signaling pathways. Curr Opin Cell Biol 1997;9:683–690.

13 Lucas JJ, Hernandez F, Gomez-Ramos P, Moran MA, Hen R, Avila J: Decreased nuclear beta-catenin, tau hyperphosphorylation and neurodegeneration in GSK-3beta conditional transgenic mice. EMBO J 2001;20:27–39.

14 Engel T, Lucas JJ, Gomez-Ramos P, Moran MA, Avila J, Hernandez F: Cooexpression of FTDP-17 tau and GSK-3beta in transgenic mice induce tau polymerization and neurodegeneration. Neurobiol Aging 2006;27:1258–1268.

15 Grundke-Iqbal I, Iqbal K, Tung YC, Quinlan M, Wisniewski HM, Binder LI: Abnormal phosphorylation of the microtubule-associated protein tau (tau) in Alzheimer cytoskeletal pathology. Proc Natl Acad Sci USA 1986;83:4913–4917.

16 Lim F, Hernandez F, Lucas JJ, Gomez-Ramos P, Moran MA, Avila J: FTDP-17 mutations in tau transgenic mice provoke lysosomal abnormalities and tau filaments in forebrain. Mol Cell Neurosci 2001;18:702–714.

Biology of Neurodegeneration

Neuro-degenerative Diseases

Neurodegenerative Dis 2010;7:16–23
DOI: 10.1159/000283477

Published online: February 13, 2010

Possible Role of Tau in Mediating Pathological Effects of apoE4 in vivo prior to and following Activation of the Amyloid Cascade

Dafna Inbar[a] Haim Belinson[a] Hanna Rosenman[b] Daniel M. Michaelson[a]

[a]Department of Neurobiology, The George S. Wise Faculty of Life Sciences, Tel Aviv University, Tel Aviv,
[b]Department of Neurology, Agnes Ginges Center for Human Genetics, the Hadassah Hebrew University Medical Center, Jerusalem, Israel

Key Words

Amyloid cascade · Apolipoprotein E · Alzheimer's disease · Neprilysin · Tau phosphorylation

Abstract

Injection of the neprilysin inhibitor thiorphan into the brain induces the accumulation of Aβ in hippocampal CA1 neurons and septal neurons in apoE4 knock-in mice but not in mice that express the corresponding Alzheimer's disease benign isoform apoE3. We investigated the possible role of tau phosphorylation in mediating this synergistic pathological cross talk between apoE4 and the amyloid cascade. This revealed that in both apoE4 and apoE3 mice, activating the amyloid cascade by inhibiting neprilysin triggers the accumulation of AT100 phosphorylated tau in the perikarya of CA1 neurons. In contrast, in the septum this treatment elevated the level of phosphorylation of the tau AT100 epitope only in the apoE4 mice. This suggests that tau-related processes by themselves do not mediate the synergistic pathological effects of apoE4 and Aβ in CA1 neurons. However, tau and cytoskeletal-related mechanisms may mediate the synergistic pathological effects of apoE4 and Aβ in the septum. The basal levels of tau phosphorylation are also affected by the apoE genotype. This effect, which is associated with hyperphosphorylation of the tau AT8 epitope, is most prominent in hippocampal CA3 neurons. This suggests that the apoE4 mice are already stressed under nonstimulated conditions and that AT8 tau phosphorylation may contribute to their increased susceptibility to brain insults.

Introduction

Alzheimer's disease (AD) is associated with genetic risk factors, of which the allele E4 of apolipoprotein E (apoE4) is the most prevalent [1, 2]. AD brain pathology is characterized by extracellular deposition of the neurotoxic peptide amyloid-β (Aβ) in senile plaques and by the intracellular deposition of hyper-phosphorylated tau in neurofibrillary tangles [3]. Importantly, Aβ deposition and the gene dose of the apoE4 allele are positively correlated [4]. A similar positive correlation was also reported between apoE4 and the densities of neurofibrillary tangles [5, 6], but this was not confirmed by others [7]. This suggests that apoE4 may be a mediator that links the amyloid plaques and the neurofibrillary tangles neuropa-

The first two authors are equal contributors to this work.

KARGER

Fax +41 61 306 12 34
E-Mail karger@karger.ch
www.karger.com

1660–2854/10/0073–0016$26.00/0

Accessible online at:
www.karger.com/ndd

Daniel M. Michaelson
Department of Neurobiology, The George S. Wise Faculty of Life Sciences
Tel Aviv University, Ramat Aviv
IL–69978 Tel Aviv (Israel)
Tel. +972 3 6409 624, E-Mail dmichael@post.tau.ac.il

thology in AD. The mechanisms that may mediate such interactions are presently not known and are an important unresolved issue in the AD field.

In order to examine the possible role of synergistic pathological interactions between apoE4 and Aβ, we recently established a novel in vivo model that is based on activating the amyloid cascade by inhibition of the Aβ-degrading enzyme neprilysin [8]. This revealed that prolonged i.c.v. injection of the neprilysin inhibitor thiorphan, induces the degeneration of hippocampal CA1 neurons and of entorhinal and septal neurons in apoE4 knock-in mice but not in corresponding mice that express the AD benign isoform apoE3 [9]. This effect is apparent within a week following initiation of treatment and is associated with the accumulation of intracellular Aβ in CA1 and septal neurons of the apoE4 but not of the corresponding apoE3 mice [9, 10].

In the present study, we examined the possibility that changes in the levels and in the intracellular compartmentation of tau in the brain and in its extent of phosphorylation play a role in the apoE4-dependent brain pathology following activation of the amyloid cascade. This was examined immunohistochemically utilizing distinct phosphorylation-insensitive (e.g. Ab H-150) and phosphorylation-sensitive anti-tau antibodies. The latter include mAb AT100, which specifically recognizes the paired helical filament-like conformation of tau [11, 12] as well as mAb AT8, which is directed at distinct phosphorylated tau epitopes whose levels of phosphorylation rise following stressful conditions and in AD [13–16].

Materials and Methods

Transgenic Mice

APOE target replacement mice [17] were purchased from Taconic. The experiments were performed with 3- to 4-month-old age-matched males and were approved by the Tel-Aviv University Animal Care Committee. Every effort was made to reduce animal stress and to minimize animal usage.

Implantation of Alzet Mini-Osmotic Pumps

Alzet mini-osmotic pumps (Alzet model 2004, which delivers its content at a rate of 0.25 μl/h), were loaded either with 0.5 mM thiorphan in artificial cerebrospinal fluid containing 1 mM ascorbic acid or with a similar solution without thiorphan. The mini-osmotic pumps were then implanted into anesthetized mice for 1 week as previously described [9].

Immunohistochemistry and Immunofluorescence Staining

Free floating coronal sections (30 cm) were prepared from these mice using a sliding microtome as previously described [9], after which the sections were immunostained as described by Matsumori et al. [18] with the following primary Abs: H-150, a Rabbit polyclonal antisera that recognizes the N-terminal of tau and is phosphorylation insensitive (1:600, Santa Cruz Biotechnology); biotinylated mAb AT100 (1:200, Innogenetics), which recognizes the phosphorylated tau T212 and S214 epitopes, and biotinylated mAb AT8, which is directed at phosphorylated S202 and T205 tau residues [15] (dilution 1:40, Innogenetics) [11, 12]. The H-150-treated sections were then washed and incubated with biotin-labeled goat anti-rabbit antibodies (1:200; Vector Labs). All of the labeled sections were then incubated with HRP-labeled Avidin (Vector Labs), after which staining was visualized with DAB (Vector Labs). The intensities of immunohistochemical staining were analyzed and quantified as the percent area stained utilizing the Image-Pro Plus system (version 5.1, Media Cybernetics, Silver Spring, Md., USA).

Results

Tau Levels and Phosphorylation in the Hippocampus

Immunohistochemical staining of the hippocampus of apoE4 and apoE3 mice with the phosphorylation-insensitive anti-tau antisera H-150 is depicted in figure 1a. As shown, staining in naïve untreated apoE3 mice was primarily in the neuritic fields and not in the cell bodies of the CA and dentate gyrus hippocampal areas. A similar pattern was observed with the naïve apoE4 mice except that the cell bodies of these mice, particularly in CA1 neurons, also contained tau. This pattern changed following inhibition of neprilysin with thiorphan, which resulted in marked accumulation of tau in the cell bodies of the CA1 neurons. This effect was similar in the apoE4 and apoE3 mice but was not observed in sham-treated mice (fig. 1a, b; $p < 0.001$ for treatment and $p < 0.02$ for group by two-way ANOVA). A similar but less pronounced effect was seen in CA3 neurons (not shown).

We next examined the extent to which the observed redistribution of tau in the apoE transgenic mice, following activation of the amyloid cascade, is related to changes in tau phosphorylation. The results thus obtained utilizing the anti-phosphorylated tau epitope AT100 are depicted in figure 2.

As shown, AT100 staining was similarly low in the hippocampi of naïve and sham-treated apoE3 and apoE4 mice but was markedly and similarly increased in these mice following inhibition of neprilysin. The increase in AT100 staining following inhibition of neprilysin was most pronounced in the cell bodies of the hippocampal CA1 neurons ($p < 0.001$ for treatment by two-way ANOVA). A similar but less pronounced effect

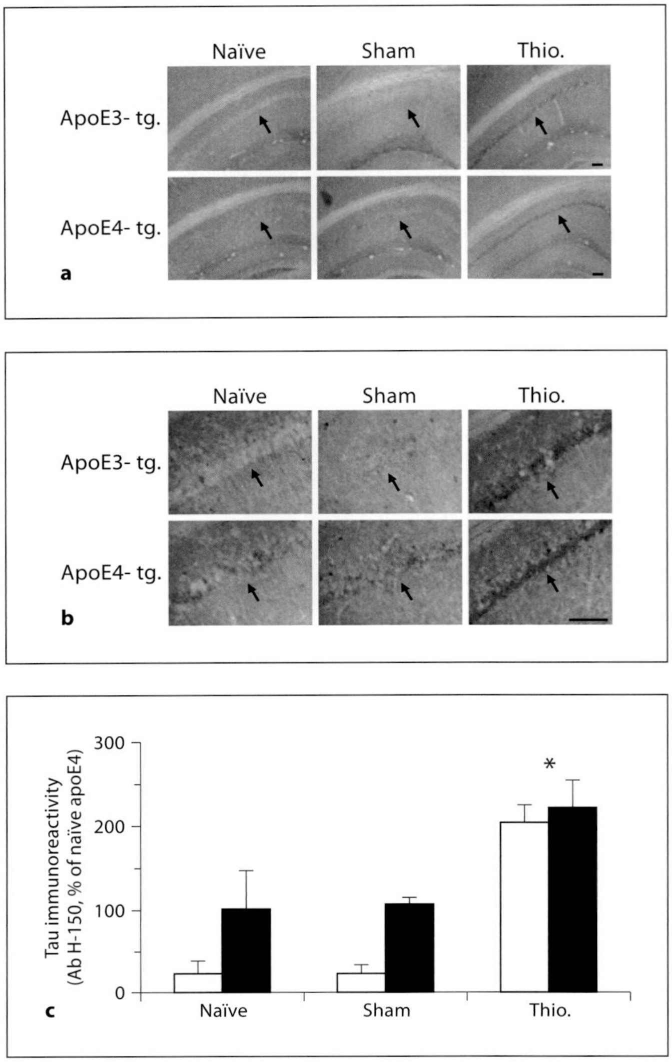

Fig. 1. Effects of apoE4 and activation of the amyloid cascade by inhibition of neprilysin on total hippocampal tau immunoreactivity. Four-month-old apoE3 and apoE4 male mice were implanted with Alzet mini-osmotic pumps that contained thiorphan or were sham treated for a week as described in Materials and Methods. These mice (n = 4 per group × treatment) and the corresponding naïve mice (n = 3 per group) were then sacrificed, after which their brains were sectioned and stained immunohistochemically with anti-tau H-150 as described in Materials and Methods. **a**, **b** Representative coronal sections of the different mouse groups immunostained with H-150 at different magnifications (scale = 100 μm). **c** Quantification of the immunostaining in CA1 neurons. Results (mean ± SD) are presented as percentage of those of naïve apoE4 mice. Empty bars denote the apoE3 mice, whereas filled bars represent the apoE4 mice. * $p < 0.001$ for the effects of treatment and $p < 0.02$ for the effect of group by two-way ANOVA.

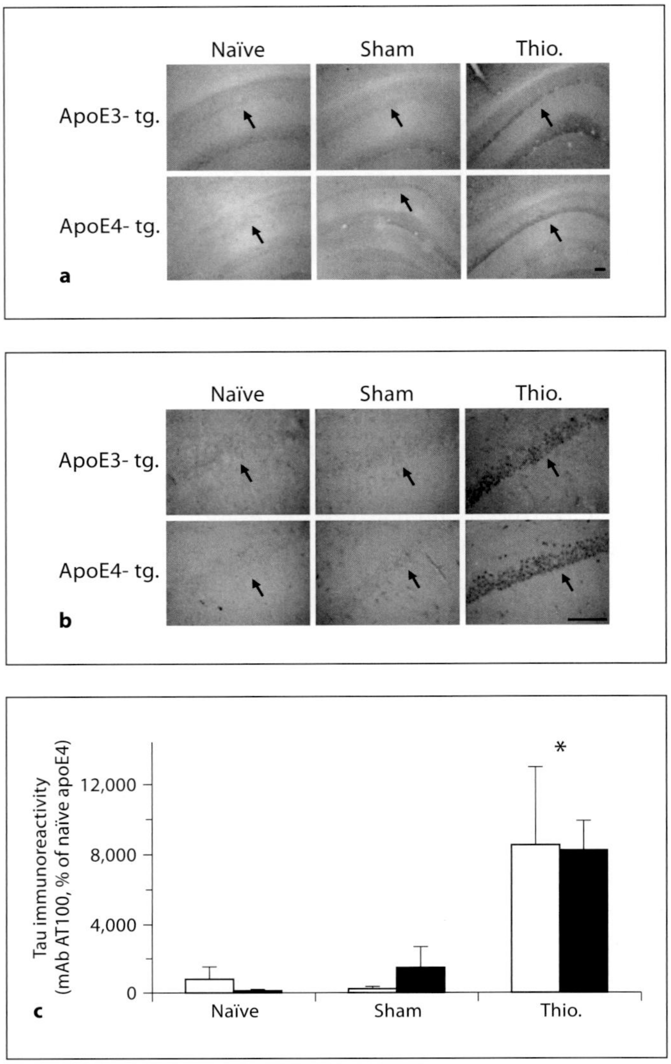

Fig. 2. Effects of apoE4 and activation of the amyloid cascade by inhibition of neprilysin on AT100 tau immunoreactivity in the hippocampus. Four-month-old apoE3 and apoE4 male mice were implanted with Alzet mini-osmotic pumps that contained thiorphan or were sham treated for a week as described in Materials and Methods. These mice (n = 4 per group × treatment) and the corresponding naïve mice (n = 3 per group) were then sacrificed, after which their brains were sectioned and stained immunohistochemically with mAb AT100, as described in Materials and Methods. **a**, **b** Representative coronal sections of the different mouse groups immunostained with mAb AT100 at different magnifications (scale = 100 μm). **c** Quantification of the immunostaining in CA1 neurons. Results (mean ± SD) are presented as the percentage of those of naïve apoE4 mice. Empty bars denote the apoE3 mice, whereas filled bars represent the apoE4 mice. * $p < 0.001$ for the effect of treatment by two-way ANOVA.

was seen in CA3 neurons. These AT100 findings are similar to those observed with the phosphorylation-insensitive anti-tau-antibody H-150 (compare fig. 1 and 2). Taken together, they suggest that inhibition of neprilysin stimulates the phosphorylation of tau and its accumulation in the perikarya of distinct hippocampal neurons, and that these effects are similar in the apoE4 and apoE3 mice. Consistent with the localized nature of this effect, the overall levels of tau in homogenates of the hippocampi of the apoE4 and apoE3 mice, as measured by H-150 immunoblot assays, were similar (data not shown).

The extent to which the observed effects are specific to the AT100 epitope was investigated utilizing mAb AT8. As shown in figure 3, AT8 staining, unlike AT100 staining, was most pronounced in the hilus and the CA3 fields and was more prominent in naïve apoE4 mice than in the corresponding apoE3 mice. Furthermore, sham treatment of the apoE4 mice resulted in a pronounced loss of the AT8 tau immunoreactivity in CA3 neurons, which was partially restored by thiorphan treatment (fig. 3). In contrast, the corresponding AT8 tau immunoreactivity of the apoE3 mice was not affected by these treatments. Importantly, the CA1 neurons of the naïve sham and thiorphan-treated apoE3 and apoE4 neurons did not stain positively for AT8. The mechanisms underlying the isoform-specific effects of apoE4 on AT8 phosphorylation of naïve apoE4 mice are not known. AT8 phosphorylation occurs in CA3 neurons that, unlike the CA1 neurons, do not seem to be affected by apoE4 and thiorphan [9, 10] and are dephosphorylated following sham treatment. These observations suggest that AT8 tau phosphorylation is not due to cross talk between apoE4 and the amyloid cascade. Furthermore, its dephosphorylation in the sham-treated mice may be related to the effects of the surgical procedure and/or of the ascorbate that is present in the artificial CSF which is infused into the mice [9].

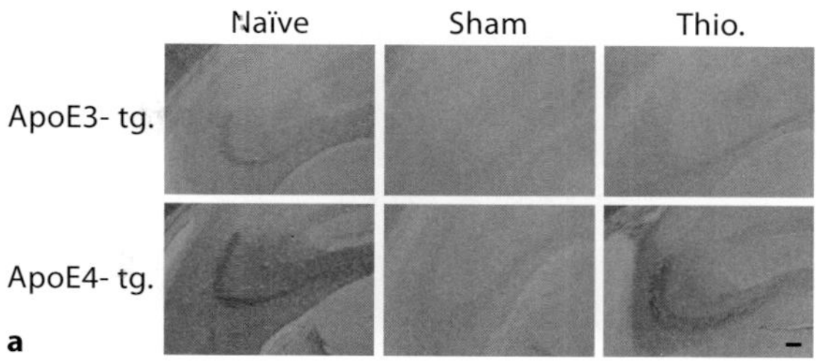

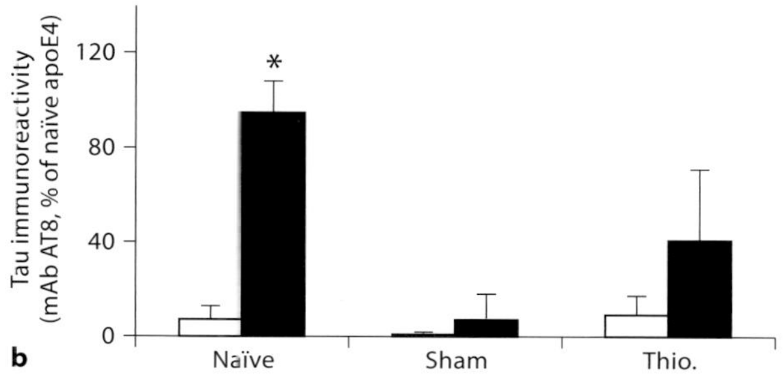

Fig. 3. Effects of apoE4 and activation of the amyloid cascade by inhibition of neprilysin on AT8 tau immunoreactivity in the hippocampus. Four-month-old apoE3 and apoE4 male mice were implanted with Alzet mini-osmotic pumps that contained thiorphan or were sham treated for a week, as described in Materials and Methods. These mice (n = 4 per group × treatment) and the corresponding naïve mice (n = 3 per group) were then sacrificed, after which their brains were sectioned and stained immunohistochemically with mAb AT8, as described in Materials and Methods. **a** Representative coronal sections of the different mouse groups immunostained with AT8 (scale = 100 μm). **b** Quantification of the immunostaining in the CA3 hippocampal subfield. Results (mean ± SD) are presented as percentage of those of the naïve apoE4 mice. Empty bars denote the apoE3 mice, whereas filled bars represent the apoE4 mice. * $p < 0.03$ for the effect of group by two-way ANOVA.

Levels and Phosphorylation of Tau in Septal Neurons

Immunohistochemical staining of the medial septum of naïve, sham- and thiorphan-treated apoE4 and apoE3 mice with the phosphorylation-insensitive tau antisera H-150 is presented in figure 4a. As shown, tau staining was similar in the apoE4 and apoE3 mice and was unaffected by either the sham or the thiorphan treatments.

Immunohistochemical staining of the medial septum of the different mouse groups with mAb AT100 is presented in figure 4b. As shown, the AT100 staining of the naïve and sham-treated apoE4 and apoE3 mice was similar and low but increased isoform-specifically in the septum of the apoE4 mice following inhibition of neprilysin. Quantification of these results revealed that group × treatment had a significant effect ($p < 0.02$ by two-way ANOVA). This was associated with a significant effect of the thiorphan treatment on the apoE4 mice ($p < 0.01$ for comparison of the sham and thiorphan-treated apoE4 mice) but not on the apoE3 mice (fig. 4c). Staining with mAb AT8 was more pronounced in the septal neurons in the naïve apoE4 mice than in the corresponding apoE3

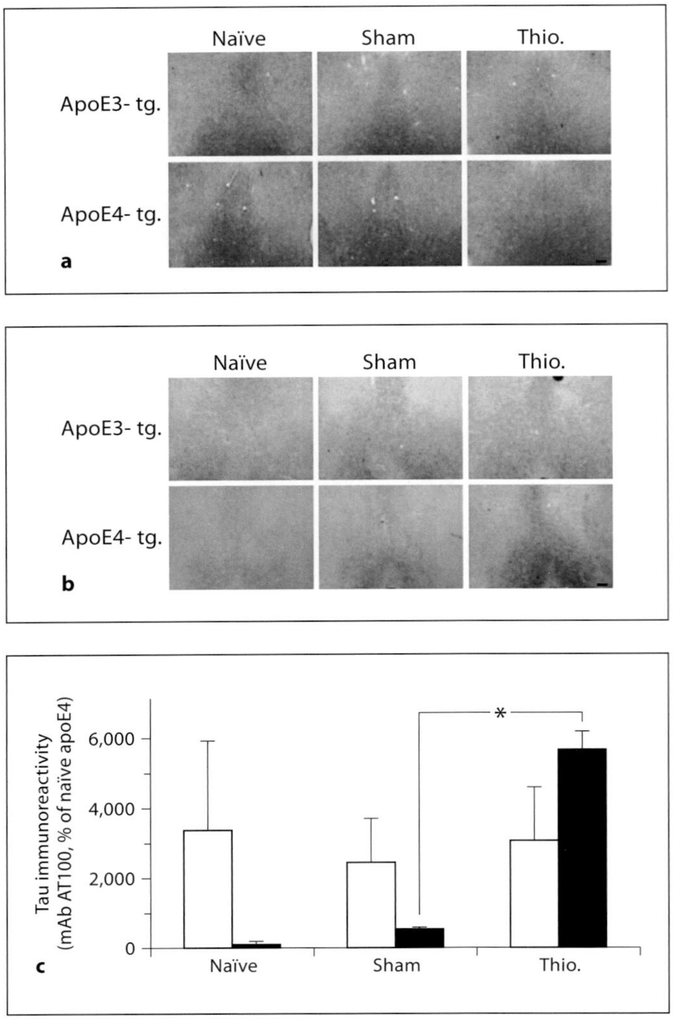

Fig. 4. Effects of apoE4 and activation of the amyloid cascade by inhibition of neprilysin on total tau and AT100 tau immunoreactivity in the septum. Four-month-old apoE3 and apoE4 male mice were implanted with Alzet mini-osmotic pumps that contained thiorphan or were sham treated for a week, as described in Materials and Methods. These mice (n = 4 per group × treatment) and the corresponding naïve mice (n = 3 per group) were then sacrificed, after which their brains were sectioned coronally and stained immunohistochemically with anti-tau Ab H-150 and with mAb AT8, as described in Materials and Methods. **a** Representative sections of the medial septum of the different mouse groups immunostained with H-150 (scale = 100 μm). Quantification of the levels of H-150 immunostaining in the medial septum revealed no effects of either group or treatment (not shown). **b** Representative coronal sections of the medial septum of the different mouse groups immunostained with mAb AT100 (scale = 100 μm). **c** Quantification of the AT100 immunostaining of the medial septum. Results (mean ± SD) are presented as percentage of those of naïve apoE4 mice. Empty bars denote the apoE3 mice, whereas filled bars represent the apoE4 mice. Two-way ANOVA group × treatment ($p = 0.02$). * $p < 0.01$ for comparison of the thiorphan and sham-treated apoE4 mice.

mice and decreased following the sham implantation of the Alzet pumps. These effects however were not statistically significant (not shown).

Discussion

The present study revealed that activation of the amyloid cascade by inhibition of the Aβ-degrading enzyme neprilysin affects the level of phosphorylation and the intracellular distribution of tau. Accordingly, in the hippocampus this treatment triggered the accumulation of tau in the perikarya of the CA1 neurons. This effect was similar in the apoE4 and apoE3 mice and was associated with parallel and similar elevations in the levels of AT100 tau phosphorylation in the CA1 perikarya (fig. 1, 2). In contrast, the phosphorylation of AT100 in septal neurons increased specifically in the apoE4 but not the apoE3 mice following inhibition of neprilysin (fig. 4). Additional experiments revealed that AT8 tau phosphorylation in the hippocampus, unlike AT100 phosphorylation, is primarily localized in the CA3 hippocampal subfields and the hilus. Furthermore, the levels of AT8 phosphorylation are markedly higher in naïve apoE4 mice than in the corresponding apoE3 mice and are markedly reduced following sham treatment (fig. 3). A similar but less pronounced effect was also seen in the septum.

The AT100 tau epitope, which is generated sequentially by several kinases [19], is associated with the paired helical filament-like conformation of tau [11, 12] and with pronounced neuronal impairments such as those found in the AD brain and in transgenic mouse models of normal and mutated human tau [20–23]. Inhibition of neprilysin elevates the levels of Aβ in the hippocampus of both the apoE3 and apoE4 mice [8] but triggers the accumulation of intraneuronal Aβ only in apoE4 mice [9, 10]. This suggests that AT100 tau phosphorylation, which is observed in the CA1 neurons of both the apoE4 and the apoE3 mice following inhibition of neprilysin, is triggered by extracellular Aβ. However, it is possible that this effect is not mediated by Aβ, but instead is due either to the accumulation of an alternative substrate of neprilysin or to the effects of thiorphan on an alternative target. The findings that in the septum the neprilysin treatment results in hyperphosphorylation of AT100 specifically in apoE4 and not apoE3 mice (fig. 4) and that this effect is associated with the accumulation of Aβ in these neurons [9, 10] suggest that AT100 tau phosphorylation and the accumulation of Aβ in apoE4 septal neurons may be related. The AT100 epitope requires the phosphorylation of tau at two distinct epitopes T212 and S214 [12]. It remains to be determined which of the kinases that play a role in this phosphorylation is affected in the septum and the hippocampus by the inhibition of neprilysin.

The mislocalization of tau into the somatodendritic compartment in hippocampal neurons and the associated hyperphosphorylation of AT100 may contribute to the observed apoE4-dependent Aβ-mediated degeneration of the CA1 neurons of the apoE4 mice following inhibition of neprilysin. However, since such tau-related effects are also observed in apoE3 mice whose CA1 neurons do not degenerate under these conditions [9, 10], we can conclude that additional effects, other than the observed tau-related changes, mediate the synergistic pathological effects of apoE4 and Aβ in the hippocampus. In the septum, the hyperphosphorylation of AT100 following inhibition of neprilysin, occurs specifically in the apoE4 mice. It is thus possible that the neurodegeneration of these neurons, unlike that of the CA1 neurons, is mediated by tau- and cytoskeletal-related pathology. Such an interpretation is consistent with recent findings that suggest that the apoE4-dependent Aβ-mediated neurodegeneration of CA1 and septal neurons are mediated via different mechanisms [10].

Neuronal impairments and stress are associated with hyperphosphorylation of AT8 [24–32]. Accordingly, the present finding that this tau epitope is hyperphosphorylated in the CA3 and hilus hippocampal subfields and in the septum of naïve apoE4 mice suggests that in these neurons apoE4 is a stressor even under regular nonchallenging conditions. This is in accordance with our previous finding that neurogenesis in the hippocampus, which is known to be affected by stress, is hyperactivated in naïve apoE4 mice [33]. Accordingly, AT8 hyperphosphorylation in naïve apoE4 may predispose these mice and contribute to their increased susceptibility to activation of the amyloid cascade [8, 9] as well as to other challenges such as exposure to environmental stimulation [33, 34], to head trauma [35] and to inflammatory stimulation [36]. The AT8 tau epitope can be phosphorylated by numerous kinases [16, 37–41], but it remains to be determined which of these enzymes mediates the effects of apoE4 on the phosphorylation of AT8 and on its neuronal distribution. Hyperphosphorylation of tau at the AT8 epitope has previously been observed in naïve apoE4 transgenic mice that express apoE under a neuronal promoter but not in those mice that express apoE4 in astrocytes [42–44]. This suggests that the effects of apoE4 on tau phosphorylation may be triggered intracellularly. However, since AT8 tau phosphorylation can also be activated via extracellular signaling [45], it is also possible that the effects of apoE4 are triggered extracellularly.

In conclusion, the present study shows that tau phosphorylation in vivo is affected by the apoE genotype and by activation of the amyloid cascade. Accordingly, activation of the amyloid cascade in both apoE4 and apoE3 mice increases the phosphorylation of the AT100 tau epitope in CA1 neurons. In contrast, in the septum this treatment elevates the levels of AT100 tau phosphorylation isoform-specifically in the apoE4 but not the apoE3 mice. This suggests that in the septum, tau phosphorylation may play a role in mediating the pathological interactions between apoE4 and the amyloid cascade. The basal levels of tau phosphorylation are also affected by the apoE genotype. This effect, which is detectable by mAb AT8, is however, most pronounced in CA3 neurons.

Acknowledgments

This work was supported in part by grants from the Israel Science Foundation (No. 487/07), and from the Joseph and Inez Eichenbaum Foundation, and by the LIPIDIDIET grant funded by the 7th Framework Program of the European Union. D.M.M. is the incumbent of the Myriam Lebach Chair in Molecular Neurodegeneration.

References

1 Corder EH, Saunders AM, Strittmatter WJ, Schmechel DE, Gaskell PC, Small GW, Roses AD, Haines JL, Pericak-Vance MA: Gene dose of apolipoprotein E type 4 allele and the risk of Alzheimer's disease in late onset families. Science 1993;261:921–923.
2 Saunders AM, Strittmatter WJ, Schmechel D, George-Hyslop PH, Pericak-Vance MA, Joo SH, Rosi BL, Gusella JF, Crapper-MacLachlan DR, Alberts MJ, et al: Association of apolipoprotein E allele epsilon 4 with late-onset familial and sporadic Alzheimer's disease. Neurology 1993;43:1467–1472.
3 Alzheimer A, Stelzmann RA, Schnitzlein HN, Murtagh FR: An English translation of Alzheimer's 1907 paper, 'Über eine eigenartige Erkankung der Hirnrinde'. Clin Anat 1995;8:429–431.
4 Schmechel DE, Saunders AM, Strittmatter WJ, Crain BJ, Hulette CM, Joo SH, Pericak-Vance MA, Goldgaber D, Roses AD: Increased amyloid beta-peptide deposition in cerebral cortex as a consequence of apolipoprotein E genotype in late-onset Alzheimer disease. Proc Natl Acad Sci USA 1993;90:9649–9653.

5 Gomez-Isla T, West HL, Rebeck GW, Harr SD, Growdon JH, Locascio JJ, Perls TT, Lipsitz LA, Hyman BT: Clinical and pathological correlates of apolipoprotein E epsilon 4 in Alzheimer's disease. Ann Neurol 1996;39:62–70.
6 Nagy Z, Esiri MM, Jobst KA, Johnston C, Litchfield S, Sim E, Smith AD: Influence of the apolipoprotein E genotype on amyloid deposition and neurofibrillary tangle formation in Alzheimer's disease. Neuroscience 1995;69:757–761.
7 Morris CM, Benjamin R, Leake A, McArthur FK, Candy JM, Ince PG, Torvik A, Bjertness E, Edwardson JA: Effect of apolipoprotein E genotype on Alzheimer's disease neuropathology in a cohort of elderly Norwegians. Neurosci Lett 1995;201:45–47.
8 Dolev I, Michaelson DM: A nontransgenic mouse model shows inducible amyloid-beta (Abeta) peptide deposition and elucidates the role of apolipoprotein E in the amyloid cascade. Proc Natl Acad Sci USA 2004;101:13909–13914.
9 Belinson H, Lev D, Masliah E, Michaelson DM: Activation of the amyloid cascade in apolipoprotein E4 transgenic mice induces lysosomal activation and neurodegeneration resulting in marked cognitive deficits. J Neurosci 2008;28:4690–4701.
10 Belinson H, Michaelson DM: Pathological synergism between amyloid-beta and apolipoprotein E4 – The most prevalent yet understudied genetic risk factor for Alzheimer's disease. J Alzheimers Dis 2009, Epub ahead of print.
11 Hoffmann R, Lee VM, Leight S, Varga I, Otvos L Jr: Unique Alzheimer's disease paired helical filament specific epitopes involve double phosphorylation at specific sites. Biochemistry 1997;36:8114–8124.
12 Zheng-Fischhofer Q, Biernat J, Mandelkow EM, Illenberger S, Godemann R, Mandelkow E: Sequential phosphorylation of Tau by glycogen synthase kinase-3beta and protein kinase A at Thr212 and Ser214 generates the Alzheimer-specific epitope of antibody AT100 and requires a paired-helical-filament-like conformation. Eur J Biochem 1998;252:542–552.
13 Augustinack JC, Schneider A, Mandelkow EM, Hyman BT: Specific tau phosphorylation sites correlate with severity of neuronal cytopathology in Alzheimer's disease. Acta Neuropathol 2002;103:26–35.
14 Frasier M, Walzer M, McCarthy L, Magnuson D, Lee JM, Haas C, Kahle P, Wolozin B: Tau phosphorylation increases in symptomatic mice overexpressing A30P alpha-synuclein. Exp Neurol 2005;192:274–287.
15 Goedert M, Jakes R, Vanmechelen E: Monoclonal antibody AT8 recognises tau protein phosphorylated at both serine 202 and threonine 205. Neurosci Lett 1995;189:167–169.
16 Korneyev AY: Stress-induced tau phosphorylation in mouse strains with different brain Erk 1 + 2 immunoreactivity. Neurochem Res 1998;23:1539–1543.
17 Sullivan PM, Mace BE, Maeda N, Schmechel DE: Marked regional differences of brain human apolipoprotein E expression in targeted replacement mice. Neuroscience 2004;124:725–733.
18 Matsumori Y, Hong SM, Fan Y, Kayama T, Hsu CY, Weinstein PR, Liu J: Enriched environment and spatial learning enhance hippocampal neurogenesis and salvages ischemic penumbra after focal cerebral ischemia. Neurobiol Dis 2006;22:187–198.
19 Yoshida H, Goedert M: Sequential phosphorylation of tau protein by cAMP-dependent protein kinase and SAPK4/p38delta or JNK2 in the presence of heparin generates the AT100 epitope. J Neurochem 2006;99:154–164.
20 Allen B, Ingram E, Takao M, Smith MJ, Jakes R, Virdee K, Yoshida H, Holzer M, Craxton M, Emson PC, Atzori C, Migheli A, Crowther RA, Ghetti B, Spillantini MG, Goedert M: Abundant tau filaments and nonapoptotic neurodegeneration in transgenic mice expressing human P301S tau protein. J Neurosci 2002;22:9340–9351.
21 Delobel P, Lavenir I, Fraser G, Ingram E, Holzer M, Ghetti B, Spillantini MG, Crowther RA, Goedert M: Analysis of tau phosphorylation and truncation in a mouse model of human tauopathy. Am J Pathol 2008;172:123–131.
22 Rosenmann H, Grigoriadis N, Eldar-Levy H, Avital A, Rozenstein L, Touloumi O, Behar L, Ben-Hur T, Avraham Y, Berry E, Segal M, Ginzburg I, Abramsky O: A novel transgenic mouse expressing double mutant tau driven by its natural promoter exhibits tauopathy characteristics. Exp Neurol 2008;212:71–84.
23 Schindowski K, Bretteville A, Leroy K, Begard S, Brion JP, Hamdane M, Buee L: Alzheimer's disease-like tau neuropathology leads to memory deficits and loss of functional synapses in a novel mutated tau transgenic mouse without any motor deficits. Am J Pathol 2006;169:599–616.
24 Bellucci A, Rosi MC, Grossi C, Fiorentini A, Luccarini I, Casamenti F: Abnormal processing of tau in the brain of aged TgCRND8 mice. Neurobiol Dis 2007;27:328–338.
25 Feng Q, Cheng B, Yang R, Sun FY, Zhu CQ: Dynamic changes of phosphorylated tau in mouse hippocampus after cold water stress. Neurosci Lett 2005;388:13–16.
26 Gotz J, Probst A, Spillantini MG, Schafer T, Jakes R, Burki K, Goedert M: Somatodendritic localization and hyperphosphorylation of tau protein in transgenic mice expressing the longest human brain tau isoform. EMBO J 1995;14:1304–1313.
27 Hu M, Waring JF, Gopalakrishnan M, Li J: Role of GSK-3beta activation and alpha7 nAChRs in Abeta(1–42)-induced tau phosphorylation in PC12 cells. J Neurochem 2008;106:1371–1377.
28 Khatoon S, Grundke-Iqbal I, Iqbal K: Levels of normal and abnormally phosphorylated tau in different cellular and regional compartments of Alzheimer disease and control brains. FEBS Lett 1994;351:80–84.
29 Masliah E, Sisk A, Mallory M, Games D: Neurofibrillary pathology in transgenic mice overexpressing V717F beta-amyloid precursor protein. J Neuropathol Exp Neurol 2001;60:357–368.
30 Oddo S, Caccamo A, Kitazawa M, Tseng BP, LaFerla FM: Amyloid deposition precedes tangle formation in a triple transgenic model of Alzheimer's disease. Neurobiol Aging 2003;24:1063–1070.
31 Otth C, Concha, II, Arendt T, Stieler J, Schliebs R, Gonzalez-Billault C, Maccioni RB: AbetaPP induces cdk5-dependent tau hyperphosphorylation in transgenic mice Tg2576. J Alzheimers Dis 2002;4:417–430.
32 Zhang YJ, Xu YF, Liu YH, Yin J, Li HL, Wang Q, Wang JZ: Peroxynitrite induces Alzheimer-like tau modifications and accumulation in rat brain and its underlying mechanisms. FASEB J 2006;20:1431–1442.
33 Levi O, Michaelson DM: Environmental enrichment stimulates neurogenesis in apolipoprotein E3 and neuronal apoptosis in apolipoprotein E4 transgenic mice. J Neurochem 2007;100:202–210.
34 Levi O, Jongen-Relo AL, Feldon J, Roses AD, Michaelson DM: ApoE4 impairs hippocampal plasticity isoform-specifically and blocks the environmental stimulation of synaptogenesis and memory. Neurobiol Dis 2003;13:273–282.
35 Sabo T, Lomnitski L, Nyska A, Beni S, Maronpot RR, Shohami E, Roses AD, Michaelson DM: Susceptibility of transgenic mice expressing human apolipoprotein E to closed head injury: the allele E3 is neuroprotective whereas E4 increases fatalities. Neuroscience 2000;101:879–884.
36 Ophir G, Amariglio N, Jacob-Hirsch J, Elkon R, Rechavi G, Michaelson DM: Apolipoprotein E4 enhances brain inflammation by modulation of the NF-kappaB signaling cascade. Neurobiol Dis 2005;20:709–718.
37 Baumann K, Mandelkow EM, Biernat J, Piwnica-Worms H, Mandelkow E: Abnormal Alzheimer-like phosphorylation of tau-protein by cyclin-dependent kinases cdk2 and cdk5. FEBS Lett 1993;336:417–424.
38 Godemann R, Biernat J, Mandelkow E, Mandelkow EM: Phosphorylation of tau protein by recombinant GSK-3beta: pronounced phosphorylation at select Ser/Thr-Pro motifs but no phosphorylation at Ser262 in the repeat domain. FEBS Lett 1999;454:157–164.

39 Illenberger S, Zheng-Fischhofer Q, Preuss U, Stamer K, Baumann K, Trinczek B, Biernat J, Godemann R, Mandelkow EM, Mandelkow E: The endogenous and cell cycle-dependent phosphorylation of tau protein in living cells: implications for Alzheimer's disease. Mol Biol Cell 1998;9:1495–1512.
40 Mandelkow EM, Drewes G, Biernat J, Gustke N, Van Lint J, Vandenheede JR, Mandelkow E: Glycogen synthase kinase-3 and the Alzheimer-like state of microtubule-associated protein tau. FEBS Lett 1992;314:315–321.
41 Sperber BR, Leight S, Goedert M, Lee VM: Glycogen synthase kinase-3 beta phosphorylates tau protein at multiple sites in intact cells. Neurosci Lett 1995;197:149–153.
42 Brecht WJ, Harris FM, Chang S, Tesseur I, Yu GQ, Xu Q, Dee Fish J, Wyss-Coray T, Buttini M, Mucke L, Mahley RW, Huang Y: Neuron-specific apolipoprotein e4 proteolysis is associated with increased tau phosphorylation in brains of transgenic mice. J Neurosci 2004;24:2527–2534.
43 Tesseur I, Van Dorpe J, Bruynseels K, Bronfman F, Sciot R, Van Lommel A, Van Leuven F: Prominent axonopathy and disruption of axonal transport in transgenic mice expressing human apolipoprotein E4 in neurons of brain and spinal cord. Am J Pathol 2000;157: 1495–1510.
44 Tesseur I, Van Dorpe J, Spittaels K, Van den Haute C, Moechars D, Van Leuven F: Expression of human apolipoprotein E4 in neurons causes hyperphosphorylation of protein tau in the brains of transgenic mice. Am J Pathol 2000;156:951–964.
45 Harris FM, Brecht WJ, Xu Q, Mahley RW, Huang Y: Increased tau phosphorylation in apolipoprotein E4 transgenic mice is associated with activation of extracellular signal-regulated kinase: modulation by zinc. J Biol Chem 2004;279:44795–44801.

Biology of Neurodegeneration

Neuro-degenerative Diseases

Neurodegenerative Dis 2010;7:24–27
DOI: 10.1159/000283478

Published online: February 13, 2010

Transition of Tau Protein from Disordered to Misordered in Alzheimer's Disease

Branislav Kovacech[a, b] Rostislav Skrabana[a, b] Michal Novak[a]

[a]Institute of Neuroimmunology, AD Centre, Slovak Academy of Sciences, Bratislava, Slovakia;
[b]Axon Neuroscience, GmbH, Vienna, Austria

Key Words
Intrinsically disordered tau · Alzheimer's disease · Conformational change · Truncation · Tau transition

Abstract
The neuronal protein tau, a member of the class of intrinsically disordered proteins, is characterized by the absence of any firm 3-D structure and high solubility when free in solution. The tau protein forms insoluble fibrils in the brain of people suffering from Alzheimer's disease (AD) and other tauopathies and plays a key role in the neurodegenerative process. Posttranslational events leading to the transition of tau from a disordered highly soluble protein to the insoluble aggregate seem to be associated with hyperphosphorylation, truncation or a combination of both. These modifications are assumed to change the native disorder of tau into a preaggregation state, which then directly initiates the fibrillization process. Conformation-specific anti-tau antibody DC11 detects pathological truncated tau forms present in AD brains but not in the normal human brain. A truncated tau protein selected from this pool of DC11-positive molecules was sufficient to initiate and drive the complete tau cascade of neurofibrillary pathology in a rat model of tauopathy. Thus, DC11 antibody recognizes the AD-specific conformation of tau not found in the normal human brain. We propose the term 'misdisordered' for this distinct conformational state of tau, which is the first step in the transition of tau from a soluble disordered protein to its insoluble, misordered aggregated form.

Intrinsically Disordered Protein Tau

Alzheimer's disease (AD) is the most frequent form of dementia. Years of research have established tau as one of the main culprits in its etiology.

The neuronal protein tau belongs to a family of microtubule-associated proteins [1]. In the adult human brain, tau exists as six major isoforms produced by alternative splicing of mRNA transcribed form a single gene [2]. Multiple phosphorylation sites further increase the diversity of tau molecules [3] resulting in multitudes of different protein forms, which are better referred to as *tau proteome* [4]. Tau plays a role in the establishment of neuronal polarity and axonal outgrowth during development and in the maintenance of axonal morphology and axonal transport in mature cells [5].

Tau is a highly soluble protein containing only limited amount of secondary or tertiary structure in solution [6] that assigns it to a group of intrinsically disordered pro-

KARGER
Fax +41 61 306 12 34
E-Mail karger@karger.ch
www.karger.com

1660–2854/10/0073–0024$26.00/0

Accessible online at:
www.karger.com/ndd

Michal Novak, MDV, PhD, DSc
Institute of Neuroimmunology, Slovak Academy of Sciences
Dubravska cesta 9
SK–84510 Bratislava (Slovak Republic)
Tel. +421 905 609 558, Fax +421 2 5477 4276, E-Mail michal.novak@savba.sk

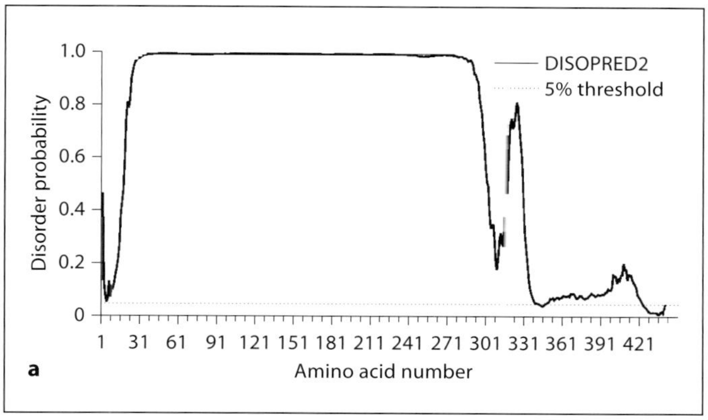

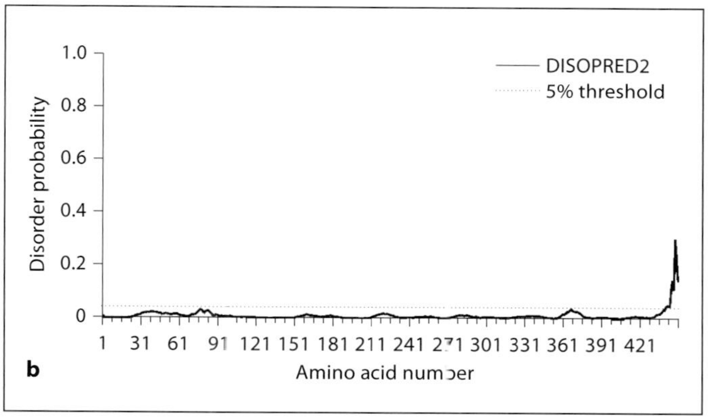

Fig. 1. In silico predictions of disorder for tau and tubulin. **a** IDP tau exhibits very high overall disorder probability. **b** Highly structured tubulin shows no sign of disorder except for the last few amino acids at its C-terminus [24]. The longest human tau isoform Tau40 and human α-tubulin (NP_006073.2) were subjected to the prediction using DISOPRED2 server at http://bioinf.cs.ucl.ac.uk/disopred/disopred.html [25]. The horizontal dotted line is the order/disorder threshold for the default false-positive rate of 5%.

teins (IDPs). The disorder probability profile of tau predicted by DISOPRED2 exhibits a high propensity for disorderedness (fig. 1). This is in striking contrast with such a profile computed for a highly structured *(ordered)* protein like α-tubulin, tau's main interacting partner. The disordered character endows tau with high binding dynamics, flexibility and promiscuity.

Disorder to Misorder Transition of Tau

In AD and other tauopathies, tau forms neurofibrillary tangles (NFTs) composed of filaments of helical or straight morphology [7]. In both kinds of filaments, tau adopts a *misordered* state characterized by a highly structured core involving distinct motifs from microtubule-binding repeats arranged in β-sheets perpendicular to the filament axis [8, 9]. The remaining sequences of tau form a disordered fuzzy coat resulting in a relatively low overall content of secondary structure in tau filaments [10, 11]. The term 'misordered' therefore describes a state of tau opposing its disordered native conformation but also distinguishes it from the misfolded state of globular proteins, which generally remains globular [12].

Thus, the formation of tau aggregates results from the *disorder* to *misorder* transition. What induces this transition? Many factors have been assumed in this process, with hyperphosphorylation and truncation being the hottest candidates.

Tau hyperphosphorylation in AD [13] has been observed soon after the discovery of tau as the structural constituent of NFTs [11, 14], and became the prime suspect in the initiation of tau pathology. Hyperphosphorylated tau isolated from AD brains sequesters normal tau and other MAP proteins, interferes with microtubule assembly, has high propensity to aggregate in vitro and to form paired and straight filaments [15, 16]. On the other hand, phosphorylation was also shown to protect tau from aggregation in an in vitro system where aggregation was induced by polyanions [17], although this might be attributed to the interaction of negative charges of the phosphate groups and those of polyanions.

Truncated tau species in AD have first been clearly documented by using a truncation-specific monoclonal antibody MN423 [18]. Tau truncation has also been proposed as an early event in neurofibrillary pathology [19, 20].

Recently, we have presented a rat model of tauopathy expressing a human truncated tau protein derived from sporadic AD [21]. This truncated tau induced the complete tau cascade of neurofibrillary degeneration (tau hyperphosphorylation, argyrophilic tangles and sarcosyl-insoluble tau formation with a typical A68 triplet), accompanied by oxidative stress, neurobehavioral impairment and premature death [22].

The truncated tau used as a transgene has been selected on the basis of its immunoreactivity with an AD-specific antibody DC11. This antibody recognizes only tau proteins that are truncated at both the N- and C-terminal ends, selectively stains tau present in the AD brain but does not react with tau present in the normal human brain [23].

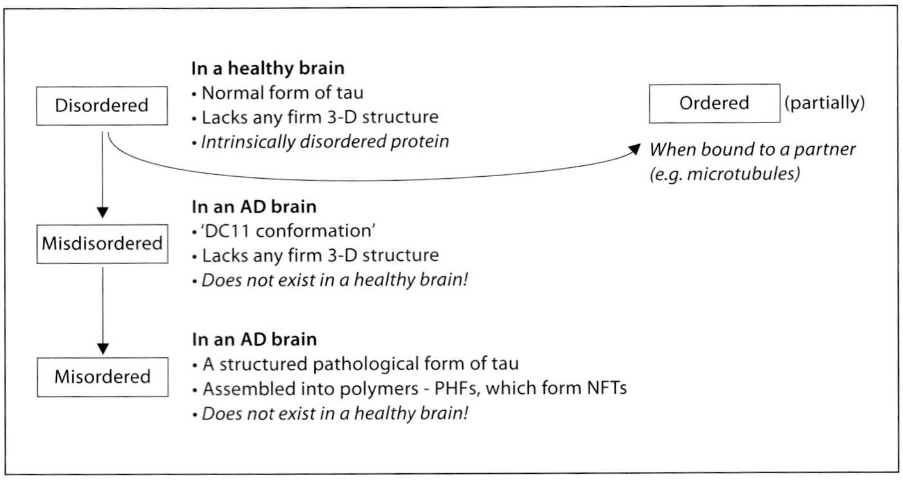

Fig. 2. Tau transition from disordered to misordered includes an intermediate stage of misdisordered tau. PHFs = Paired helical filaments.

This unique feature of the truly conformational antibody DC11 revealed that truncated tau species possess specific pathological conformation distinct from that of full-length tau. Thus, the antibody helped us to uncover an important step in the tau transition from disordered to misordered. Pathological 'DC11 conformation' of tau generated by truncation represents a prefibrillar form of tau directly preceding its polymerization into misordered filaments (fig. 2). Furthermore, using a panel of monoclonal antibodies with epitopes distributed along the truncated tau we observed that the main characteristic of the truncated tau was the higher accessibility of its microtubule-binding region in comparison with full-length tau [unpubl. obs.]. Therefore, this form of tau conformationally differs from normal disordered tau, but does not have a firm structure, yet. We named this status 'misdisordered' to specifically underline these conformational characteristics.

Since the misdisordered truncated tau is able to induce neurofibrillary degeneration in vivo [21], it is a promising target for AD therapy or prevention.

Acknowledgment

This work was supported by research grants APVV 0603-06, APVV 0621-07, APVV 0471-06, LPP-0326-06 and LPP-0363-06.

References

1 Weingarten MD, Lockwood AH, Hwo SY, Kirschner MW: A protein factor essential for microtubule assembly. Proc Natl Acad Sci USA 1975;72:1858–1862.
2 Goedert M, Spillantini MG, Jakes R, Rutherford D, Crowther RA: Multiple isoforms of human microtubule-associated protein tau: sequences and localization in neurofibrillary tangles of Alzheimer's disease. Neuron 1989;3:519–526.
3 Hanger DP, Byers HL, Wray S, Leung KY, Saxton MJ, Seereeram A, Reynolds CH, Ward MA, Anderton BH: Novel phosphorylation sites in tau from Alzheimer brain support a role for casein kinase 1 in disease pathogenesis. J Biol Chem 2007;282:23645–23654.
4 Hanes J, Zilka N, Bartkova M, Caletkova M, Dobrota D, Novak M: Rat tau proteome consists of six tau isoforms: implication for animal models of human tauopathies. J Neurochem 2009;108:1167–1176.
5 Garcia ML, Cleveland DW: Going new places using an old map: Tau, microtubules and human neurodegenerative disease. Curr Opin Cell Biol 2001;13:41–48.
6 Schweers O, Schonbrunn-Hanebeck E, Marx A, Mandelkow E: Structural studies of tau protein and Alzheimer paired helical filaments show no evidence for beta-structure. J Biol Chem 1994;269:24290–24297.
7 Iqbal K, Liu F, Gong CX, Alonso Adel C, Grundke-Iqbal I: Mechanisms of tau-induced neurodegeneration. Acta Neuropathol 2009;118:53–69.
8 Mandelkow E, von Bergen M, Biernat J, Mandelkow EM: Structural principles of tau and the paired helical filaments of Alzheimer's disease. Brain Pathol 2007;17:83–90.
9 Skrabana R, Sevcik J, Novak M: Intrinsically disordered proteins in the neurodegenerative processes: formation of tau protein paired helical filaments and their analysis. Cell Mol Neurobiol 2006;26:1085–1097.
10 Barghorn S, Davies P, Mandelkow E: Tau paired helical filaments from Alzheimer's disease brain and assembled in vitro are based on beta-structure in the core domain. Biochemistry 2004;43:1694–1703.
11 Wischik CM, Novak M, Edwards PC, Klug A, Tichelaar W, Crowther RA: Structural characterization of the core of the paired helical filament of Alzheimer disease. Proc Natl Acad Sci USA 1988;85:4884–4888.

12 Chiti F, Dobson CM: Protein misfolding, functional amyloid, and human disease. Annu Rev Biochem 2006;75:333–366.
13 Grundke-Iqbal I, Iqbal K, Tung YC, Quinlan M, Wisniewski HM, Binder LI: Abnormal phosphorylation of the microtubule-associated protein tau (tau) in Alzheimer cytoskeletal pathology. Proc Natl Acad Sci USA 1986; 83:4913–4917.
14 Ihara Y, Nukina N, Miura R, Ogawara M: Phosphorylated tau protein is integrated into paired helical filaments in Alzheimer's disease. J Biochem (Tokyo) 1986;99:1807–1810.
15 Alonso AC, Li B, Grundke-Iqbal I, Iqbal K: Mechanism of tau-induced neurodegeneration in Alzheimer disease and related tauopathies. Curr Alzheimer Res 2008;5:375–384.
16 Alonso A, Zaidi T, Novak M, Grundke-Iqbal I, Iqbal K: Hyperphosphorylation induces self-assembly of tau into tangles of paired helical filaments/straight filaments. Proc Natl Acad Sci USA 2001;98:6923–6928.
17 Schneider A, Biernat J, von Bergen M, Mandelkow E, Mandelkow EM: Phosphorylation that detaches tau protein from microtubules (ser262, ser214) also protects it against aggregation into Alzheimer paired helical filaments. Biochemistry 1999;38:3549–3558.
18 Novak M, Wischik CM, Edwards P, Pannell R, Milstein C: Characterisation of the first monoclonal antibody against the pronase resistant core of the Alzheimer PHF. Prog Clin Biol Res 1989;317:755–761.
19 Novak M, Kabat J, Wischik CM: Molecular characterization of the minimal protease resistant tau unit of the Alzheimer's disease paired helical filament. EMBO J 1993;12: 365–370.
20 Rissman RA, Poon WW, Blurton-Jones M, Oddo S, Torp R, Vitek MP, LaFerla FM, Rohn TT, Cotman CW: Caspase-cleavage of tau is an early event in Alzheimer disease tangle pathology. J Clin Invest 2004;114:121–130.
21 Zilka N, Filipcik P, Koson P, Fialova L, Skrabana R, Zilkova M, Rolkova G, Kontsekova E, Novak M: Truncated tau from sporadic Alzheimer's disease suffices to drive neurofibrillary degeneration in vivo. FEBS Lett 2006;580:3582–3588.
22 Zilka N, Korenova M, Novak M: Misfolded tau protein and disease modifying pathways in transgenic rodent models of human tauopathies. Acta Neuropathol 2009;118:71–86.
23 Vechterova L, Kontsekova E, Zilka N, Ferencik M, Ravid R, Novak M: DC11: a novel monoclonal antibody revealing Alzheimer's disease-specific tau epitope. Neuroreport 2003;14:87–91.
24 Nogales E, Wolf SG, Downing KH: Structure of the alpha beta tubulin dimer by electron crystallography. Nature 1998;391:199–203.
25 Ward JJ, Sodhi JS, McGuffin LJ, Buxton BF, Jones DT: Prediction and functional analysis of native disorder in proteins from the three kingdoms of life. J Mol Biol 2004;337:635–645.

Biology of Neurodegeneration

Neuro-degenerative Diseases

Neurodegenerative Dis 2010;7:28–31
DOI: 10.1159/000283479

Published online: February 13, 2010

'Prion-Like' Propagation of Mouse and Human Tau Aggregates in an Inducible Mouse Model of Tauopathy

Astrid Sydow Eva-Maria Mandelkow

Max-Planck-Unit for Structural Molecular Biology, Hamburg, Germany

Key Words
Alzheimer's disease · Tau · Aggregation · Transgenic mouse models · Tauopathy

Abstract
Background: Aggregates of the tau protein are a hallmark of Alzheimer's and several other neurodegenerative diseases. Various transgenic mouse models have been generated to study the aggregation process. Since wild-type tau is highly soluble and does not aggregate readily, most models make use of tau mutations that occur in human frontotemporal dementias and are more prone to aggregate. These mouse models show neurofibrillary tangles similar to those of Alzheimer's disease. However, since the mice contain both endogenous wild-type mouse tau and exogenous human mutant tau, the relative contribution of these components to the aggregates has been a matter of debate. ***Objective:*** Using a new set of regulatable transgenic mouse models, we sought to determine whether mouse tau coaggregates with human tau when it is switched on. Furthermore, we asked what type of tau remains in the aggregates after switching off the expression of exogenous tau. ***Methods:*** We generated doxycycline-inducible transgenic mice expressing either full-length human tau or the tau repeat domain (tau_{RD}). In addition, both types of human tau derivatives were expressed in a 'proaggregant' form (with the frontotemporal dementia with parkinsonism linked to chromosome 17 mutation ΔK280), or in an 'antiaggregant' form (with additional proline mutations to block β-structure and aggregation). ***Results:*** The proaggregant tau_{RD} mice develop tangles rapidly after induction, the antiaggregant mice do not. Analysis by biochemistry and immunohistology reveals that the tangles contain both exogenous and endogenous mouse tau. After switching off the proaggregant tau_{RD}, tangles persist for extended periods. However, they are composed entirely of mouse tau. ***Conclusions:*** Mouse tau and exogenous human tau can coaggregate in transgenic models of tauopathy. The aggregates are in dynamic equilibrium with their subunits, so that exogenous tau disappears when its expression is switched off. Once the seeds of aggregation are generated by the foreign tau species, they propagate in a 'prion-like' fashion within the cell even after the foreign tau has disappeared.

Introduction

Tau is a microtubule-associated protein which occurs mainly in neuronal axons and stabilizes microtubules as tracks for axonal transport. Tau is a highly soluble, natively unfolded protein, yet it forms pathological 'paired-helical filaments' in neurodegenerative diseases such as Alzheimer's disease (AD), frontotemporal dementia with parkinsonism linked to chromosome 17 (FTDP17), PSP, Pick's disease and others. The tau-microtubule interaction is based on tau's 'repeat domain' of ~100 residues which also forms the core of Alzheimer paired helical filaments (fig. 1). This illustrates the close relationship be-

KARGER

Fax +41 61 306 12 34
E-Mail karger@karger.ch
www.karger.com

1660–2854/10/0073–0028$26.00/0

Accessible online at:
www.karger.com/ndd

Eva-Maria Mandelkow
Max-Planck-Unit for Structural Molecular Biology
Notkestrasse 85
DE–22607 Hamburg (Germany)
Tel. +49 40 899 828 10, Fax +49 40 897 168 22, E-Mail mandelkow@mpasmb.desy.de

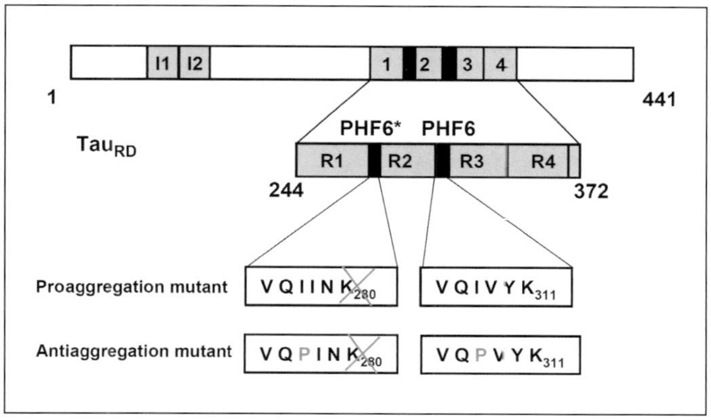

Fig. 1. Constructs of tau derived from tau repeat domain. The top bar diagram represents the longest isoform of the human tau40 (441 residues). The bottom diagram shows the four-repeat construct tau$_{RD}$ derived from htau40. One of the constructs used here contains the FTDP17 mutation ΔK280 in order to accelerate aggregation by promoting β-structure (proaggregant mutant). The second mutant has additionally two proline mutations (I277P and I308P in the hexapeptide motifs) in order to inhibit the aggregation by disrupting β-structure (antiaggregant mutant).

tween physiological and pathological functions of tau [for reviews, see 1, 2]. Because of the good solubility of tau, it has been difficult to design cell or mouse models of tau pathology; overexpression of tau alone generally does not yield aggregation. Researchers have therefore made use of tau mutations that occur in cases of FTDP17 and tend to be more prone to aggregation than wild-type tau. A well-known example is the mutation P301L [3]. In our work, we have chosen the mutant ΔK280 because of its rapid aggregation in vitro [4].

We generated several transgenic mouse lines based on this mutation, expressing either the repeat domain of human tau (tau$_{RD}$), or full-length human tau [5, 6]. The expression was made regulatable by doxycycline using the tetracycline-responsive transactivator (tet-off system [7]). Expression was restricted to the forebrain by means of the CaMKIIα-promoter [8]. In the presence of doxycycline, no expression of tau$_{RD}$ and no aggregation were detected after 5 months, indicating that the system was tightly regulated. In order to distinguish the effects of tau expression from aggregation, we designed two types of protein, containing either the ΔK280 mutation alone, or in combination with two prolines in the hexapeptide motifs that control the transition to β-structure and therefore the aggregation of tau [9]. In the latter case, no aggregation occurs because prolines are not compatible with β-structure. These two forms are termed 'proaggregant' or 'antiaggregant' tau.

When expressing human tau in a mouse, one has to consider the relationship with endogenous mouse tau. Both types of protein are very similar, especially in their microtubule-binding and repeat domains. In vitro, both bind tightly to microtubules, and both are able to copolymerize into paired helical filaments, regardless of isoform [10]. One would therefore expect this to happen in vivo as well. However, this has been a matter of debate for several reasons. One is that wild-type mouse tau does not aggregate by itself (e.g., in models of AD based on APP mutations), and wild-type human tau, even when expressed at high levels, does not aggregate either [11]. This has led to the assumption that endogenous mouse tau or the environment in a mouse neuron is protective against aggregation. In apparent support of this view, human wild-type tau (comprising all isoforms) was shown to aggregate only when mouse tau was eliminated [12]. A second problem was the detectability. Both mouse and human tau exist as multiple isoforms (3 and 6, respectively) which approach each other closely on an SDS gel, especially since all of them can be phosphorylated at multiple sites, with shifts in MR values causing overlaps of bands. Thus, the analysis of the composition by immunoblotting is ambiguous because most tau antibodies cross-react between human and mouse tau.

In this report, we show that these ambiguities can be circumvented by expressing human tau$_{RD}$ variants in transgenic mice which differ in their aggregation propensity and are clearly distinguishable from mouse tau by their lower molecular weight. The results show that pro-aggregant human tau$_{RD}$ can induce normal mouse tau to coaggregate when they are coexpressed within a neuronal cell, and that the aggregation can be propagated within the cell even when the foreign tau disappears.

Results and Discussion

In the mouse model used here [5], we chose to express a human tau construct (the four-repeat domain, tau$_{RD}$) that is much smaller than the endogenous mouse isoforms (fig. 1). It is therefore readily distinguished in biochemical assays. Nevertheless, tau$_{RD}$ contains all the sequence motifs required for aggregation (the hexapeptide motifs in R2 and R3). Furthermore, since most of the AD-diagnostic antibody epitopes lie outside the repeat domain, the composition of aggregates in brain sections and immunoblots can be readily determined.

These tools allow one to demonstrate that exogenous human tau and mouse tau can indeed coaggregate. The

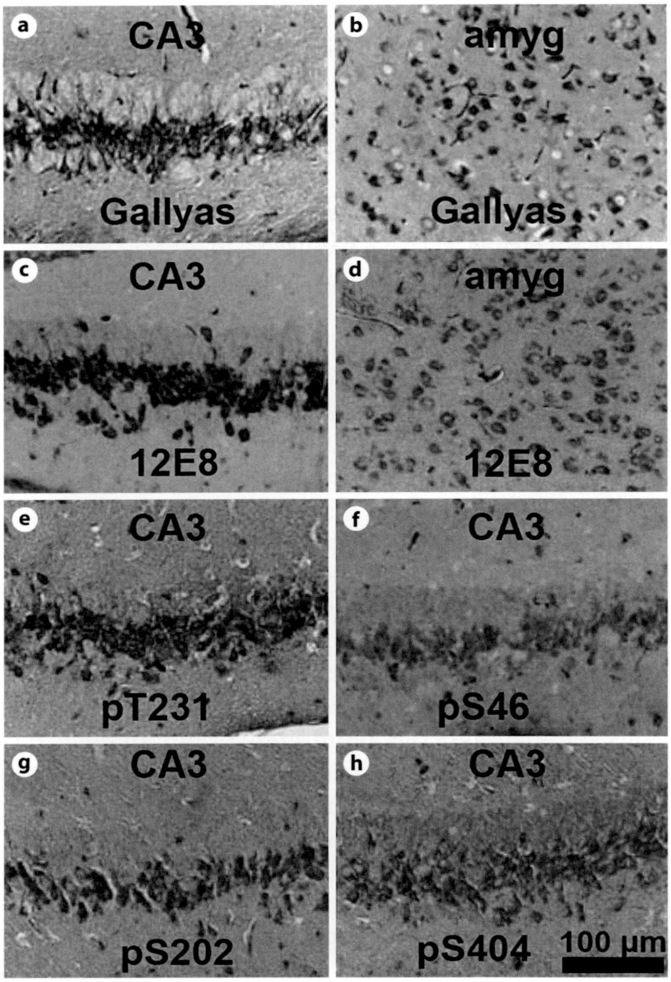

Fig. 2. Coaggregation and phosphorylation of endogenous and exogenous tau in proaggregant mutant mice. Images from CA3 region and amygdala. **a**, **b** Gallyas silver staining for NFTs. **c–h** Immunostaining with antibodies against different phosphoepitopes of tau. Note that pT231, pS46, pS202, and pS404 lie outside the repeats. This demonstrates that full-length mouse tau is incorporated into the tangles. Scale bars = 100 μm.

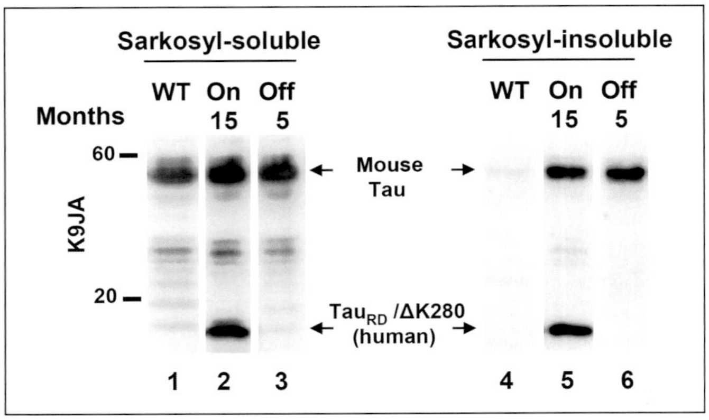

Fig. 3. Tangles of mouse tau persist after switching off the expression of proaggregant tau_{RD}. Immunoblot analysis of sarkosyl-soluble fractions (lanes 1–3) and sarkosyl-insoluble fractions (lanes 4–6) from cortex homogenates. Lanes 1 and 4 show wild type, lanes 2 and 5 proaggregation mutant 15 months expression on, lanes 3 and 6 proaggregation mutant 9 months on and 5 months off. Lanes 1–3 show additional weak bands representing fragments of mouse tau. Note that after the switch-off for 5 months the soluble and insoluble proaggregant tau_{RD} disappears and the remaining aggregates consist only of mouse tau.

mutant tau_{RD} appears in Western blots as a band of 12–14 kDa, clearly distinct from the endogenous mouse tau [see also 5]. This allows one to determine the ratios of the proteins. Both the proaggregant and antiaggregant mouse lines had similar levels of exogenous tau, ~70% of endogenous tau protein. The aggregation can be evaluated by the sarkosyl extraction method [13] which reveals tangles as well as pretangle aggregates. Most exogenous tau_{RD} proteins and the three adult mouse tau isoforms are in the soluble fraction, both for pro- and antiaggregation mutants. Sarkosyl-insoluble fractions contain pronounced tau only in the proaggregation mouse line. The ratio of tau_{RD} to endogenous tau in the sarkosyl-insoluble and soluble fractions is similar (0.4–0.5), showing that endogenous mouse tau is incorporated into the aggregates. By contrast, the antiaggregation mouse line, like the wild-type line, shows no or very little tau in the sarkosyl-insoluble pellet.

Immunohistochemistry of the brains yields a similar picture. In the proaggregant mice, tangle formation starts at ~2 months of gene expression, and Gallyas-positive neurons appear in the entorhinal cortex and amygdala. At 12–15 months, neurofibrillary tangle (NFT) pathology spreads across the entorhinal cortex and neocortex [see also 5]. By contrast, the antiaggregation tau mice show no NFTs even at 22 months. The aggregates of the proaggregant mice can be immunostained with antibodies whose epitopes lie outside the repeat domain and occur only in mouse tau; this provides confirmation of the coaggregation between endogenous tau and exogenous proaggregant tau_{RD} (fig. 2).

A key question in the AD field is whether the aggregation of tau is reversible. When the expression of proaggregant tau_{RD} is switched on for 9 months, and then off for 5 months, the exogenous sarkosyl-soluble and insoluble protein nearly disappears (fig. 3). As shown elsewhere, the degradation of aggregated tau is largely dependent on macroautophagy [14]. By contrast, the aggregated endogenous mouse tau in the sarkosyl-insoluble fractions decreases only moderately, indicating that the tangles formed from mouse tau persist. This can be explained by the continued synthesis of endogenous mouse tau and the presence of seeds of aggregation once they have been generated within a cell.

Several conclusions can be drawn from these experiments:

- The beta propensity of tau in the repeat domain determines its aggregation behavior in transgenic mice. Thus, proaggregant tau_{RD} aggregates, antiaggregant tau_{RD} does not.
- Once the seeding of aggregates is achieved by proaggregant tau species within a cell, aggregation can spread to the pool of normal endogenous tau that is neither elevated nor mutated. In other words, the 'poisonous' conformation can be propagated to 'healthy' endogenous tau in a fashion reminiscent of prion propagation. As a result, mouse tau coaggregates with human tau_{RD}.
- Aggregation is surprisingly persistent once it has been initiated. Tau aggregates survive long after the initial proaggregant culprit (tau_{RD}) has been switched off and disappeared. The remaining aggregates consist entirely of wild-type mouse tau (which cannot be switched off). The result has several implications:
- The neuron's self-defense mechanisms are still active, even after harboring tau aggregates for several months, i.e., when tau_{RD} is switched off, it can be eliminated from the soluble and insoluble pool of proteins.
- Since tau_{RD} is gradually released from the aggregates and eliminated, the aggregates must be in a dynamic equilibrium with their subunits.

An important consequence of the last point is that it should be possible to shift the equilibrium between aggregates and subunits by low molecular weight compounds that lock tau in a nonaggregating conformation. A number of such tau inhibitor compounds have been developed and are currently examined for their therapeutic potential [for a review, see 15].

Acknowledgements

We thank Dagmar Drexler, Olga Petrova and Anne Hofmann for excellent technical assistance, Dr. Jacek Biernat and Dr. Eckhard Mandelkow for stimulating discussions. This research was supported by the Max-Planck Society, Deutsche Forschungsgemeinschaft, Breuer Foundation, and EU/Memosad.

References

1 Goedert M, Klug A, Crowther RA: Tau protein, the paired helical filament and Alzheimer's disease. J Alzheimers Dis 2006;9: 195–207.
2 Schneider A, Mandelkow E: Tau-based treatment strategies in neurodegenerative diseases. Neurotherapeutics 2008;5:443–457.
3 Lewis J, Dickson DW, Lin WL, Chisholm L, Corral A, Jones G, Yen SH, Sahara N, Skipper L, Yager D, Eckman C, Hardy J, Hutton M, McGowan E: Enhanced neurofibrillary degeneration in transgenic mice expressing mutant tau and APP. Science 2001;293:1487–1491.
4 Barghorn S, Zheng-Fischhofer Q, Ackmann M, Biernat J, von Bergen M, Mandelkow EM, Mandelkow E: Structure, microtubule interactions, and paired helical filament aggregation by tau mutants of frontotemporal dementias. Biochemistry 2000;39:11714–11721.
5 Mocanu MM, Nissen A, Eckermann K, Khlistunova I, Biernat J, Drexler D, Petrova O, Schönig K, Bujard H, Mandelkow E, Zhou L, Rune G, Mandelkow EM: The potential for beta-structure in the repeat domain of tau protein determines aggregation, synaptic decay, neuronal loss, and coassembly with endogenous Tau in inducible mouse models of tauopathy. J Neurosci 2008;28: 737–748.
6 Eckermann K, Mocanu MM, Khlistunova I, Biernat J, Nissen A, Hofmann A, Schönig K, Bujard H, Haemisch, A, Mandelkow E, Zhou L, Rune G, Mandelkow EM: The beta-propensity of Tau determines aggregation and synaptic loss in inducible mouse models of Alzheimer tauopathy. J Biol Chem 2007;282: 31755–31765.
7 Gossen M, Bujard H: Studying gene function in eukaryotes by conditional gene inactivation. Annu Rev Genet 2002;36:153–173.
8 Mayford M, Bach ME, Huang YY, Wang L, Hawkins RD, Kandel ER: Control of memory formation through regulated expression of a CaMKII transgene. Science 1996;274: 1678–1683.
9 von Bergen M, Barghorn S, Li L, Marx A, Biernat J, Mandelkow EM, Mandelkow E: Mutations of tau protein in frontotemporal dementia promote aggregation of paired helical filaments by enhancing local beta-structure. J Biol Chem 2001;276:48165–48174.
10 Kampers T, Pangalos M, Geerts H, Wiech H, Mandelkow E: Assembly of paired helical filaments from mouse tau: implications for the neurofibrillary pathology in transgenic mouse models for Alzheimer's disease. FEBS Lett 1999;451:39–44.
11 Götz J, Ittner LM: Animal models of Alzheimer's disease and frontotemporal dementia. Nat Rev Neurosci 2008;9:532–544.
12 Andorfer C, Kress Y, Espinoza M, de Silva R, Tucker KL, Barde YA, Duff K, Davies P: Hyperphosphorylation and aggregation of tau in mice expressing normal human tau isoforms. J Neurochem 2003;86:582–590.
13 Greenberg SG, Davies P: A preparation of Alzheimer paired helical filaments that displays distinct tau proteins by polyacrylamide gel electrophoresis. Proc Natl Acad Sci USA 1990;87:5827–5831.
14 Wang YP, Martinez-Vincente M, Krüger U, Kaushik S, Wong E, Mandelkow EM, Cuervo AM, Mandelkow E: Tau fragmentation, aggregation and clearance: the dual role of lysosomal processing. Human Molec Gen 2009;18:4153–4170.
15 Bulic B, Pickhardt M, Schmidt B, Mandelkow EM, Waldmann H, Mandelkow E: Development of tau aggregation inhibitors for Alzheimer's disease. Angew Chem Int Ed Engl 2009;48:1740–1752.

Biology of Neurodegeneration

Neuro-degenerative Diseases

Neurodegenerative Dis 2010;7:32–37
DOI: 10.1159/000266476

Published online: February 13, 2010

Are Aβ and Its Derivatives Causative Agents or Innocent Bystanders in AD?

Nikolaos K. Robakis

Center for Molecular Biology and Genetics of Neurodegeneration, Mount Sinai School of Medicine, New York University, New York, N.Y., USA

Key Words
Alzheimer's disease · Aβ peptides · Amyloid precursor protein · Neuronal loss

Abstract
Alzheimer's disease (AD) is characterized by neurodegeneration in neocortical regions of the brain. Currently, Aβ-based theories, including amyloid depositions and soluble Aβ, form the basis of most therapeutic approaches to AD. It remains unclear, however, whether Aβ and its derivatives are the primary causative agents of neuronal loss in AD. Reported studies show no significant correlations between brain amyloid depositions and either degree of dementia or loss of neurons, and brain amyloid loads similar to AD are often found in normal individuals. Furthermore, behavioral abnormalities in animal models overexpressing amyloid precursor protein seem independent of amyloid depositions. Soluble Aβ theories propose toxic Aβ42 or its oligomers as the agents that promote cell death in AD. Aβ peptides, however, are normal components of human serum and CSF, and it is unclear under what conditions these peptides become toxic. Presently, there is little evidence of disease-associated abnormalities in soluble Aβ and no toxic oligomers specific to AD have been found. That familial AD mutations of amyloid precursor protein, PS1 and PS2 promote neurodegeneration suggests the biological functions of these proteins play critical roles in neuronal survival. Evidence shows that the PS/γ-secretase system promotes production of peptides involved in cell surface-to-nucleus signaling and gene expression, providing support for the hypothesis that familial AD mutations may contribute to neurodegeneration by inhibiting PS-dependent signaling pathways.

Introduction

Alzheimer's disease (AD) is defined by large numbers of neuritic plaques (NPs) and neurofibrillary tangles (NFTs) in neocortical regions of the brain, but it is now accepted that dementia is caused by extensive neuronal and synapse losses in the hippocampus and neocortex. NPs are complex extracellular structures containing a core of amyloid depositions of fibrillar Aβ-proteins surrounded by reactive astrocytes, microglia, and dystrophic neurites. NFTs accumulate intracellularly and consist mainly of paired helical filaments of overphosphorylated tau protein [1]. Most AD cases occur after the age of

Part of this review was presented in the CME-certified symposium 'Targeting the Molecular Pathways of AD: Rationale and Outcomes for Disease Modification Strategies' held in conjunction with the 9th International Conference on AD/PD 2009 in Prague, Czech Republic, on March 12, 2009.

KARGER

Fax +41 61 306 12 34
E-Mail karger@karger.ch
www.karger.com

Accessible online at:
www.karger.com/ndd

Nikolaos K. Robakis
Center for Molecular Biology and Genetics of Neurodegeneration
Mount Sinai School of Medicine, New York University
One Gustave Levy Place, Box 1229, New York, NY 10029 (USA)
Tel. +1 212 241 9380, Fax +1 212 831 1947, E-Mail nikos.robakis@mssm.edu

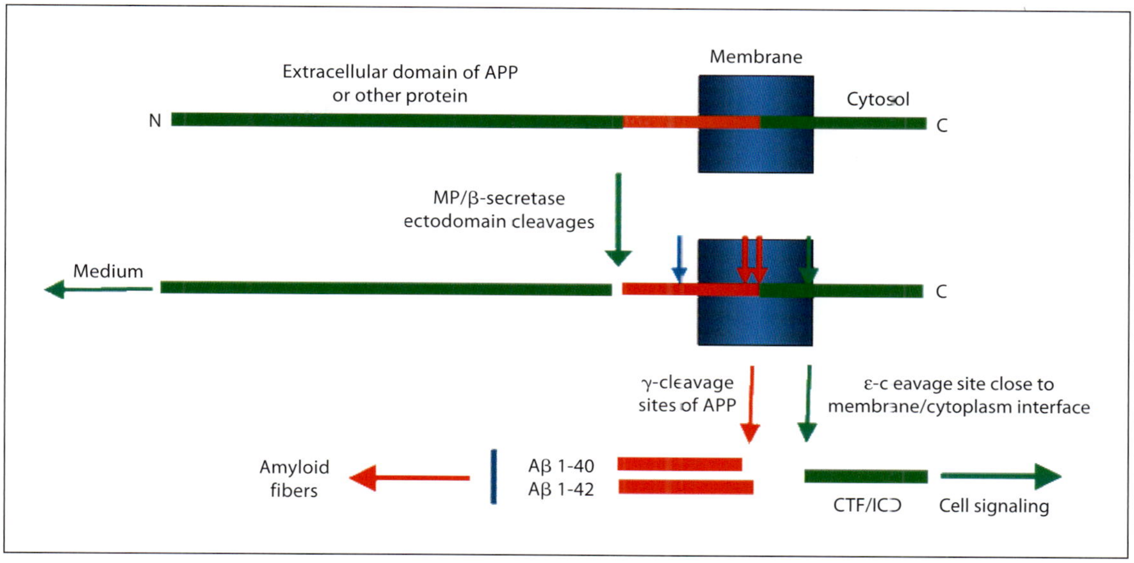

Fig. 1. Amyloidogenic and signaling cleavages of APP are distinct but closely related. Both depend on the PS1/γ-secretase system. β- and γ-secretase cleavages promote production of Aβ peptides. APP and other cell surface receptors are cleaved extracellularly by metalloproteinases (MPs) and then by γ-secretase at the ε-site to promote production of biologically active CTFs (ICDs). In the nonamyloidogenic processing, APP is cleaved by α-secretase close to the extracellular face of the plasma membrane (blue arrow, see [37]). This cleavage inhibits production of Aβ peptides.

65 or 70 and are termed sporadic because they lack a clear genetic etiology, but a small percent of all cases display clear genetic linkages and are classified as familial AD (FAD). Three genetic loci have been linked to FAD including the genes encoding the amyloid precursor protein (APP), the precursor of the Aβ peptides, PS1 and PS2. Despite intense research efforts in the last 25 years, it is still unclear what causes the accelerated neuronal cell death of sporadic AD although aging and apoE alleles are risk factors. In contrast, FAD is driven by specific genetic mutations although the biological mechanisms by which these mutations promote neurodegeneration remain unclear.

Processing of APP and Production of Aβ

In the last quarter of a century, much attention has been focused on Aβ peptides and their derivatives including soluble Aβ oligomers and fibrilar amyloid depositions as the main causative agents of AD. Aβ peptides are a family of small proteins ranging in length from 39 to 43 amino acids. Under conditions that favor aggregation, soluble Aβ peptide chains form extended β-pleated sheet structures held together in oligomeric arrangements by hydrogen bonds [2]. These Aβ oligomers aggregate further to precipitate as amyloid fibrils in NPs and blood vessels (cerebrovascular amyloid, CVA). Aβ peptides are derived from the amyloidogenic processing of APP through the sequential cleavages by β- and γ-secretases. β-Secretase cleaves first at the extracellular N-terminus of the Aβ sequence of APP to produce a membrane-bound fragment termed C99 that contains the Aβ sequence plus the transmembrane and cytoplasmic domains of APP (fig. 1). C99 peptide is then processed by the PS/γ-secretase complex at the γ-sites located in the middle of the transmembrane sequence producing Aβ peptides with distinct C-terminal ends (fig. 1).

Recent evidence shows that in addition to the amyloidogenic γ-cleavages of APP, the PS/γ-secretase system promotes the ε-cleavage of a large number of cell surface type I transmembrane proteins, including APP, Notch1 receptor, E-cadherin, N-cadherin and CD44 [reviewed in 3]. This alternative cleavage takes place downstream from the γ-cleavages at the end of the transmemebrane sequence of the substrate (fig. 1). Cleavage at the ε-site follows a metalloproteinase cleavage at the extracellular domain of the substrate and results in the release of soluble cytosolic peptides containing the intracellular domains (ICDs or C-terminal fragments, CTFs) of cleaved substrate. Similar to γ-cleavages, the ε-cleavage is also sensitive to γ-secretase inhibitors. To date, at least 20 cell surface proteins have been shown to be cleaved at the ε-sites by γ-secretase producing soluble peptides containing the CTFs of the cleaved substrates. Research in the last several years showed that these peptides may migrate to the nucleus where they act as regulators of gene expression or they may remain in the cytoplasm where they regulate the metabolism of transcription factors [3].

Amyloid Depositions Cannot Explain the Neurodegeneration Responsible for Dementia

In 1987, it was suggested that CVA depositions promote AD by compromising the blood-brain barrier allowing neurotoxic serum products into the neuropil [4]. This serum-born toxicity promotes neurodegeneration and formation of NFTs. This was an important concept as it raised for the first time the possibility that amyloid depositions of Aβ may be causally related to AD. Subsequent work however, indicated that many AD patients had little cerebrovascular damage, suggesting that AD neurodegeneration can develop in the absence of significant CVA depositions. The amyloid cascade hypothesis of AD, a variant of the CVA theory, suggested that depositions of Aβ amyloid fibrils in NPs trigger a neurotoxic cascade causing neurodegeneration and dementia [1, 5]. In the last two decades, many workers concentrated on the specific mechanism(s) by which NPs may promote neuronal cell death, but presently there is not a clear mechanism that could explain the proposed neurotoxicity of amyloid depositions, and many workers doubt these depositions are the main causative agents of AD [6, 7]. Although amyloid pathology may contribute secondarily to the neuronal dysfunction of AD, it seems unlikely that amyloid plaques constitute the main pathological agent as a number of studies failed to show significant correlations between concentration or brain distribution of NPs and degree of dementia, loss of neurons, distribution of dystrophic neurites, or cytoskeletal abnormalities [8, 9]. Furthermore, amyloid depositions at levels similar to those seen in AD are often detected in normal individuals [10, 11], and transgenic (Tg) mouse models constructed to develop high levels of brain amyloid deposits failed to show significant neurodegeneration. Interestingly, several of these models showed synaptic and electrophysiological abnormalities before detection of amyloid deposits, probably as a result of the abnormally high levels of exogenous APP [12, 13] expressed by these animals. Finally, recent studies in humans showed that clearance of amyloid depositions resulted neither in cognitive improvement nor in decreased rate of mental deterioration [14], suggesting that NPs are probably not the driving force of the neurodegeneration and cognitive decline of AD. It seems therefore unlikely that clearance of brain amyloid depositions will result in significant improvements of the cognitive functions of AD patients.

AD Neurodegeneration May Be Independent of Aβ and Oligomers

The inability of the amyloid plaque theories to explain the neurodegeneration of AD prompted the development of the soluble oligomer Aβ theories which posit that soluble oligomers of extracellular or intracellular Aβ42 represent the neurotoxic forms of Aβ. Indeed, recent reports suggest that soluble oligomeric Aβ may interfere with synaptic plasticity of cell cultures or memory function in experimental animal models [15, 16]. Most of these models however, are based on Tg animals or cell lines constructed to overexpress exogenous APP, an artificial condition that does not apply to AD where there is no evidence of APP overexpression [17]. More important, behavioral abnormalities in animal models overexpressing APP cannot be unambiguously assigned to soluble Aβ oligomers because in addition to Aβ, APP is metabolized to a large number of derivatives, some of which, including CTFs, have been reported to be neurotoxic. It is important to note that overexpression of proteins in animal brain often results in neurotoxicity due to, among other factors, trafficking abnormalities driven by the overexpressed protein. It is thus unclear whether the behavioral abnormalities detected in Tg APP mice are due to specific Aβ species or to additional toxicities of the overexpressed exogenous APP.

Soluble Aβ peptides are produced by most cells and are found in all people. Apparently, these peptides are normal components of human serum and CSF, and it has been proposed that they have useful biological functions [18]. Efforts to show AD-associated abnormalities in soluble Aβ have failed, and it is thus unclear under what conditions these normal peptides become toxic, especially in sporadic AD where no significant disease-associated abnormalities have been detected in their production or degradation. Similarly, there is no evidence of a soluble toxic Aβ oligomeric species specific to AD (detection of such a species would also be important to the diagnosis of this disease). Without such evidence, it is hard to accept the concept that Aβ oligomers identified in animal models overexpressing APP are relevant to AD, a disease that displays no significant overexpression of APP. Regarding the in vitro neurotoxicity of Aβ42, it is important to note that this neurotoxicity becomes detectable when Aβ is used at concentrations which are at least ten thousand times higher than the peptide concentrations found in vivo (usually less than 500 pM). Repeated attempts in our laboratory to show neurotoxicity for either the monomeric or aggregated forms of Aβ42 at concentrations below 1 μM have been unsuccessful [Famer and Robakis, unpubl. obs.].

Reports that FAD mutants of PS1 invariably increase production of neurotoxic Aβ42 by causing a gain of γ-secretase function seemed to support a causative role of Aβ in AD. Based on these reports, it was proposed that FAD mutations promote dementia by increasing production of Aβ42 (gain of function) and, by extrapolation, this mechanism may also be central to other forms of AD [19, 20]. Additional work, however, showed that many FAD mutations of PS1 inhibit the γ-secretase cleavage at the ε-site of several substrates including cadherins, ephrin B and APP, suggesting that PS1 FAD mutants may cause a loss, rather than a gain, of γ-secretase activity [21–23]. These findings seemed inconsistent with the suggestion that all PS1 FAD mutations cause a gain of γ-secretase cleavage activity. Furthermore, such a specific gain of function is rather unexpected for a large number of mutations distributed throughout the PS1 polypeptide. More recent work from our [24] and other [25–27] laboratories showed that many PS1 FAD mutants fail to increase production of Aβ42, indicating that not all FAD mutations increase the amyloidogenic processing of APP.

It has been suggested that although a number of PS FAD mutations are unable to increase production of neurotoxic Aβ42, these mutants cause an increase in the ratio of Aβ42/40 and this increase may somehow cause neurodegeneration and the AD phenotype [27, 28]. Our data [24], however, show that although some PS1 FAD mutations may cause an increase in this ratio, others do not. Five FAD mutants tested in two different cell systems failed to show a significant increase in Aβ42/40 ratio. Our data are similar to reports that several PS2 FAD mutants [25] have no significant effects on the production of Aβ42 or on the ratio of Aβ42/40. Additional studies have failed to show a significant correlation between age of FAD onset induced by PS mutations and the increase in either Aβ42 or the Aβ42/40 ratio induced by these mutants. Importantly, brain Aβ42 levels do not correlate with the age of disease onset [27], and although the APP Swedish FAD mutation induces a robust increase in both Aβ42 and Aβ40, it does not significantly change the Aβ40/42 ratio [28]. Finally, there is no known mechanism to drive the postulated change in the 40/42 ratio in sporadic AD.

The lack of disease-associated increases in soluble Aβ peptides or their oligomeric forms makes it unclear what drives aggregation and precipitation of Aβ amyloid in AD. Since there is no evidence of Aβ overexpression in AD, a plausible explanation is that neurodegeneration affects the ability of the brain to keep the Aβ peptides soluble. For example, healthy neurons may produce a factor that inhibits aggregation of Aβ. Neurons compromised by the disease may produce lower levels of this hypothetical factor thus promoting aggregation and precipitation of the soluble Aβ. This explanation is in agreement with a relatively small but consistent decrease in soluble Aβ found in AD brains. In contrast, amyloidosis in experimental animal models is driven by high levels of Aβ produced by the overexpressed exogenous APP.

Effects of PS FAD Mutants on Neurodegeneration May Be Independent of Their Effects on Aβ42 or the Aβ Ratio

That many FAD mutations have no significant effect on the production of Aβ42 supports the suggestion that the effects of these mutations on neurodegeneration and AD may be distinct from their effects on Aβ [24]. This suggestion is supported by reports that PS mutations can cause neurodegeneration in the absence of either amyloid depositions or increased Aβ and that loss of PS1 may result in neurodegeneration and cognitive decline through amyloid-independent mechanisms [29]. A specific APP mutation rescued neurodegeneration and behavioral abnormalities in Tg animals without affecting Aβ production or amyloid deposits [30], and patients of an Italian family carrying a PS1 mutant associated with FAD showed no abnormalities in either the in vivo levels of soluble Aβ peptides or in the Aβ 42/40 ratio [31]. In summary, a large number of experimental observations seem inconsistent with the theory that FAD mutations promote neurodegeneration by increasing production of neurotoxic Aβ42. Similarly, there is no evidence of any Aβ oligomers specific to AD, neither are there any AD-specific changes in the concentration of these oligomers.

Such evidence is necessary to support the hypothesis that oligomers are causally involved in AD and would also be valuable findings for the diagnosis of the disease.

Although for the last quarter of a century Aβ-based theories have been the leading explanation for the dementia of AD, it is still unclear that these peptides are the primary causative agents of AD. In contrast, a number of data suggest that the ability of FAD mutations to promote neurodegeneration may be independent of their effects on the production of Aβ or the ratio of Aβ species. The FAD mutations of APP, PS1 and PS2 suggest that the biological function of these proteins play critical roles in neuronal survival and function. A recent report indicates that APP interacts with cell death receptor 6 (DR6) and triggers neuronal degeneration. The data suggest that a secreted extracellular fragment of APP binds to and activates DR6 stimulating cell death. Based on these observations, it was hypothesized that the APP-DR6 system may contribute to the neuronal cell death of AD [32]. Interestingly, this report may explain how overexpression of APP stimulates neurodegeneration in animal models as increased production of the DR6-binding secreted APP fragment will stimulate neurodegeneration. Evidence from other groups support the hypothesis that the functions of PS1 in cell survival [33, 34] may be involved in the effects of the FAD mutations on neurodegeneration. Additional evidence indicates that the PS FAD mutants affect γ-secretase-dependent transcriptional pathways independently of Aβ and that these effects may contribute to neurodegeneration and AD [35, 36]. It is now clear for example, that the ε-cleavage of many cell surface receptors including Notch1, cadherins, EphB receptors and even APP, catalyzed by the γ-secretase proteolytic system, promotes release of ICD peptides (fig. 1), which may act as transcriptional factors, suggesting that this system plays central roles in diverse signaling pathways leading to transcriptional regulation [3]. Importantly, recent reports show that FAD mutations inhibit the ε-cleavage of cell surface receptors, and this inhibition results in a dramatic decrease in the production of ICDs involved in signal transduction and gene expression [21, 22]. Together, these data provide support for the hypothesis that transcriptional dysregulation may be another mechanism by which FAD mutations contribute to the neurodegeneration and memory defects characteristic of AD [35].

Acknowledgement

This study was supported by Alzheimer's Association grant IIRG-06-26751.

References

1 Selkoe DJ: Alzheimer's disease: genes, proteins, and therapy. Physiol Rev 2001;81:741–766.
2 Glenner G: A retrospective and prospective overview of the investigations on amyloid and amyloidosis – the β fibrilloses; in Glenner GG, Costa PP, Freitas FD (eds): Amyloid and Amyloidosis. Amsterdam, Excerpta Medica, 1980, pp 3–13.
3 Marambaud P, Robakis NK: Genetic and molecular aspects of Alzheimer's disease shed light on new mechanisms of transcriptional regulation. Genes Brain Behav 2005;4:134–146.
4 Glenner GG, Wong CW: Amyloidogenesis in Alzheimer's disease and Down's syndrome. Banbury Report 27: Mol Neuropath of Aging. Cold Spring Harbor, Cold Spring Harbor Press, 1987, pp 53–265.
5 Hardy J, Higgins GA: Alzheimer's disease: the amyloid cascade hypothesis. Science 1992;256:184–185.
6 Neve RL, Robakis NK: Alzheimer's disease: a reexamination of the amyloid hypothesis. Trends Neurosci 1998;21:15–19.
7 Smith MA, Joseph JA, Perry G: Arson: Tracking the culprit in Alzheimer's disease. Ann NY Acad Sci 2000;924:35–38.
8 Arriagada PV, Growdon JH, Hedley-Whyte ET, Hyman BT: Neurofibrillary tangles but not senile plaques parallel duration and severity of Alzheimer's disease. Neurology 1992;42:631–639.
9 Bouras C, Kövari E, Herrmann FR, et al: Stereologic analysis of microvascular morphology in the elderly: Alzheimer disease pathology and cognitive status. J Neuropathol Exp Neurol 2006;65:235–244.
10 Crystal H, Dickson D, Fuld P, et al: Clinicopathologic studies in dementia: nondemented subjects with pathologically confirmed Alzheimer's disease. Neurology 1988;38:1682–1687.
11 Davis DG, Schmitt FA, Wekstein DR, Markesbery WR: Alzheimer neuropathologic alterations in aged cognitively normal subjects. J Neuropathol Exp Neurol 1999;58:376–388.
12 Hsia AY, Masliah E, McConlogue L, et al: Plaque-independent disruption of neural circuits in Alzheimer's disease mouse models. Proc Natl Acad Sci USA 1999;96:3228–3233.
13 Mucke L, Masliah E, Yu GQ, Mallory M, Rockenstein EM, Tatsuno G, Hu K, Kholodenko D, Johnson-Wood K, McConlogue L: High-level neuronal expression of abeta 1–42 in wild-type human amyloid protein precursor transgenic mice: synaptotoxicity without plaque formation. J Neurosci 2000;20:4050–4058.
14 Holmes C, Boche D, Wilkinson D, et al: Long-term effects of Aβ42 immunisation in Alzheimer's disease: follow-up of a randomised, placebo-controlled phase I trial. Lancet 2008;372:216–223.
15 Cleary JP, Walsh DM, Hofmeister JJ, et al: Natural oligomers of the amyloid-beta protein specifically disrupt cognitive function. Nat Neurosci 2005;8:79–84.
16 Walsh DM, Klyubin I, Fadeeva JV, et al: Naturally secreted oligomers of amyloid beta protein potently inhibit hippocampal long-term potentiation in vivo. Nature 2002;416:535–539.

17 Robakis NK, Ramakrishna N, Wolfe G, Wisniewski HM: Molecular cloning and characterization of a cDNA encoding the cerebrovascular and the neuritic plaque amyloid peptides. Proc Natl Acad Sci USA 1987;84: 4190–4194.
18 Robinson SR, Bishop GM: Aβ as a bioflocculant: implications for the amyloid hypothesis of Alzheimer's disease. Neurobiol Aging 2002;23:1051–1072.
19 Hardy J, Selkoe DJ: The amyloid hypothesis of Alzheimer's disease: progress and problems on the road to therapeutics. Science 2002;297:353–356.
20 Klein WL, Krafft GA, Finch CE: Targeting small Abeta oligomers: the solution to an Alzheimer's disease conundrum? Trends Neurosci 2001;24:219–224.
21 Marambaud P, Wen PH, Dutt A, et al: A CBP binding transcriptional repressor produced by the PS1/epsilon-cleavage of N-cadherin is inhibited by PS1 FAD mutations. Cell 2003; 114:635–645.
22 Georgakopoulos A, Litterst C, Ghersi E, et al: Metalloproteinase/presenilin 1 processing of ephrinB regulates EphB-induced Src phosphorylation and signaling. EMBO J 2006;25:1242–1252.
23 Chen F, Gu Y, Hasegawa H, et al: Presenilin 1 mutations activate gamma 42-secretase but reciprocally inhibit epsilon-secretase cleavage of amyloid precursor protein (APP) and S3-cleavage of notch. J Biol Chem 2002;277: 36521–36526.
24 Shioi J, Georgakopoulos A, Mehta P, et al: FAD mutants unable to increase neurotoxic Aβ 42 suggest that mutation effects on neurodegeneration may be independent of effects on Aβ. J Neurochem 2007;101:674–681.
25 Walker ES, Martinez M, Brunkan AL, Goate A: Presenilin 2 familial Alzheimer's disease mutations result in partial loss of function and dramatic changes in Abeta 42/40 ratios. J Neurochem 2005;92:294–301.
26 Bentahir M, Nyabi O, Verhamme J, et al: Presenilin clinical mutations can affect gamma-secretase activity by different mechanisms. J Neurochem 2006;96:732–742.
27 Kumar-Singh S, Theuns J, Van Broeck B, et al: Mean age-of-onset of familial Alzheimer disease caused by presenilin mutations correlates with both increased Abeta42 and decreased Abeta40. Hum Mutat 2006;27:686–695.
28 Duering M, Grimm MO, Grimm HS, Schroder J, Hartmann T: Mean age of onset in familial Alzheimer's disease is determined by amyloid beta 42. Neurobiol Aging 2005;26: 785–788.
29 Saura CA, Choi SY, Beglopoulos V, et al: Loss of presenilin function causes impairments of memory and synaptic plasticity followed by age-dependent neurodegeneration. Neuron 2004;42:23–36.
30 Galvan V, Gorostiza OF, Banwait S, et al: Reversal of Alzheimer's-like pathology and behavior in human APP transgenic mice by mutation of Asp664. Proc Natl Acad Sci USA 2006;103:7130–7135.
31 Batelli S, Albani D, Prato F, et al: Early-onset Alzheimer disease in an Italian family with presenilin-1 double mutation E318G and G394V. Alzheimer Dis Soc Disord 2008;22: 184–187.
32 Nikolaev A, McLaughlin T, O'Leary DDM, Tessier-Lavigne M: APP binds DR6 to trigger axon pruning and neuron death via distinct caspases. Nature 2009;457:981–989.
33 Baki L, Shioi J, Wen P, et al: PS1 activates PI3K thus inhibiting GSK-3 activity and tau overphosphorylation: effects of FAD mutations. EMBO J 2004;23:2586–2596.
34 Kang DE, Yoon IS, Repetto E, et al: Presenilins mediate phosphatidylinositol 3-kinase/AKT and ERK activation via select signaling receptors. Selectivity of PS2 in platelet-derived growth factor signaling. J Biol Chem 2005;280:31537–31547.
35 Robakis NK: An Alzheimer's disease hypothesis based on transcriptional dysregulation. Amyloid 2003;10:80–85.
36 Seidner GA, Ye Y, Faraday MM, Alvord WG, Fortini ME: Modeling clinically heterogeneous presenilin mutations with transgenic Drosophila. Curr Biol 2006;16:1026–1033.
37 Anderson JP, Esch FS, Keim PS, Sambamurti K, Lieberburg I, Robakis NK: Exact cleavage site of Alzheimer amyloid precursor in neuronal PC-12 cells. Neurosci Lett 1991; 128:126–128.

Biology of Neurodegeneration

Neuro-degenerative Diseases

Neurodegenerative Dis 2010;7:38–41
DOI: 10.1159/000283480

Published online: February 13, 2010

Neuroinflammation – An Early Event in Both the History and Pathogenesis of Alzheimer's Disease

Piet Eikelenboom[a, b] Erik van Exel[b] Jeroen J.M. Hoozemans[c] Rob Veerhuis[b, d] Annemieke J.M. Rozemuller[c] Willem A. van Gool[a]

[a]Department of Neurology, Academic Medical Center, University of Amsterdam, Departments of [b]Psychiatry, [c]Pathology, and [d]Clinical Chemistry and Alzheimer's Center, VU University Medical Center, Amsterdam, The Netherlands

Key Words

β-Amyloid · Alzheimer's disease · Cytokines · Acute phase reactants · Innate immunity · Microglia · Inflammaging

Abstract

Background: About hundred years ago, Oskar Fischer proposed that the senile plaques are the consequence of the deposition of a foreign substance that could induce an inflammatory response leading to an abnormal neuritic response of the surrounding neurons. ***Objectives:*** To show that the interest in inflammation in Alzheimer's disease (AD) is not only an early event in the history of AD but that inflammation is also an early event in the pathogenesis of AD. ***Methods:*** Evaluation of the neuropathological, epidemiological and genetic evidence for a role of inflammation early in the pathogenesis of AD. ***Results:*** Neuropathological studies show presence of activated microglia and inflammation-related mediators in the cerebral neocortex of autopsied patients with a low Braak stage for AD pathology. Prospective population-based cohort studies indicate that higher serum levels of acute phase proteins predict dementia. On a genetic level, it was found that the production capacity of proinflammatory cytokines after stimulation with lipopolysaccharide (a process that is under strong genetic control) is higher in offspring with a parental history of late-onset AD. ***Conclusion:*** Neuropathological studies show that a neuroinflammatory response in the cerebral neocortex parallels the early stages of AD pathology and precedes the late stage, tau-related pathology. Epidemiological and genetic studies indicate that systemic markers of the innate immunity are risk factors for late-onset AD.

Introduction

The idea that inflammation could be involved in the pathogenesis of Alzheimer's disease (AD) goes back to the days when Alois Alzheimer published a case study with a disorder that was named after him later on. Oskar Fischer from the Charles University of Prague described at that time that plaque formation could be the result of deposition of a foreign substance that provokes a local inflammatory response, followed by a regenerative response of the surrounding nerve fibers [1, 2]. However, Fischer could not find morphological characteristics of an inflammatory response around plaques and he reported also that complement-binding studies for the plaques were negative. Eighty years later immunohistochemical studies revealed that amyloid plaques are indeed colocalized with a broad variety of inflammation-related pro-

KARGER

Fax +41 61 306 12 34
E-Mail karger@karger.ch
www.karger.com

1660–2854/10/0073–0038$26.00/0

Accessible online at:
www.karger.com/ndd

Piet Eikelenboom
Valeriuskliniek
Valeriusplein 9
NL–1075 Amsterdam BG (The Netherlands)
Tel. +31 20 788 5666, Fax +31 20 673 7458, E-Mail p.eikelenboom@ggzingeest.nl

teins (complement factors, acute-phase proteins, proinflammatory cytokines), and clusters of activated microglia and reactive astrocytes. These findings have led to the view that the amyloid plaque is the nidus of a chronic inflammatory response that is induced locally by fibrillar Aβ peptides which activate innate immunity [3]. Experimental animal studies have shown that fibrillar Aβ interacts with the LPS receptor CD14, the key receptor for the activation of the innate immunity [4]. The interest for inflammation is not only an early event in the history of Alzheimer's research, recent findings suggest that inflammation may be also an early event in the pathogenesis of AD. In this paper, we will review the neuropathological, epidemiological and genetic evidence relevant to this hypothesis.

Neuropathological Evidence

Neuropathological studies performed on patients in different stages of AD pathology show increased neuronal expression of cyclooxygenase-2, expression of cell cycle proteins, microglial and astroglial activation in the cerebral neocortex of patients with low Braak scores for AD pathology [5, 6]. Gene expression microarrays show that inflammatory changes parallel the early stages of AD pathology. The main categories of upregulated genes include genes encoding for complement factors, major histocompatibility complex proteins II, cell adhesion molecules and enzymes involved in prostaglandin synthesis [7, 8]. Clinical work using positron emission tomography (PET) with the peripheral benzodiazepine receptor ligand PK-11195 as marker for activated microglia indicates that activation of microglia precedes cerebral atrophy in AD patients [9]. A recent PET study using the Pittsburg compound B for visualization of fibrillar β-amyloid and the PK-11195 ligand for microglia activation shows that amyloid deposition and microglia activation can be detected in vivo in around 50% of the patients with mild cognitive impairment [10]. Thus, neuropathological and neuroradiological studies indicate that inflammatory changes are a relatively early pathogenic event that precedes the process of neuropil destruction in AD.

Epidemiological Evidence

Prospective population studies show that higher serum levels of systemic inflammation markers, particularly C-reactive protein, interleukin-6 and α_1-antichymotrypsin can predict cognitive decline or dementia [11–14]. Studies performed in the past decade have shown that ageing is accompanied by a low-grade upregulation of certain inflammatory responses of the innate immunity. Franceschi et al. [15] have coined the term 'inflammaging' for this age-related, chronic, low-grade and systemic state of inflammation [16]. While the age-related overactive innate immunity may remain subclinical in many elderly, a proportion of individuals may shift from a state of 'normal' or 'subclinical' inflammaging to one or more of any age-associated diseases. There is some evidence that the process of inflammaging is under genetic control, and for this reason it is postulated that these individuals could have a 'high responder inflammatory genotype'.

Genetic Evidence

Some evidence has been reported that certain polymorphisms of the proinflammatory cytokines such as interleukin-1β and tumor necrosis factor-α, and of the acute phase proteins such as α_2-macroglobulin and α_1-antichymotrypsin are risk factors for AD. However, at the moment these findings are inconclusive to consider them as established genetic markers of AD. Twin studies have shown that the heritability of circulating inflammatory mediators of the innate immunity is modest (about 20%). In contrast to the circulating inflammatory mediators, the cytokine production upon stimulation with endotoxin is under strong genetic control and the heritability estimates of the production of the various cytokines ranges from 53 to 86% in nondiseased populations [17]. To identify inflammation-heritable traits for AD we have recently performed a study comparing middle-aged offspring (mean age about 50 years) from parents with and without a history of late-onset AD [18]. The innate proinflammatory responsiveness was determined by the incubation of whole blood samples with lipopolysaccharide stimulated ex vivo, followed by the determination of the various cytokines using ELISA techniques. In offspring with a parental history of AD, the capacity to produce proinflammatory cytokines was increased, resulting in significantly higher levels of interleukin-1β, tumor necrosis factor-α, interleukin-6, interferon-γ and interleukin-1β/interleukin-1ra ratio. All these positive associations were independent of ApoE4 genotype.

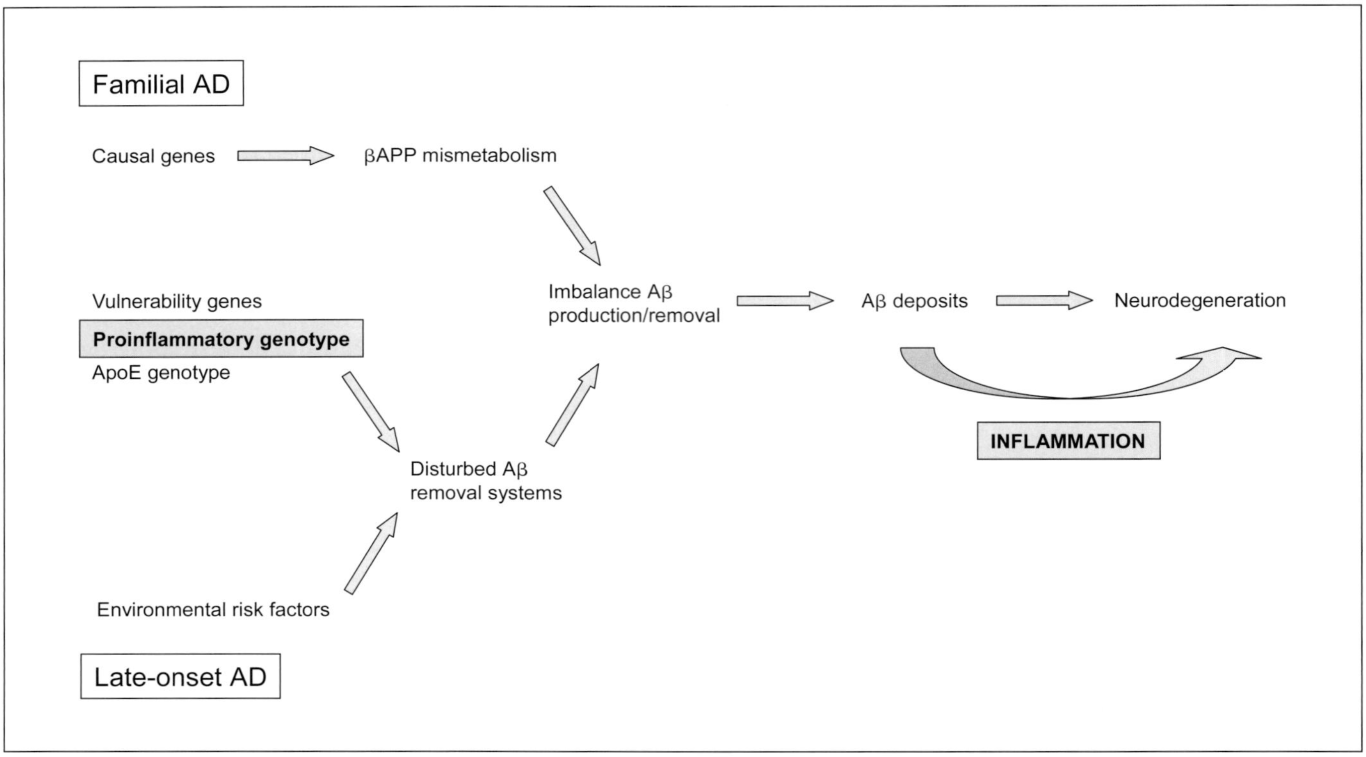

Fig. 1. Schematic presentation of the relationships between the etiology of AD, Aβ metabolism and inflammation. Modified from Eikelenboom and van Gool [19].

Conclusions

The etiology of AD is heterogeneous, but the underlying pathological cascade is homogeneous. Neuropathological studies show that the Aβ-associated neuroinflammatory response starts in the early stages of AD pathology preceding the stages that are associated with the clinical dementia syndrome. Epidemiological and genetic studies indicate that inflammation-related mechanisms can contribute to the multifactorial etiology of the sporadic late-onset form of AD. The relationships between the etiology, Aβ metabolism and inflammation for the different subtypes are presented in a hypothetical scheme (fig. 1). An altered balance between the production and removal of Aβ has been considered as the crucial step in AD pathogenesis. The autosomal dominant forms of AD are characterized by an increased production of Aβ, while the sporadic late-onset AD could be the consequence of disturbances of the Aβ removal system.

References

1 Fischer O: Miliare Nekrosen mit drusigen Wucherungen der Neurofibrillen, eine regelmässige Veränderung der Hirnrinde bei seniler Demenz. Monatsschr Psychiatr Neurol 1907;22:361–372.

2 Fischer O: Die presbyofrene Demenz, deren anatomischen Grundlage und klinische Abgrenzung. Z Ges Neurol Psychiatr 1910;3:371–471.

3 Eikelenboom P, Veerhuis R, Scheper W, Rozemuller AJM, van Gool WA, Hoozemans JJM: The significance of neuroinflammation in understanding Alzheimer's disease. J Neural Transm 2006;113:1685–1695.

4 Fassbender K, Walter S, Kühl S, Landmann R, Ishii K, Bertsch T, Stalder K, Muelhauser F, Liu Y, Ulmer AJ, Rivest T, Lentschat T, Gulbins E, Jucker M, Staufenbiel M, Brechtel K, Walter J, Multhaup G, Penke B, Adachi Y, Hartmann T, Beyreuther K: The LPS receptor (CD14) links innate immunity with Alzheimer's disease. FASEB J 2004;18:2003–2005.

5 Hoozemans JJM, Veerhuis R, Rozemuller JM, Eikelenboom P: Neuroinflammation and regeneration in early stages of Alzheimer's disease pathology. Int J Dev Neurosci 2006;24:157–165.

6 Webster B, Hansen L, Adame A, Crews L, Torrance M, Thal L, Masliah E: Astroglial activation of extracellular-regulated kinase in early stages of Alzheimer's disease. J Neuropathol Exp Neurol 2006;65:142–151.
7 Blalock EM, Geddes JW, Chen KC, Porter NM, Markesbery WR, Landfield PW: Incipient Alzheimer's disease: microarray correlation reveal major transcriptional and tumor supressor responses. Proc Natl Acad Sci USA 2004;101:2713–2718.
8 Parachikova A, Agadjanyan MG, Cribss DH, Blurton-Jones M, Perreau, Rogers J, Beach TG, Cotman CW: Inflammatory changes parallel the early stages of Alzheimer disease. Neurobiol Aging 2007;28:1821–1833.
9 Cagnin A, Brooks DJ, Kennedy AM, Gunn RN, Myers R, Turkheimer FE, Jones T, Banati RB: In vivo-measurement of activated microglia in dementia. Lancet 2001;358:461–467.
10 Okello A, Edison P, Archer HA, Turkheimer FE, Kennedy J, Bullock R, Walker Z, Kennedy A, Fox N, Rossor M, Brooks DJ: Microglial activation and amyloid deposition in mild cognitive impairment: a PET study. Neurology 2009;72:56–62.
11 Schmidt R, Schmidt H, Curb JD, Masaki K, White LR, Launer LJ: Early inflammation in dementia: a 25-years follow-up of the Honolulu-Asia Aging Study. Ann Neurol 2002;52:168–174.
12 Yaffe K, Lindquist K, Penninx BWH, Simsonsick EM, Pahor M, Krichchevsky S, Launer L, Kuller L, Rubin S, Harris T: Inflammatory markers and cognition in well-functioning African-American and white elders. Neurology 2003;61:76–80.
13 Dik MG, Jonker G, Hack CE, Smit JH, Comijs HC, Eikelenboom P: Serum inflammatory proteins and cognitive decline in older persons. Neurology 2005;64:1371–1377.
14 Porcellini E, Davis EJ, Chiappelli M, Ianni E, Di Stefano G, Forti P, Ravaglia G, Licastro F: Elevated plasma levels of α1-antichymotrypsin in age-related cognitive decline and Alzheimer's disease: a potential therapeutic target. Curr Pharm Des 2008;14:2659–2664.
15 Franceschi C, Capri M, Monti D, Giunta S, Olivieri F, Sevini F, Panourgia MP, Invidia L, Celani L, Scurti M, Cevenini E, Castellani GC, Salvioli S: Inflammaging and anti-inflammaging: a systemic perspective on aging and longevity emerged from studies in humans. Mech Ageing Dev 2007;128:92–105.
16 Fernandez F, Nikolic WV, Obregon D, Rrapo E, Town T, Tan J: Inflammaging as a prodrome to Alzheimer's disease. J Neuroinflammation 2008;5:51.
17 de Craen AJ, Posthuma D, Remarque EJ, van den Biggelaar AH, Westendorp RGJ, Boomsma DI: Heritabili estimates of the innate immunity: an extended twin study. Genes Immun 2005;6:167–170.
18 van Exel E, Eikelenboom P, Comijs H, Frohlich M, Smit JH, Stek ML, Scheltens P, Eefsting JE, Westendorp RGJ: Vascular factors and markers of inflammation in offspring with a parental history of late-onset Alzheimer's disease. Arch Gen Psychiatry 2009;66:1263–1270.
19 Eikelenboom P, van Gool WA: Neuroinflammatory perspectives on the two faces of Alzheimer's disease. J Neural Transm 2004;113:1685–1695.

Biology of Neurodegeneration

Neuro-degenerative Diseases

Neurodegenerative Dis 2010;7:42–45
DOI: 10.1159/000283481

Published online: February 13, 2010

Analysis of APL1β28, a Surrogate Marker for Alzheimer Aβ42, Indicates Altered Precision of γ-Cleavage in the Brains of Alzheimer Disease Patients

Masayasu Okochi Shinji Tagami Masatoshi Takeda

Psychiatry, Department of Integrated Medicine, Division of Internal Medicine, Osaka University Graduate School of Medicine, Osaka, Japan

Key Words

Alzheimer disease biomarker · Amyloid-β peptide 42 · Amyloid precursor-like protein 1 · Cerebrospinal fluid

Abstract

Alzheimer's disease (AD) is the most common cause of dementia in the elderly. Currently, therapeutic intervention after the disease onset is difficult because progressive neuronal death precedes clinical symptoms. Available medicines for AD, such as AchE inhibitors, transiently slow the progression of the dementia symptoms, but they do not inhibit the pathological process. At present, next generation anti-AD drugs are in development in many pharmaceutical companies. Importantly, most of them are to inhibit the progress of the pathological process and, thus, at the same time, the establishment of a highly probable prediction of future AD onset is inseparable. AD is now diagnosed using clinical criteria coupled with brain imaging systems such as SPECT and PET. To diagnose AD cases before the appearance of clinical symptoms, it will be necessary to (a) establish new, more sensitive clinical criteria, (b) develop methods for detecting the pathological accumulation of proteins (e.g. Aβ) in the brain, or (c) develop biomarkers for predicting the accumulation of Aβ/tau in the brain. Our recent discovery of APL1β28, a possible biomarker of AD, may help in the development of early detection methods for AD.

Amyloid-β peptide 42 (Aβ42) is a major constituent of senile plaques and is thought to induce Alzheimer's disease (AD) [1, 2]. Thus, the level of Aβ42 production in the brain, especially relative to total Aβ production, is a potential biomarker of the pathological process in AD. However, the relative ratio of Aβ42 in cerebrospinal fluid (CSF) is reduced in patients with AD [3–5], presumably because cerebral Aβ42 is highly aggregatable (fig. 1). To date, surrogate markers for estimating Aβ42 generation in the brain have not been identified.

We have recently reported that human CSF contains three species of 'Aβ-like peptides' [6] derived from APLP1 (i.e. APL1β25, -27 and -28) that are generated by β- and γ-cleavages (fig. 2) [7]. In contrast to Aβ, the APL1β peptides are not amyloidogenic and do not accumulate in the AD brain (fig. 1). Most γ-secretase modulators (GSMs) that upregulate the relative production of Aβ42 cause a parallel increase in the production of APL1β28 in cultured cells. Interestingly, the relative APL1β28 levels are higher in the CSF of sporadic AD patients than in that of non-AD controls. These findings indicate that (a) the novel APL1β28 peptide, an elongated form of APLP1-derived Aβ-like peptide, is a long-sought surrogate marker for AD Aβ42 and (b) the relative APL1β28 level in CSF is a candidate presymptomatic diagnostic marker for AD [7].

KARGER

Fax +41 61 306 12 34
E-Mail karger@karger.ch
www.karger.com

1660–2854/10/0073–0042$26.00/0

Accessible online at:
www.karger.com/ndd

Masayasu Okochi, MD
Psychiatry, Department of Integrated Medicine
Division of Internal Medicine, Osaka University Graduate School of Medicine
D3, Yamada-oka 2-2, Suita, Osaka 565-0871 (Japan)
Tel. +81 6 6879 3053, Fax +81 6 6879 3059, E-Mail mokochi@psy.med.osaka-u.ac.jp

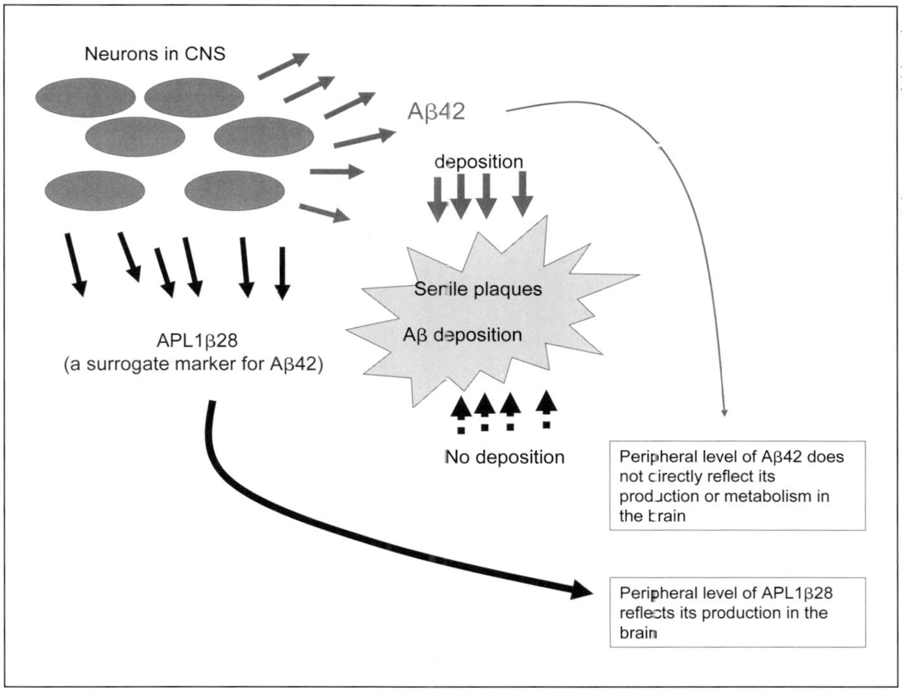

Fig. 1. CSF level of nonamyloidogenic APL1β28, but not amyloidogenic Aβ42, reflects its generation in the brain.

The reverse relationship of Aβ42 levels can be used as a biomarker to some extent after disease onset. Combining the values of relative APL1β28 level and Aβ42 level in CSF may be more useful to AD diagnosis at the presymptomatic stage. It is true that, so far, in peripheral blood we have not succeeded in detecting the surrogate marker for Aβ42. However, we hope that the detection of Aβ-like peptides will supplant expensive and time-consuming methods, such as PET, in the initial screening and detection of AD.

An increase in the ratio of Aβ42 to total Aβ has been widely accepted as a pathological 'gain of function' that determines the onset of familial AD. However, it is not yet known whether the increase in the Aβ42:Aβ ratio plays a role in the pathological process of sporadic AD, the most common form of AD. Instead, many studies have examined Aβ degradation and metabolism in sporadic AD. These studies have indicated that the mechanism of Aβ degradation is important in the pathogenesis of AD [8, 9]. To understand this trend, it is important to consider the highly aggregatable biochemical feature of Aβ42 (see also fig. 1). In the CSF of sporadic AD patients, the relative Aβ42 level does not correspond to its generation in the brain. In sporadic AD brains, levels of insoluble Aβ42 are extremely high, and soluble Aβ42 levels tend to decrease. Therefore, to date, there have been no plans to study whether the level of Aβ42 production changes in sporadic AD brains. One of the most important issues has remained unsolved.

Using one of the APLP1-derived 'Aβ-like peptide' [6] species, APL1β28, as a nonamyloidogenic CSF surrogate marker of Aβ42 (see fig. 1 and 2), we indicated that the ratio of Aβ42 to Aβ production might increase in brains of sporadic AD patients bearing wild-type βAPP and presenilins [7]. To our knowledge, this is the first in vivo human study suggesting that sporadic AD can be caused by an upregulation of the relative level of Aβ42 to total Aβ in the central nervous system.

Considering the usefulness and limitation of symptomatic drugs for AD [10–13], Aβ-targeting compounds are currently being developed for the treatment of AD. These include a group of compounds that lower the production of Aβ, or more specifically, Aβ42. Such drugs inhibit progression of the pathological process but do not restore the normal process. Moreover, expensive, long-term cohort studies are necessary to study the effects of these drugs. To simplify the process, it would be useful to know whether a single administration can decrease Aβ production in vivo. As Aβ42 levels in the CSF often do not reflect their levels in the brain, a surrogate marker such as APL1β28 could be useful for evaluating the effects of drugs targeting Aβ. It is expected that compounds

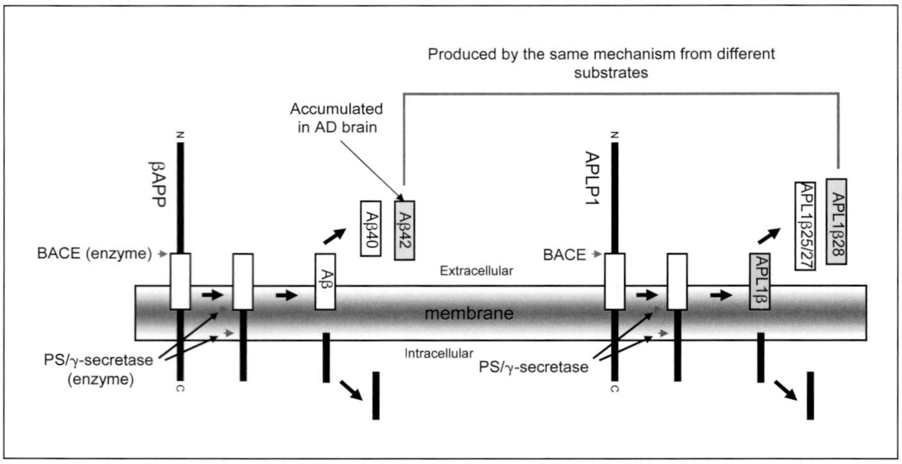

Color version available online

Fig. 2. APL1β and Aβ are produced by the sequential cleavages by BACE and PS/γ-secretase. APL1β28 and Aβ42, longer species of 'Aβ-like peptides' derived from APLP1 and βAPP, are produced very similarly.

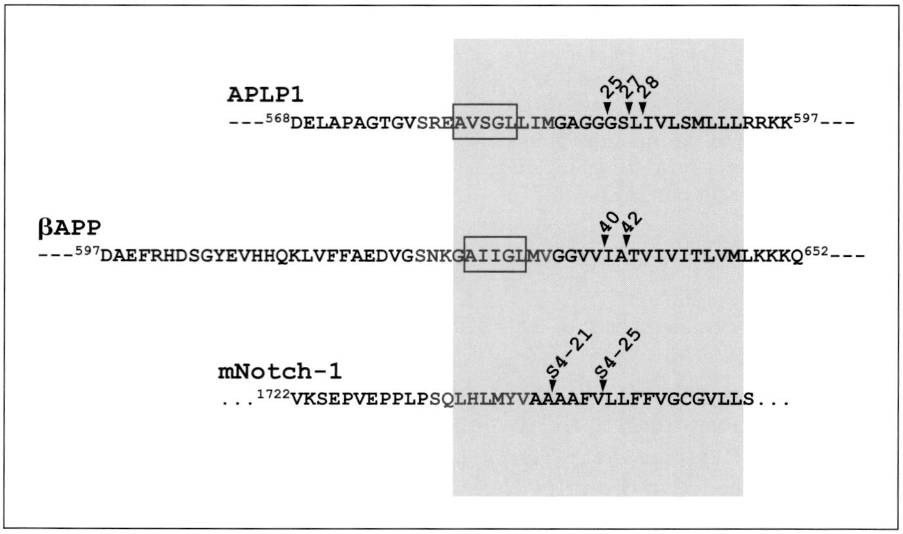

Color version available online

Fig. 3. The AXXGL motif in transmembrane domains of APLP1 and βAPP. In our analysis using βAPP, mNotch-1 and APLP1 as substrates, the effects of the GSMs including fenofibrate and S2474 were found on γ-cleavages of pleural substrates including APLP1 and full-length mouse Notch-1 (not TM swap chimera).

lowering Aβ will be administered in the hope of preventing the future onset of AD. Prior to commencing preventive medication, patients will want to have clear evidence that it is needed. We propose that an increase in the ratio of APL1β28 to total APLP1 will serve as the rationale for such preventive medication.

Recently, Kukar et al. [14] reported that a few GSMs target βAPP but not PS/γ-secretase. This report and their review [15] suggest that GSMs can change the relative ratio of Aβ42 to total Aβ production by specifically binding to βAPP. However, our results indicate that GSMs affect not only βAPP but also mNotch1 and APLP1 (fig. 3) [7, 16]. This implies that GSMs do not bind only βAPP. Although the results of Kukar et al. [9] demonstrate that some GSMs bind to βAPP, it is not clear whether the binding is responsible for the modulation of γ-cleavage. Moreover, whether all GSMs act by a unique process is not clear. Thus, further studies are needed to determine whether other GSMs, for example those with IC50s in the nanomolar range, act by the same mechanism as GSMs that bind βAPP.

Pathological mutations in presenilins and βAPP are thought to cause familial AD by increasing the relative level of Aβ42 to Aβ production. Until 10 years ago, the relative level of Aβ42 production was thought to be constant and, therefore, not upregulated in the absence of mutations. However, in 2001, Weggen et al. [17] reported that a subset of NSAIDs modulates the cleavage precision of presenilin/γ-secretase and changes the relative level of Aβ42 production. This indicated that the relative level of Aβ42 production can be changed, even in people with wild-type presenilin and βAPP. Moreover, Serneels et al.

[18] recently showed that the relative level of Aβ42 produced by Aph1B-containing presenilin/γ-secretase may be higher than that produced by Aph1A-containing presenilin/γ-secretase. Furthermore, our results indicate that the ratio of Aβ42 to Aβ may be upregulated in the CSF of sporadic AD patients [7]. Collectively, these findings might suggest that there is an endogenous mechanism for regulating the precision of cleavage by presenilin/γ-secretase that could play a role in the pathogenesis of AD. Alternatively, the relative ratio of APL1β28 to APLP1 in CSF may be unchangeable and specific to individuals, so that the CSF APL1β28:APLP1 ratio would be a risk factor for AD.

Acknowledgements

We are grateful for funding from the 'Program for the Promotion of Fundamental Studies in Health Sciences of the National Institute of Biomedical Innovation (05-26)', grants-in-Aid for 'Scientific Research on Priority Areas – Advanced Brain Science Project' and 'KAKEN-HI' from the Ministry of Education, Culture, Sports, Science, and Technology, and grants-in-aid from the Japanese Ministry of Health, Labor and Welfare in Japan.

References

1 Masters CL, Simms G, Weinman NA, Multhaup G, McDonald BL, Beyreuther K: Amyloid plaque core protein in Alzheimer disease and Down syndrome. Proc Natl Acad Sci USA 1985;82:4245–4249.
2 Selkoe DJ: Alzheimer's disease: genes, proteins, and therapy. Physiol Rev 2001;81:741–766.
3 Motter R, Vigo-Pelfrey C, Kholodenko D, Barbour R, Johnson-Wood K, Galasko D, Chang L, Miller B, Clark C, Green R, et al: Reduction of beta-amyloid peptide42 in the cerebrospinal fluid of patients with Alzheimer's disease. Ann Neurol 1995;38:643–648.
4 Jensen M, Schroder J, Blomberg M, Engvall B, Pantel J, Ida N, Basun H, Wahlund LO, Werle E, Jauss M, Beyreuther K, Lannfelt L, Hartmann T: Cerebrospinal fluid A beta42 is increased early in sporadic Alzheimer's disease and declines with disease progression. Ann Neurol 1999;45:504–511.
5 Andreasen N, Hesse C, Davidsson P, Minthon L, Wallin A, Winblad B, Vanderstichele H, Vanmechelen E, Blennow K: Cerebrospinal fluid beta-amyloid(1–42) in Alzheimer disease: differences between early- and late-onset Alzheimer disease and stability during the course of disease. Arch Neurol 1999;56: 673–680.
6 Okochi M, Steiner H, Fukumori A, Tanii H, Tomita T, Tanaka T, Iwatsubo T, Kudo T, Takeda M, Haass C: Presenilins mediate a dual intramembranous gamma-secretase cleavage of Notch-1. EMBO J 2002;21:5408–5416.
7 Yanagida K, Okochi M, Tagami S, Nakayama T, Kodama TS, Nishitomi K, Jiang J, Mori K, Tatsumi S, Arai T, Ikeuchi T, Kasuga K, Tokuda T, Kondo M, Ikeda M, Deguchi K, Kazui H, Tanaka T, Morihara T, Hashimoto R, Kudo T, Steiner H, Haass C, Tsuchiya K, Akiyama H, Kuwano R, Takeda M: The 28-amino acid form of an APLP1-derived A beta-like peptide is a surrogate marker for A beta42 production in the central nervous system. EMBO Mol Med 2009;1:223–235.
8 Saido TC, Iwata N: Metabolism of amyloid beta peptide and pathogenesis of Alzheimer's disease. Towards presymptomatic diagnosis, prevention and therapy. Neurosci Res 2006;54:235–253.
9 Jingwei J, Okochi M, Tagami S, Nishitomi K, Yanagida K, Nakayama T, Tatsimi S, Mori K, Takeda M: Macrophage colony stimulating factor is associated with excretion of amyloid-β peptides from cerebrospinal fluid to peripheral blood. Psychogeriatrics 2008;8: 188–195.
10 Kumagai R, Matsumlya M, Tada Y, Miyakawa K, Ichimlya Y, Arai H: Long-term effect of donepezil for Alzheimer's disease: Retrospective clinical evaluation of drug efficacy in Japanese patients. Psychogeriatrics 2008; 8:19–23.
11 Tanaka T, Kazui H, Morihara T, Sadik G, Kudo T, Takeda M: Post-marketing survey of donepezil hydrochloride in Japanese patients with Alzheimer's disease with BPSD. Psychogeriatrics 2008;8:114–123.
12 Inoue J, Hoshino R, Nojima H, Okamoto N: Investigation of the short- and long-term effects of donepezil on cognitive function in Alzheimer's disease. Pyschogeriatrics 2009; 9:27–33.
13 Nozawa M, Ichikawa Y, Nozawa E, Utumi Y, Sugiyama H, Murayama N, Iseki E, Arai H: Clinical effects of high oral dose of donepezil for patients with Alzheimer's disease in Japan. Psychogeriatrics 2009;9:50–55.
14 Kukar TL, Ladd TB, Bann MA, Fraering PC, Narlawar R, Maharvi GM, Healy B, Chapman R, Welzel AT, Price RW, Moore B, Rangachari V, Cusack B, Eriksen J, Jansen-West K, Verbeeck C, Yager D, Eckman C, Ye W, Sagi S, Cottrell BA, Torpey J, Rosenberry TL, Fauq A, Wolfe MS, Schmidt B, Walsh DM, Koo EH, Golde TE: Substrate-targeting gamma-secretase modulators. Nature 2008;453: 925–929.
15 Golde TE, Kukar TL: Medicine. Avoiding unintended toxicity. Science 2009;324:603–604.
16 Okochi M, Fukumori A, Jiang J, Itoh N, Kimura R, Steiner H, Haass C, Tagami S, Takeda M: Secretion of the Notch-1 Abeta-like peptide during Notch signaling. J Biol Chem 2006;281:7890–7898.
17 Weggen S, Eriksen JL, Das P, Sagi SA, Wang R, Pietrzik CU, Findlay KA, Smith TE, Murphy MP, Bulter T, Kang DE, Marquez-Sterling N, Golde TE, Koo EH: A subset of NSAIDs lower amyloidogenic Abeta42 independently of cyclooxygenase activity. Nature 2001;414:212–216.
18 Serneels L, Van Biervliet J, Craessaerts K, Dejaegere T, Horre K, Van Houtvin T, Esselmann H, Paul S, Schafer MK, Berezovska O, Hyman BT, Sprangers B, Sciot R, Moons L, Jucker M, Yang Z, May PC, Karran E, Wiltfang J, D'Hooge R, De Strooper B: Gamma-Secretase heterogeneity in the Aph1 subunit: relevance for Alzheimer's disease. Science 2009;324:639–642.

Neuro-degenerative Diseases

Biology of Neurodegeneration

Neurodegenerative Dis 2010;7:46–49
DOI: 10.1159/000283482

Published online: February 13, 2010

Expression of Familial Alzheimer's Disease-Linked Human Presenilin 1 Variants Impair Enrichment-Induced Adult Hippocampal Neurogenesis

Karthikeyan Veeraraghavalu[a] Se Hoon Choi[b] Sangram S. Sisodia[a, b]

[a]Department of Neurobiology, and [b]Committee on Neurobiology, University of Chicago, Chicago, Ill., USA

Key Words

Presenilin 1 · Adult hippocampal neurogenesis · Microglia · Enriched environment

Abstract

Presenilin 1 (PS1) plays a critical role in neurogenesis both during development and in the adult. We recently reported that ubiquitous expression of familial, early-onset Alzheimer's disease-linked PS1 mutants impairs enrichment-induced proliferation and neurogenesis of hippocampal neural progenitor cells (NPCs) in a non-cell autonomous manner. The impairments in proliferation and neurogenesis are, at least in part, due to alterations in the levels of specific chemokines and growth factors secreted from microglia expressing familial Alzheimer's disease-linked PS1 variants. To test our hypothesis that the fate of hippocampal NPCs in PS1 mutant mice is largely determined by cellular factors produced within the niche itself, we are examining the fate of NPCs from hippocampi of wild-type human PS1 or PS1 mutant mice that are marked with green fluorescent protein and BrdU following transplantation into heterologous hosts. In parallel, we have generated transgenic mice that harbor a transgene encoding the PS1ΔE9 variant flanked with *loxP* sites that can be conditionally deleted in a temporal and/or spatial manner using specific cre driver lines. These studies will allow us to assess the contributions of varying cell types within the hippocampal stem cell niche that express mutant PS1 to NPC proliferation and differentiation.

Alzheimer's disease (AD) is a progressive neurodegenerative disease characterized by neuronal loss, deposition of β-amyloid peptides (Aβ), and cognitive dysfunction. Familial, early-onset, autosomal-dominant forms of AD (FAD) are caused by expression of mutant genes encoding presenilin 1 (PS1), presenilin 2 (PS2), and amyloid precursor protein. While the molecular mechanism(s) by which PS mutants cause FAD are not fully understood, expression of these polypeptides enhances the ratio of Aβ42/Aβ40 peptides, leading to selective deposition of the Aβ42.

It is now well established that stem cell-like populations (termed neural progenitor cells, NPCs) in the subgranular layer of the dentate gyrus (DG) continue to proliferate and differentiate into neuronal and astroglial cells throughout adulthood. Adult-born neurons are electrically active and capable of firing action potentials and receiving synaptic inputs, suggesting that these cells are integrated into the existing neural circuitry of the hippocampal formation. Indeed, studies have correlated

KARGER

Fax +41 61 306 12 34
E-Mail karger@karger.ch
www.karger.com

1660–2854/10/0073–0046$26.00/0

Accessible online at:
www.karger.com/ndd

Sangram S. Sisodia
The University of Chicago, Department of Neurobiology
947 E. 58th Street, AB 308
Chicago, IL 60637 (USA)
Tel. +1 773 834 3015, Fax +1 773 702 3774, E-Mail ssisodia@bsd.uchicago.edu

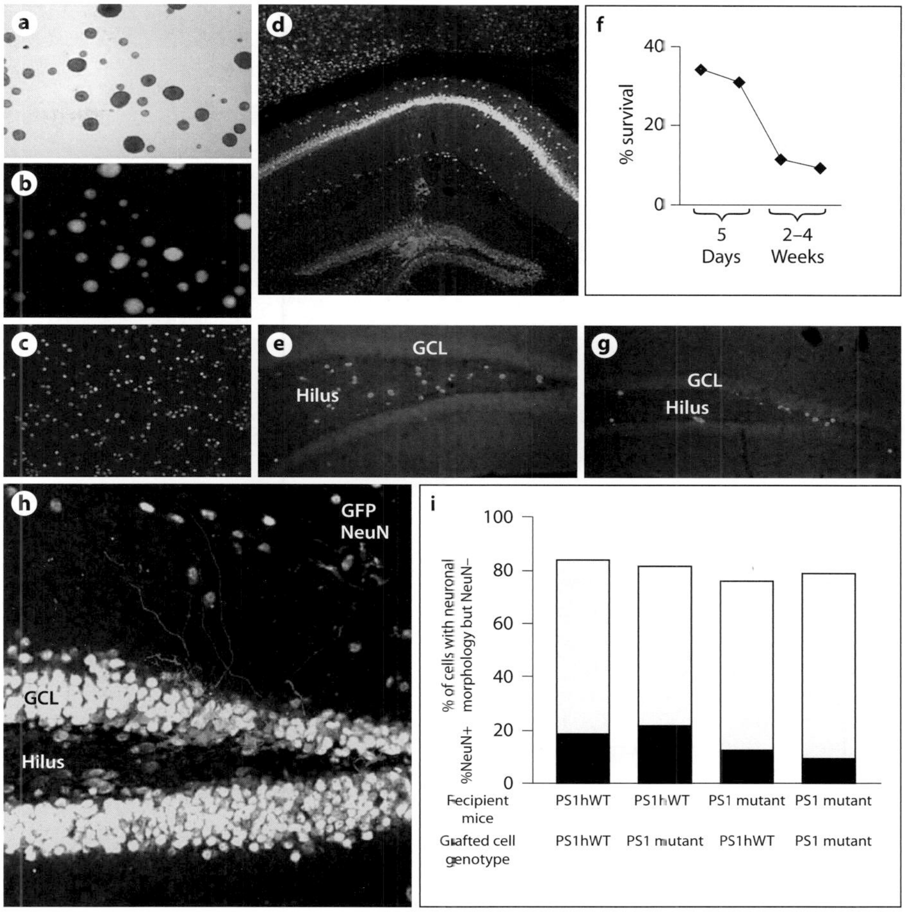

Color version available online

Fig. 1. a, **b** Images of GFP-positive neurospheres. **c** Images of BrdU-loaded single cell suspension of NPCs. **d** Grafted GFP-positive NPCs in the DG. **e** Grafted BrdU-loaded NPCs in the DG. **f** Survival efficacy of grafted NPCs. **g** Grafted NPCs migrated to the SGL. **h** Images of GFP-positive NPCs co-labeled with NeuN. **i** Percentage of GFP-positive NPCs co-labeled with NeuN (n = 3–4 per group). GCL = Granule cell layer.

increased neurogenesis in the DG with improved performance on hippocampal learning tasks, suggesting that adult-generated neurons can positively impact on adult hippocampal function. In this regard, exposure of adult rodents to an enriched environment (EE) paradigm leads to enhanced proliferation of hippocampal NPCs and elevated production of neurons that populate the DG.

While PS1 has an established role as the catalytic subunit of γ-secretase, an enzyme complex that is responsible for intramembranous processing of amyloid precursor protein, Notch and other type I membrane proteins, it has become increasingly evident that PS1 plays other physiological roles. For example, we and others have shown that genetic reduction in PS leads to neurodegeneration in an age-dependent manner [1, 2] that is paralleled by progressive, age-dependent transcriptome alterations in genes related to neurodegeneration [3]. In addition, we have previously reported that PS1 plays a pivotal role in adult hippocampal neurogenesis by showing that mice in which the endogenous *PSEN1* gene was conditionally deleted in the adult forebrain showed impaired progenitor proliferation and reduced numbers of newly generated neurons following EE, when compared to mice in which the *PSEN1* gene is intact [4]. More recently, we reported that enrichment-induced proliferation and neuronal differentiation of NPCs in the DG of transgenic mice harboring ubiquitously expressed, mouse prion protein (Mo.PrP) promoter-driven transgenes encoding FAD-linked PS1 variants (PS1ΔE9 or PS1M146L) are significantly impaired compared to enriched mice expressing wild-type human PS1 (PS1hWT) [5]. Interestingly, our in vitro studies of NPCs isolated from the hippocampi of PS1hWT or PS1 mutant mice failed to reveal any differences in either the proliferation or differentiation of these progenitors, findings that would argue against a cell-intrinsic function of mutant PS1 in NPC physiology.

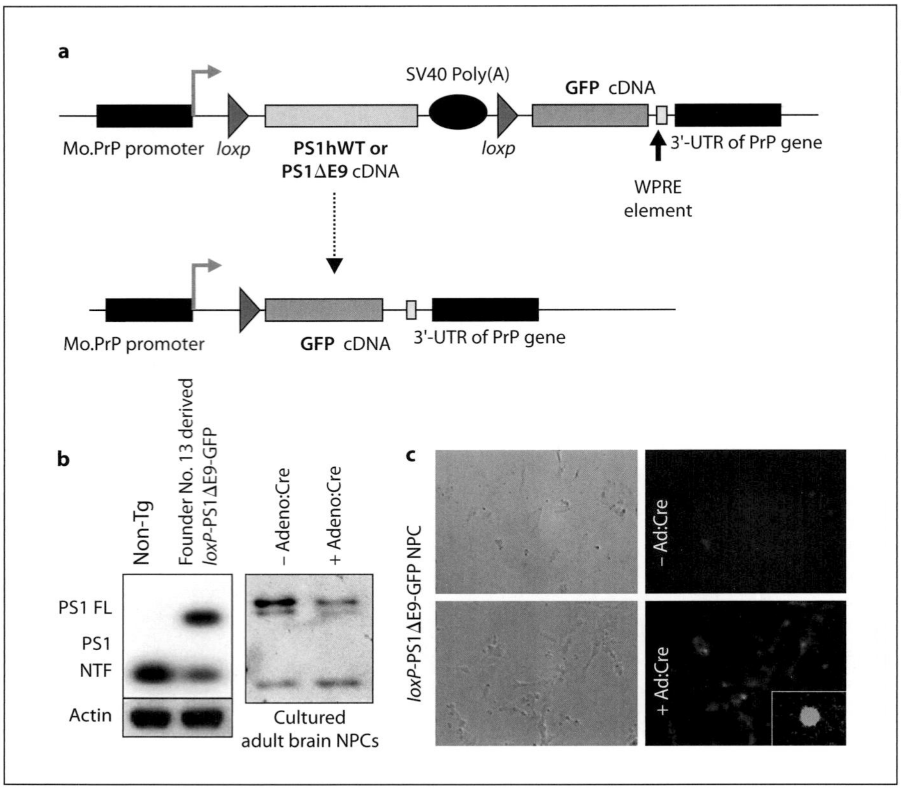

Color version available online

Fig. 2. **a** Schematic shows the mouse PrP.XhoI vector encoding *loxP*-flanked PS1ΔE9 transgene. **b** Expression of PS1-ΔE9 polypeptide in total brain lysate prepared from F1s derived from founder line No. 13. **c** Cre-induced excision of PS1ΔE9 transgene and concomitant expression of GFP were observed in NPCs following transduction with adenovirus:cre. Insert shows a GFP-positive neurosphere.

In an attempt to examine non-cell autonomous mechanisms that may effect NPC proliferation and differentiation, we first turned our attention to microglial cells, the immune-competent cells of the brain that are present within the hippocampal stem cell niche. Importantly, enrichment-induced neurogenesis is correlated with a dramatic increase in the presence of activated microglia [6]; blocking enrichment-enhanced microglial activation by immunosuppression also impairs neuronal differentiation of NPCs. We co-cultured interleukin-4-activated primary microglia from mice expressing either PS1hWT or PS1 mutants with cultured PS1hWT NPCs and observed that mutant microglia markedly inhibited proliferation and neuronal lineage commitment of wild-type neurospheres. Moreover, the conditioned media from microglia expressing FAD-linked PS1 variants also impair the neurogenenic potential of PS1hWT neurospheres or newly born progenitors in organotypic slices from PS1hWT mice. Extending these analyses, we observed considerable differences in the profile of secreted soluble factors between microglia expressing PS1hWT or FAD-linked PS1 variants. The altered protein levels were paralleled by differences in mRNAs encoding these polypeptides. Remarkably, we observed differences in the levels of many of these mRNAs in microglia isolated from enriched adult PS1hWT versus PS1 mutant mice. Taken together, these results lead us to conclude that soluble factors released from microglia, at least in part, are responsible for the defective EE-induced neurogenesis observed in transgenic mice.

To test our hypothesis that the fate of hippocampal NPCs in mice expressing FAD-linked PS1 variants is determined by cellular factors produced within multiple cell types present in the niche, we are currently performing two series of experiments. In the first, we have transplanted either PS1hWT or mutant PS1 NPCs that were retrovirally transduced to constitutively express green fluorescent protein (GFP) or co-labeled with BrdU into the hippocampus of heterologous mice maintained in enriched conditions in order to assess the survival and differentiation of the engrafted cells. We grafted single cell suspensions of GFP- or BrdU-labeled NPCs (fig. 1a–c) into the DG of heterologous hosts and, after a 7-day recovery period, subjected these animals to EE for 5 weeks. Six weeks following transplantation, animals were sacrificed and sections were stained with anti-BrdU antibodies. Representative images shown in figure 1d and e reveal that we are able to detect the transplanted GFP-positive or BrdU-positive NPCs, respectively. Our preliminary studies revealed that the survival efficiency of PS1hWT NPCs in the PS1hWT host is ~32% after 5 days, and 10% after 4 weeks (fig. 1f). Remarkably, a fraction of the surviving NPCs seemed to migrate to the subgranular cell layer (SGL) of the DG (fig. 1g), findings consistent with other studies [7]. Preliminary quantification of the number of transplanted NPCs co-labeled with NeuN that are localized in the SGL or granule cell layer (fig. 1h) revealed that less than 20% of grafted NPCs are co-labeled with NeuN, but more importantly, that the host has a marked effect on the neurogenenic potential of the engrafted NPCs (fig. 1i).

Our second strategy is to characterize hippocampal NPC proliferation and neurogenesis in mice that express a mouse prion promoter-driven transgene encoding FAD-linked PS1ΔE9 that can be conditionally inactivated in a cell-specific and/or temporal manner using *cre-loxP* approaches. To score the efficacy of cre-driven recombination, a cDNA encoding a GFP marker fluorescent protein was introduced after the second *loxP* site. We now show that in a mouse line that harbors the Mo.PrP-*loxP*-PS1ΔE9-GFP transgene, Western blot analysis of total brain lysates reveals overexpression of PS1ΔE9 polypeptides and significant 'replacement' of endogenous mouse PS1, as observed earlier (fig. 2b) [8]. More importantly, transduction of NPCs established from adult *loxP*-PS1ΔE9-GFP mice with an adenovirus expressing cre recombinase resulted in loss of PS1ΔE9 expression with concomitant appearance of GFP fluorescence signal (fig. 2c). These observations reveal that the line carrying the *loxP*-PS1ΔE9-GFP cassette is amenable to cre-dependent excision of the PS1ΔE9 transgene, and hence is best suited to explore cell type-specific effects of the PS1ΔE9 mutant on enrichment-mediated neurogenesis.

In summary, our findings offer a paradigm shift in understanding the impact of FAD-linked PS1 variants on the pathogenesis of FAD and the effects on circuits involved in memory formation and plasticity in the adult brain.

References

1 Chen Q, Nakajima A, Choi SH, Xiong X, Tang YP: Loss of presenilin function causes Alzheimer's disease-like neurodegeneration in the mouse. J Neurosci Res 2008;86:1615–1625.

2 Saura CA, Choi SY, Beglopoulos V, Malkani S, Zhang D, Shankaranarayana Rao BS, Chattarji S, Kelleher RJ 3rd, Kandel ER, Duff K, Kirkwood A, Shen J: Loss of presenilin function causes impairments of memory and synaptic plasticity followed by age-dependent neurodegeneration. Neuron 2004;42:23–36.

3 Mirnics K, Norstrom EM, Garbett K, Choi SH, Zhang X, Ebert P, Sisodia SS: Molecular signatures of neurodegeneration in the cortex of PS1/PS2 double knockout mice. Mol Neurodegener 2008;3:14–25.

4 Feng R, Rampon C, Tang YP, Shrom D, Jin J, Kyin M, Sopher B, Miller MW, Ware CB, Martin GM, Kim SH, Langdon RB, Sisodia SS, Tsien JZ: Deficient neurogenesis in forebrain-specific presenilin-1 knockout mice is associated with reduced clearance of hippocampal memory traces. Neuron 2001;32:911–926.

5 Choi SH, Veeraraghavalu K, Lazarov O, Marler S, Ransohoff RM, Ramirez JM, Sisodia SS: Non-cell-autonomous effects of presenilin 1 variants on enrichment-mediated hippocampal progenitor cell proliferation and differentiation. Neuron 2008;59:568–580.

6 Ziv Y, Ron N, Butovsky O, Landa G, Sudai E, Greenberg N, Cohen H, Kipnis J, Schwartz M: Immune cells contribute to the maintenance of neurogenesis and spatial learning abilities in adulthood. Nat Neurosci 2006;9:268–275.

7 Fricker RA, Carpenter MK, Winkler C, Greco C, Gates MA, Bjorklund A: Site-specific migration and neuronal differentiation of human neural progenitor cells after transplantation in the adult rat brain. J Neurosci 1999;19:5990–6005.

8 Thinakaran G, Borchelt DR, Lee MK, Slunt HH, Spitzer L, Kim G, Ratovitsky T, Davenport F, Nordstedt C, Seeger M, Hardy J, Levey AI, Gandy SE, Jenkins NA, Copeland NG, Price DL, Sisodia SS: Endoproteolysis of presenilin 1 and accumulation of processed derivatives in vivo. Neuron 1996;17:181–190.

Biology of Neurodegeneration

Neuro-
degenerative
Diseases

Neurodegenerative Dis 2010;7:50–55
DOI: 10.1159/000283483

Published online: February 13, 2010

p53 Is Regulated by and Regulates Members of the γ-Secretase Complex

Frédéric Checler Julie Dunys Raphaelle Pardossi-Piquard
Cristine Alves da Costa

Institut de Pharmacologie Moléculaire et Cellulaire et Institut de NeuroMédecine Moléculaire, UMR6097 CNRS/UNSA, Valbonne, France

Key Words
Amyloid β-peptides · Alzheimer's disease · Presenilin · Tumor suppressor p53 · γ-Secretase complex

Abstract
Amyloid β-peptides is the generic term for a set of hydrophobic peptides that accumulate in Alzheimer's disease (AD)-affected brains. These amyloid-β peptide fragments are mainly generated by an enzymatic machinery referred to as γ-secretase complex that is built up by the association of four distinct proteins, namely presenilin 1 (PS1) or PS2, nicastrin, Aph-1 and Pen-2. AD is also characterized by exacerbated cell death that appears linked to the tumor suppressor p53. Interestingly, all members of the γ-secretase complex control p53-dependent cell death. On the other hand, p53 appears to be able to regulate directly or indirectly the expression and transcription of PS1, PS2 and Pen-2. This review will focus on the functional cross-talk between the members of the γ-secretase complex and p53 and will discuss the putative implication of this oncogene in AD pathology.

Introduction

Alzheimer's disease (AD)-affected brains are characterized by senile plaques, neurofibrillary tangles, and synaptic loss and are also often accompanied by apoptotic stigmata. Whether these distinct histological hallmarks are topologically, kinetically and mechanistically linked is still a matter of debate. At first sight, two lesions could be theoretically linked. Thus, amyloid-β peptides (Aβ) that invade cortical and subcortical brain areas and that are the main components of senile plaques were reported to affect the transcription of p53 [1], an oncogene, the expression of which appears clearly enhanced in AD brains [1–4] and which likely accounts for AD-related neuronal cell death [5–7].

Aβ peptides derive from the sequential proteolytic attacks of a longer precursor protein βAPP (β-amyloid precursor protein) by β- and γ-secretases, respectively [8]. The latter activity conditions the C-terminal end of Aβ peptides and, therefore, is responsible for the final step leading to Aβ42, the most toxic Aβ species [9] that accumulates at early stages of AD pathology. γ-Secretase is likely a generic term referring to both presenilin (PS)-independent [10–13] and PS-dependent activities [14]. The latter activity is borne by a multiproteic complex composed of either PS1 or PS2, one of the anterior pharynx defective Aph-1 isoforms, Pen-2 and nicastrin (Nct) [15–

KARGER
Fax +41 61 306 12 34
E-Mail karger@karger.ch
www.karger.com

1660–2854/10/0073–0050$26.00/0

Accessible online at:
www.karger.com/ndd

Frédéric Checler
Institut de Pharmacologie Moléculaire et Cellulaire et
Institut de NeuroMédecine Moléculaire, UMR6097 CNRS/UNSA
660 route des lucioles, FR–06560 Valbonne (France)
Tel. +33 49 395 3460, Fax +33 49 395 7708, E-Mail checler@ipmc.cnrs.fr

17]. Interestingly, previous studies indicated that PS1 and PS2 could differently control neuronal cell death [18–20] and that PS2 triggered p53-dependent apoptosis [21–23]. On the other hand, p53 was reported to transcriptionally downregulate PS1 expression [24, 25]. This very interesting cross-talk between PS and p53 linking the γ-secretase complex with the tumor suppressor has been reinforced recently by several papers showing a functional relationship between p53 and other members of the γ-secretase complex. Thus, both Aph-1a/b, Pen-2 and Nct trigger antiapoptotic phenotypes by downregulating p53 via γ-secretase activity-dependent and -independent mechanisms [26, 27], while the oncogene was recently shown to affect Pen-2 transcription [28].

Materials and Methods

Cells and Transfections

Telencephalon-specific murine cells (TSM1) overexpressing myc-tagged Pen-2 were obtained and cultured as previously described [26].

PS Promoter Transactivation Assays

The murine PS1 (mPS1) and human PS2 (hPS2) promoters in frame with luciferase reporter gene have been previously described [29–31]. Stably transfected TSM1 cells expressing Pen-2 were cotransfected with 1.0 μg of either mPS1-luciferase or hPS2-luciferase cDNA and 0.5 μg of a β-galactosidase transfection vector (to normalize transfection efficiency) by means of the Lipofectamine 2000 reagent (Invitrogen); then, luciferase and β-galactosidase activities were analyzed according to the manufacturer's recommendations (Promega).

Statistical Analysis

Statistical analyses were performed using Prism Software (Graphpad Software, San Diego, Calif., USA) by means of the Neumans-Keuls multiple comparison test.

Results and Discussion

All Members of the γ-Secretase Complex Regulate p53-Dependent Cell Death

Initial evidence that PS1 could modulate cell death came from Bursztajn et al. [18] who demonstrated that overexpressed PS1 could lower the neuronal susceptibility to apoptotic stimuli, and that this phenotype could be abolished by pathogenic mutations. As a matter of confirmation, PS1 reduction by either knockout or antisense targeting increased the vulnerability of hippocampal neurons and cell death [19]. It is interesting that the PS1 congener PS2 triggers a proapoptotic phenotype [32–35] that is exacerbated by AD-associated familial mutations [36, 37]. We clearly demonstrated that PS2-associated cell death was due to an increased p53-dependent caspase-3 activity [21]. Thus, PS2 overexpression enhances expression and transactivation of p53 as well as that of one of its downstream targeted gene p21waf-1, while p53 antisense downregulation reduces PS2-induced caspase-3 activation [21]. That PS1 and PS2 trigger opposite phenotypes appeared at first glance puzzling. However, we demonstrated that PS2 overexpression/knockout could drastically lower/enhance PS1 expression [21] in agreement with Kang et al. [38] who showed that mutated PS1 drastically reduced PS2 fragments. Furthermore, Roperch et al. [24] established that PS1 expression was reduced during p53-induced apoptosis. Finally, p53 was reported to act as a direct transcriptional repressor of PS1 promoter transactivation [24, 25]. Therefore, one could envision that PS2-associated enhancement of p53 could indirectly lead to the reduction of PS1. We recently established that the other members of the γ-secretase complex could also modulate cell death in a p53-dependent manner. Thus, we showed that Aph-1a, Aph-1b, Pen-2 and Nct all reduced staurosporine-induced caspase-3 activation in various cell systems including neurons [26]. This agreed well with studies showing that selective apoptosis was observed in the neuronal tube of Aph-1a knockout mice [39] and that depletion of Pen-2 and Nct led to neuronal loss and cell death in the zebrafish and apoptosis in the heart and brain of mouse embryos, respectively [40, 41]. Interestingly, we showed that the antiapoptotic phenotypes displayed by these proteins were also fully abolished by p53 deficiency [26]. PS have been proposed to harbor the catalytic site of the γ-secretase complex [42]. It was therefore important to establish whether the enzymatic activity linked to the complex could be involved in the PS-associated control of p53-dependent cell death. This was indeed the case since both mutations of catalytic aspartyl residues of PS and γ-secretase inhibitors lowered p53 expression in wild-type fibroblasts but not in PS-deficient cells [43]. Four lines of evidence suggested that AICD (βAPP IntraCellular Domain), the C-terminal fragment released in the cytosol upon γ-secretase attack of βAPP, indeed controlled p53 transcription and expression [43]. First, AICD controls p53 at a transcriptional level. Second, AICD triggers p53-dependent caspase-3 activation and cell death. Third, AICD-induced cell death is abolished by p53 deficiency. Fourth, βAPP deficiency affects p53 levels in vitro and in vivo [44]. Interestingly, PS1 and PS2 triggered clear opposite effects on p53 transactivation. Thus, PS1 and PS2 overexpressions lower and increase p53 transactivation,

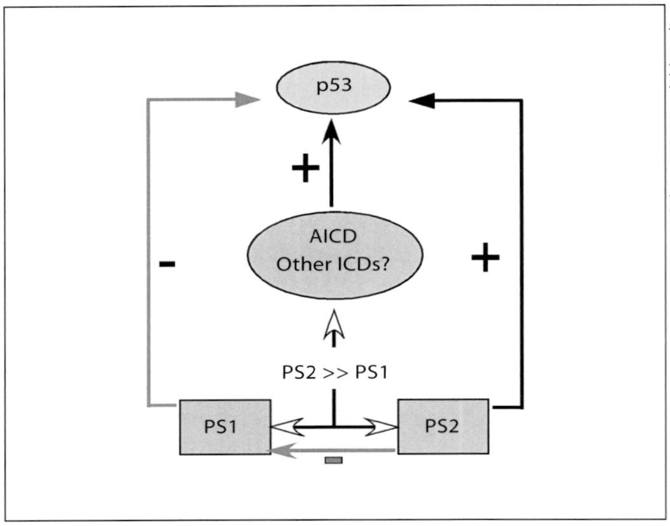

Color version available online

Fig. 1. Schematic representation of the control of p53 by PS. Schematic representation of the pathways linking PS1, PS2, ICDs and p53. As we previously described [43], PS1 lowers p53 while PS2 increases p53. Both proteins functionally interact, but PS2 is dominant for the p53-dependent proapoptotic phenotype (PS2 >> PS1) [43]. γ-Secretase activities associated with PS1 and PS2 generate AICD and likely other ICDs that positively modulate p53 [43].

Table 1. Influence of the members of the γ-secretase complex on p53 and requirement for complex structure and catalytic activity

	Effect on p53	Requirement for γ-secretase complex	Requirement for γ-secretase activity	References
PS1	↘	yes	yes	40
PS2	↗	yes	yes	21, 22, 40
Aph-1	↘	yes	no	26
Pen-2	↘	yes	no	26, 38
Nicastrin	↘	no	no	27

respectively, while invalidation of the genes encoding these proteins elicits opposite phenotypes [43]. It is important to note that the phenotype harbored by cells devoid of both PS1 and PS2 mimics that observed with PS2 knockout cells [43], indicating that PS2 was clearly 'dominant' for the control of p53. One hypothesis could be that PS2 displays higher affinity/efficiency for other substrates, the cleavage of which gives rise to fragments also able to control p53 (fig. 1). As a matter of fact, we showed that the members of the βAPP family amyloid precursor like-protein (APLP) 1 and APLP2, which undergoes γ-secretase cleavages, produce intracellular fragments (ALIDs) that are also able to control p53 [43]. It is also interesting to note that the N141I mutation on PS2 potentiates p53-dependent staurosporine-stimulated caspase-3 activity [see suppl. fig. 2 in 43]. Whether PS1 mutations abolish the protective effect of wild-type PS1 is not yet demonstrated, but it is rather tempting to speculate that in both PS1- and PS2-related mutations responsible for familial cases of AD, a common trigger corresponds to activation of the p53 pathway. Whether Aph-1a, Pen-2 and Nct control p53 through their participation in the γ-secretase complex remained a matter of interrogation. Interestingly, these proteins control p53 by apparently distinct mechanisms. Thus, Aph-1a/b and Pen-2 require the complex formation to exert their function since their protective phenotype was abolished by PS deficiency, i.e. when the structure of the γ-secretase complex was disrupted [26]. However, Aph-1a/b and Pen-2-induced phenotypes remained insensitive to γ-secretase inhibitors, indicating that Aph-1a/b and Pen-2 elicit their antiapoptotic function within the γ-secretase complex but independent of the associated γ-secretase catalytic activity [26]. Recently, we showed that Nct triggers its p53-dependent protective function independent of the γ-secretase structure and activity [27]. Thus, Nct-associated phenotype was not sensitive to γ-secretase inhibitors and remained unaffected by Nct mutations that alter Aβ production [27]. Furthermore, Nct still lowers caspase-3 activation in cells devoid of PS [27]. Overall, the above data summarized in table 1 indicate that although all proteins identified as members of the γ-secretase control p53-dependent cell death, this could be via both γ-secretase complex-dependent and independent mechanisms.

p53 Regulates PS1 and Pen-2 Transcription

The first indication that p53 could control the promoter transactivation of proteins involved in the γ-secretase complex came from previous reports that showed that p53 functioned as a transcriptional repressor of PS1 [24, 25]. Since, no additional evidence of the involvement of p53 in the control of other members of the γ-secretase complex had been released. Recently, we demonstrated that p53 deficiency downregulated Pen-2 expression, promoter transactivation and mRNA levels and that p53 expression rescued Pen-2 expression and promoter transactivation in p53-deficient cells [28]. Such regulation occurs likely via indirect mechanisms since Pen-2 promoter sequence did not reveal canonical consensus sequences

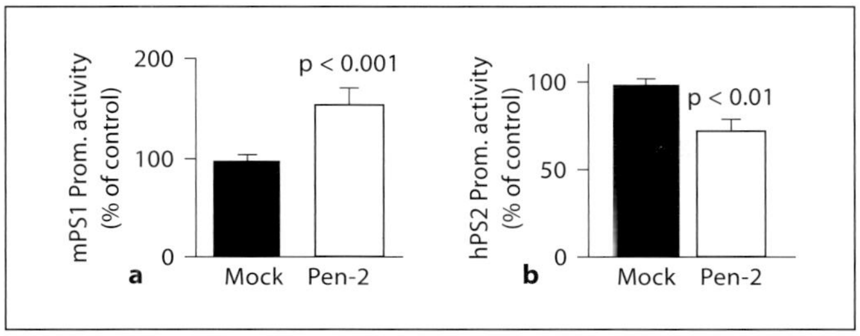

Fig. 2. Pen-2 overexpression triggers opposite effects on PS1 and PS2 promoter transactivation in neurons. Stably transfected TSM1 neurons overexpressing Pen-2 or empty vector (Mock) were transiently transfected with PS1 (**a**) or PS2 (**b**) promoter-luciferase reporter gene constructs. Twenty-four hours after transfection, promoter transactivations were analyzed as described in 'Materials and Methods'. Bars are the means of four (**a**) or six (**b**) independent determinations for promoter and real-time PCR analyses, respectively. p values compare luciferase activity with that obtained in Mock-transfected cells.

targeted by p53 [28]. Therefore, these data show that p53 is regulated by, and regulates several members of the γ-secretase complex.

p53, a Pivotal Intermediate in the Cross-Talk of γ-Secretase Members

The pivotal role of p53 allows envisioning that this oncogene could behave as a molecular intermediate responsible for a cross-talk between members of the γ-secretase complex. For example, as Pen-2 decreases p53 expression, this should thereby directly influence p53-dependent control of PS1 and PS2 promoter. This was indeed the case since we showed that Pen-2 overexpression increased PS1 promoter transactivation while it reduced that of PS2 (fig. 2). This was in agreement with the above-described influence of p53 on PS1 and PS2. Thus, Pen-2 reduces p53 and therefore lowers p53-associated repression of PS1, thereby resulting in increased PS1 promoter transactivation. In the case of PS2, p53 reduction ultimately resulted in decreased *PS2* promoter transactivation. The fact that Pen-2 lowered *PS2* transcription is in agreement with a study by Placanica et al. [45] showing that Pen-2 overexpression decreased total PS2 expression levels. Since PS control AICD production and thereby p53 expression, one should also expect that PS could ultimately control p53-dependent expression of Pen-2. This is indeed the case. We showed that PS depletion drastically reduced Pen-2 expression, promoter transactivation and mRNA levels [28]. We also showed that overexpression of AICD was sufficient to trigger Pen-2 promoter transactivation

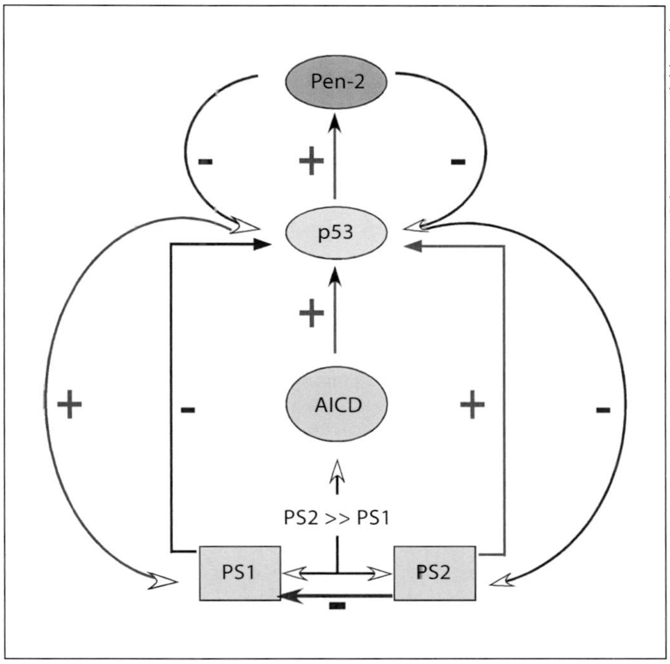

Fig. 3. Schematic representation of cross-regulation between PS, p53 and Pen-2. As we previously described [43], PS1 lowers p53 while PS2 increases p53. Both proteins functionally interact, but PS2 is dominant for the p53-dependent proapoptotic phenotype (PS2 >> PS1) [43]. AICD positively modulates p53 [43], and p53 increases Pen-2 transcription [26]. Conversely, there exists a feedback loop by which Pen-2 downregulates p53 [26]. Thus, when Pen-2 expression is increased, p53 is lowered. Because p53 is a transcriptional repressor of PS1, Pen-2-induced lowering of p53 leads to increased levels of PS1 and concomitantly enhances the transcription of PS1 promoter (present study).

Color version available online

[28]. That this effect was due to AICD-associated control of p53 was demonstrated by the fact that AICD was unable to modulate Pen-2 transactivation in p53-deficient cells [28]. The functional interaction between PS and Pen-2 is summarized in figure 3. Altogether, our data show that p53 plays a central role in the regulation of the expression and transactivation of the members of the γ-secretase complex and unravel the fact that there exists a functional cross-talk between members of the complex where p53 plays a pivotal role.

Acknowledgements

We wish to sincerely thank Drs. Vitek, Renbaum and Levy-Lahad for providing us with the PS2 and PS1 promoter constructs. This work was supported by the Fondation pour la Recherche Médicale and by the Conseil Général des Alpes Maritimes.

References

1 Ohyagi Y, Asahara H, Chui DH, Tsuruta Y, Sakae N, Miyoshi K, Yamada T, Kikuchi H, Taniwaki T, Murai H, Ikezoe K, Furuya H, Kawarabayashi T, Shoji M, Checler F, Iwaki T, Makifuchi T, Takeda K, Kira J, Tabira T: Intracellular Abeta42 activates p53 promoter: a pathway to neurodegeneration in Alzheimer's disease. FASEB J 2005;19:255–257.

2 de la Monte S, Sohn YK, Ganju YK, Wands JR: p53- and CD95-associated apoptosis in neurodegenerative diseases. Lab Invest 1998; 78:401–411.

3 Kitamura Y, Shimohama S, Kamoshima W, Matsuoka Y, Nomura Y, Taniguchi T: Changes of p53 in the brains patients with Alzheimer disease. Biochem Biophys Res Commun 1997;232:418–421.

4 Garcia-Ospina GP, Ginenez-del Rio M, Lopera F, Velez-Pardo C: Neuronal DNA damage correlates with a positive detection of c-Jun, nuclear factor κB, p53 and Par-4 transcription factors in Alzheimer's disease. Rev Neurol 2003;36:1004–1010.

5 Cotman CW, Anderson AJ: A potential role for apoptosis in neurodegeneration and Alzheimer's disease. Mol Neurobiol 1995;10: 19–45.

6 Shimohama S: Apoptosis in Alzheimers' disease – an update. Apoptosis 2000;5:9–16.

7 Marx J: Neuroscience. New leads on the 'how' of Alzheimer's. Science 2001;293: 2192–2194.

8 Checler F: Processing of the β-amyloid precursor protein and its regulation in Alzheimer's disease. J Neurochem 1995;65:1431–1444.

9 Burdick D, Soreghan B, Kwon M, Kosmoski J, Knauer M, Henschen A, Yates J, Cotman C, Glabe C: Assembly and aggregation properties of synthetic Alzheimer's A4/β amyloid peptide analogs. J Biol Chem 1992;267:546–554.

10 Armogida M, Petit A, Vincent B, Scarzello S, da Costa CA, Checler F: Endogenous beta-amyloid production in presenilin-deficient embryonic mouse fibroblasts. Nat Cell Biol 2001;3:1030–1033.

11 Wilson CA, Doms RW, Lee VM-Y: Distinct presenilin-dependent and presenilin-independent γ-secretases are responsible for total cellular Aβ production. J Neurosci Res 2003;74:361–369.

12 Lai MT, Crouthamel MC, DiMuzio J, Pietrak BL, Donoviel DB, Bernstein A, Gardell SJ, Li YM, Hazuda D: A presenilin-independent aspartyl protease prefers the gamma-42 site cleavage. J Neurochem 2006;96:118–125.

13 Yagishita S, Futai E, Ishiura S: In vitro reconstitution of gamma-secretase activity using yeast microsomes. Biochem Biophys Res Commun 2008;377:141–145.

14 De Strooper B, Saftig P, Craessaerts K, Vanderstichele H, Guhde G, Annaert W, Von Figura K, Van Leuven F: Deficiency of presenilin-1 inhibits the normal cleavage of amyloid precursor protein. Nature 1998;391:387–390.

15 Takasugi N, Tomita T, Hayashi I, Tsuruoka M, Niimura M, Takahashi Y, Thinakaran G, Iwatsubo T: The role of presenilin cofactors in the γ-secretase complex. Nature 2003;422: 438–441.

16 Edbauer D, Winkler E, Regula JT, Pesold B, Steiner H, Haass C: Reconstitution of γ-secretase activity. Nat Cell Biol 2003;5:486–488.

17 Kimberly WT, LaVoie MJ, Ostaszewski B, Ye W, Wolfe MS, Selkoe DJ: γ-Secretase is a membrane protein complex comprised presenilin, nicastrin, Aph 1, and Pen2. Proc Natl Acad Sci 2003;100:6382–6387.

18 Bursztajn S, DeSouza R, McPhie DL, Berman SA, Shioi J, Robakis NK, Neve RL: Overexpression in neurons of human presenilin-1 or a presenilin-1 familial Alzheimer's disease mutant does not enhance apoptosis. J Neurosci 1998;18:9790–9799.

19 Guo Q, Fu W, Sopher BL, Miller MW, Ware CB, Martin GM, Mattson MP: Increased vulnerability of hippocampal neurons to excitotoxic necrosis in presenilin-1mutant knock-in mice. Nat Med 1999;5:101–106.

20 Hong C-S, Caromille L, Nomata Y, Mori H, Bredesen DE, Koo EH: Contrasting role of presenilin-1 and presenilin-2 in neuronal differentiation in vitro. J Neurosci 1999;19: 637–643.

21 Alves da Costa C, Paitel E, Mattson MP, Amson R, Telerman A, Ancolio K, Checler F: Wild-type and mutated presenilins 2 trigger p53-dependent apoptosis and down-regulate presenilin 1 expression in HEK293 human cells and in murine neurons. Proc Natl Acad Sci USA 2002;99:4043–4048.

22 Alves da Costa C, Mattson MP, Ancolio K, Checler F: The C-terminal fragment of presenilin 2 triggers p53-mediated staurosporine-induced apoptosis, a function independent of the presenilinase-derived N-terminal counterpart. J Biol Chem 2003;278:12064–12069.

23 Alves da Costa C: Recent insights on the pro-apoptotic phenotype elicited by presenilin 2 and its caspase and presenilinase-derived fragments. Curr Alz Res 2005;2:507–514.

24 Roperch JP, Alvaro V, Prieur S, Tyunder M, Nemani M, Lethrosne F, Piouffre L, Gendron MC, Israeli D, Dausset J, Oren M, Amson R, Telerman A: Inhibition of presenilin1 expression is promoted by p53 and p21WAF-1 and results in apoptosis and tumor suppression. Nat Med 1998;4:835–838.

25 Pastorcic M, Das HK: Regulation of transcription of the human presenilin-1 gene by Ets transcription factor and the p53 protooncogene. J Biol Chem 2000;275:34938–34945.

26 Dunys J, Kawarai T, Sevalle J, Dolcini V, St George-Hyslop P, Alves da Costa C, Checler F: p53-dependent Aph-1 and Pen-2 anti-apoptotic phenotype requires the integrity of the gamma-secretase complex but is independent of its activity. J Biol Chem 2007;282: 10516–10525.

27 Pardossi-Piquard R, Dunys J, Giaime E, Guillot-Sestier MV, St George-Hyslop P, Checler F, Alves da Costa C: p53-dependent control of cell death by nicastrin: lack of requirement for presenilin-dependent gamma-secretase complex. J Neurochem 2009; 109:225–237.

28 Dunys J, Sevalle J, Giaime E, Pardossi-Piquard R, Vitek M, Renbaum P, Levy-Lahad E, Zhang YW, Xu H, Checler F, Alves da Costa C: p53-dependent control of Pen-2 promoter transactivation by presenilins. J Cell Sci 2009, in press.

29 Mitsuda N, Roses AD, Vitek MP: Transcriptional regulation of the mouse presenilin-1 gene. J Biol Chem 1997;272:23489–23497.

30 Renbaum P, Beeri R, Gabai E, Amiel M, Gal M, Ehrengruber MU, Levy-Lahad E: Egr-1 upregulates the Alzheimer's disease presenilin-2 gene in neuronal cells. Gene 2003;318: 113–124.

31 Wang R, Zhang YW, Sun P, Liu R, Zhang X, Xia K, Xia J, Xu H, Zhang Z: Transcriptional regulation of PEN-2, a key component of the gamma-secretase complex, by CREB. Mol Cell Biol 2006;26:1347–1354.

32 Wolozin B, Iwasaki K, Vito P, Ganjei JK, Lacana E, Sunderland T, Zhao B, Kusiak J, W, Wasco W, D'Adamio L: Participation of presenilin 2 in apoptosis: enhanced basal activity conferred by an Alzheimer mutation. Science 1996;274:1710–1713.

33 Vito P, Lacana E, D'Adamio L: Interfering with apoptosis: Ca^{2+}-binding protein ALG-2 and Alzheimer's disease gene ALG-3. Science 1996;271:521–525.

34 Kim TW, Pettingell WH, Jung YK, Kovacs DM, Tanzi RE: Alternative cleavage of Alzheimer-associated presenilins during apoptosis by a caspase-3 family protease. Science 1997;277:373–376.

35 Araki W, Yuasa K, Takeda S, Shirotani K, Takahashi K, Tabira T: Overexpression of presenilin-2 enhances apoptotic death of cultured cortical neurons. ANYAS 2000; 920:241–244.

36 Janicki S, Monteiro M: Increased apoptosis arising from increased expression of Alzheimer's disease associates presenilin-2 mutation (N141I). J Cell Biol 1997;139:485–495.

37 Deng G, Pike CJ, Cotman CW: Alzheimer-associated presenilin-2 confers increased sensitivity to apoptosis in PC12 cells. FEBS Lett 1996;397:50–54.

38 Kang DE, Yoon IS, Repetto E, Busse T, Yermian N, Ie L, Koo EH: Presenilins mediate PI3K/AKT and ERK activation via select signaling receptors: selectivity of PS2 in PDGF signaling. J Biol Chem 2005;280:31537–31547.

39 Serneels L, Dejaegere T, Craessaerts K, Horré K, Jorissen E, Tousseyn T, Hébert S, Coolen M, Martens G, Zwijsen A, Annaert W, Hartmann D, De Strooper B: Differential contribution of the three Aph1 genes to γ-secretase activity in vivo. Proc Natl Acad Sci USA 2005;102:1719–1724.

40 Campbell WA, Yang H, Zetterberg H, Baulac S, Sears JA, Liu T, Wong STC, Zhong TP, Xia W: Zebrafish lacking Alzheimer presenilin enhancer 2 (Pen-2) demonstrate excessive p53-dependent apoptosis and neuronal loss. J Neurochem 2006;96:1423–1440.

41 Van Nguyen V, Hawkins C, Bergeron C, Supala A, Huang J, Westaway D, St George-Hyslop P, Rozmahel R: Loss of nicastrin elicits an apoptotic phenotype in mouse embryos. Brain Res 2006;1086:76–84.

42 Wolfe MS, Xia W, Ostaszewski BL, Diehl TS, Kimberly WT, Selkoe DJ: Two transmembrane aspartates in presenilin-1 required for presenilin endoproteolysis and γ-secretase activity. Nature 1999;398:513–517.

43 Alves da Costa C, Sunyach C, Pardossi-Piquard R, Sevalle J, Vincent B, Boyer N, Kawarai T, Girardot N, St George-Hyslop P, Checler F: Presenilin-dependent gamma-secretase-mediated control of p53-associated cell death in Alzheimer's disease. J Neurosci 2006;26:6377–6385.

44 Checler F, Sunyach C, Pardossi-Piquard R, Sevalle J, Vincent B, Kawarai T, Girardot N, St George-Hyslop P, da Costa CA: The gamma/epsilon-secretase-derived APP intracellular domain fragments regulate p53. Curr Alzheimer Res 2007;4:423–426.

45 Placanica L, Tarassishin L, Yang G, Peethumnongsin E, Kim SH, Zheng H, Sisodia S, Li YM: PEN2 and presenilin-1 modulate the dynamic equilibrium of presenilin-1 and presenilin-2 gamma-secretase complexes. J Biol Chem 2008;284:2967–2977.

Biology of Neurodegeneration

Neuro-degenerative Diseases

Neurodegenerative Dis 2010;7:56–59
DOI: 10.1159/000283484

Published online: February 13, 2010

Amyloid-β-Derived Diffusible Ligands Cause Impaired Axonal Transport of Mitochondria in Neurons

Xinglong Wang[a] George Perry[a, b] Mark A. Smith[a] Xiongwei Zhu[a]

[a]Department of Pathology, Case Western Reserve University, Cleveland, Ohio, and
[b]College of Sciences, University of Texas at San Antonio, San Antonio, Tex., USA

Key Words
Aβ-derived diffusible ligands · Mitochondria · Axonal transport · Alzheimer's disease

Abstract
Background: Alzheimer's disease (AD) is the most prevalent form of dementia predominantly affecting the elderly. It is believed that soluble amyloid-β (Aβ) oligomers are involved in the pathogenesis of AD, yet the underlying mechanisms remain elusive. ***Objectives:*** Emerging evidence suggests that mitochondrial dysfunction likely plays a critical role in Aβ-induced neuronal degeneration. Previously, we demonstrated that Aβ-derived diffusible ligands (ADDLs) induce reduced mitochondrial density in neurites, and we suspect that an impaired mitochondrial trafficking might be involved, which is tested in this study. ***Methods:*** Using live cell imaging, anterograde and retrograde transport of mitochondria in primary hippocampal neurons treated with sublethal doses of ADDLs was measured. ***Results:*** We found that ADDLs induced significant impairment in both anterograde and retrograde transport of mitochondria along axons. ***Conclusion:*** These results suggest that an impaired mitochondrial transport likely contributes to ADDL-induced abnormal mitochondrial distribution and dysfunction and also reinforce the idea that axonal transport is likely involved in AD pathogenesis.

Introduction

Alzheimer's disease (AD) is the most common neurodegenerative disorder in the aged population and is characterized by two pathological hallmarks, i.e., senile plaques and neurofibrillary tangles, along with extensive neuronal death in selected brain regions [1]. Despite extensive research efforts, the mechanisms underlying neurodegeneration in AD remain elusive. Largely due to the fact that AD-causing mutations found in amyloid-β (Aβ) precursor protein (APP) and presenilin 1 and 2 have a primary effect on Aβ processing and plaque formation, a myriad of studies have focused on the central role of Aβ in the pathogenesis and progression of AD, and it is generally believed that the soluble oligomers of Aβ are the major toxic species. Emerging evidence suggest that mi-

KARGER
Fax +41 61 306 12 34
E-Mail karger@karger.ch
www.karger.com

Accessible online at:
www.karger.com/ndd

Xiongwei Zhu, PhD
Department of Pathology, Case Western Reserve University
2103 Cornell Road
Cleveland, OH 44106 (USA)
Tel. +1 216 368 5903, Fax +1 216 368 8964, E-Mail xiongwei.zhu@case.edu

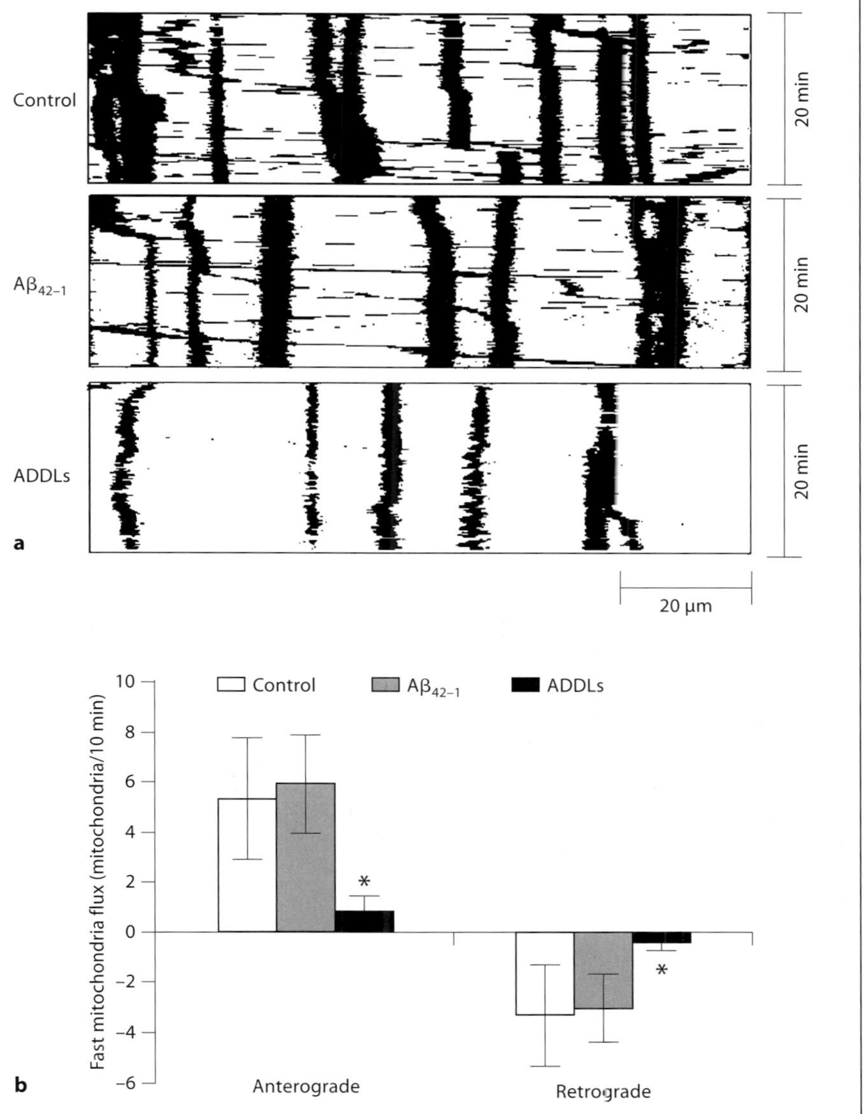

Fig. 1. Effect of ADDLs on FAT of mitochondria. Rat E18 hippocampal neurons (DIV 9) were transfected with Mito-DsRed2. 24 h after incubation with or without 800 nM ADDLs at DIV 11, neurons were imaged in time-lapse (10 s interval, 20 min). **a** Representative kymographs showing transport of mitochondria in the segment of axon around 100 μm in length beginning 300 μm from the cell body of control neurons or neurons treated with Aβ42–1 and ADDLs. **b** Quantification of mitochondria flux (number mitochondria/10 min) revealed that both anterograde and retrograde FAT of mitochondria were greatly impaired by ADDLs rather than negative control or Aβ42–1. At least 20 neurons were analyzed in three independent experiments (* $p < 0.05$, Student's t test).

tochondria are a major intracellular target of soluble Aβ oligomers [2]. Interestingly, we found abnormal mitochondrial dynamics in AD fibroblasts [3] and demonstrated that APP overexpression, likely through Aβ production, induced abnormal mitochondrial dynamics in neuronal cells [4]. Most recently, we confirmed abnormal mitochondrial dynamics in AD neurons and demonstrated that Aβ-derived diffusible ligand (ADDLs) induced abnormal mitochondrial dynamics in neurons [5]. One of the common features in all these models demonstrating abnormal mitochondrial dynamics is an abnormal mitochondrial distribution, i.e., perinuclear accumulation of mitochondria in AD fibroblasts or M17 cells overexpressing mutant APP or reduced mitochondrial density in neurites of primary hippocampal neurons. Since fast axonal transport (FAT) of mitochondria underlies the uniform distribution of mitochondria along the axon [6], these findings prompted us to question whether an abnormal mitochondrial transport is involved. In this study, by using live cell imaging, we investigated axonal transport in ADDL-treated primary hippocampal neurons.

Materials and Methods

Cell Culture and Transfection

Primary neurons from E18 rat hippocampus (BrainBits) were seeded at 30,000–40,000 cells per well on 35 × 10 mm culture dishes coated with poly-D-lysine/laminin in neurobasal medium supplemented with 2% B27 (Invitrogen)/0.5 mM glutamine/25 mM glutamate. Half the culture medium was changed every 3 days with neurobasal medium supplemented with 2% B27 (Invitrogen) and 0.5 mM glutamine. All cultures were kept at 37°C in a humidified 5% CO_2-containing atmosphere. More than 90% of cells were neurons after they were cultured for 12 days in vitro (DIV), verified by positive staining for neuronal specific markers microtubule-associated protein-2 (MAP2, dendritic marker) and Tau-1 (axonal marker). At DIV 9, neurons were transfected with Mito-DsRed2 construct (Clontech) using Neurofect (Genlantis) according to the manufacturer's protocol.

Time-Lapse Imaging and Image Analysis

ADDLs were prepared as previously described [5]. Two days after transfection with Mito-DsRed2, neurons were treated with ADDLs and then put in a well-equipped environmental chamber with controlled CO_2 content, humidity and temperature. Time-lapse images were captured with an inverted Leica DMI6000 fluorescence microscope (Leica) with a fully automated scanning stage and Leica EL6000 alignment-free metal halide bulb. The microscope was driven by MetaMorph software (Version 7.04, Molecular Devices). Images were acquired using a ×40 1.24 NA objective and a Retiga-EXi CCD digital camera (QImaging). Positive transfected neurons were identified by their expression of red fluorescence, and three different neurons were selected for time-lapse imaging at the same time. Images were acquired every 10 s for a total of 121 images (20 min) without apparent phototoxicity or photobleaching. Kymographs were generated using MetaMorph software (Molecular Devices). Image analysis was performed with WCIF ImageJ (developed by W. Rasband) and MetaMorph software (Molecular Devices).

Results

To investigate FAT of mitochondria, rat E18 hippocampal neurons were plated on poly-D-lysine/laminin-coated glass dishes and transfected with Mito-DsRed2 to label mitochondria at DIV 9. 48 h after transfection, neurons were treated with 800 nM ADDLs or 10 μM Aβ42–1. 24 h after treatment, mitochondria movement in neurons was imaged for up to 20 min under fluorescent microscope for time-lapse recordings. No cell death was observed under these conditions as determined by LDH assay (not shown). Because of high mitochondria density in the proximal segment of axon, we just measured FAT of mitochondria in the relative distal segment of axon (around 100 μm in length beginning 300 μm from the cell body of neurons; fig. 1a). Consistent with our prior report [5], ADDL treatment led to less mitochondria in axons. FAT of mitochondria included anterograde and retrograde movements, and mitochondria with velocity less than 0.1 μm/s were classified as stationary. The mitochondria flux that passed a single point in the center of kymographs was counted as described before [7]. Notably, in ADDL-treated neurons, both anterograde (0.80 ± 0.67) and retrograde FAT (0.44 ± 0.21) of mitochondria were significantly reduced compared to nontreated control neurons (5.34 ± 2.47 for anterograde and 3.31 ± 2.02 for retrograde transport of mitochondria; fig. 1b). Neurons treated with Aβ42–1 demonstrated similar FAT of mitochondria to control neurons.

Discussion

Previously, it was demonstrated that acute treatment of Aβ monomers and fibrils induces significant reduction in motile mitochondria [8]. In this study, we performed a more detailed study on axonal transport of mitochondria and found that soluble Aβ oligomers induced significantly reduced mitochondrial axonal transport, suggesting that impaired axonal transport of mitochondria likely contributes to ADDL-induced abnormal mitochondrial distribution in neurites. This is consistent with a recent study demonstrating an overall disruption of FAT induced by soluble Aβ oligomers in isolated squid axoplasms [9]. In fact, deficits in axonal transport may represent an early step in AD pathogenesis since axonal swelling and reduced axonal transport were observed before apparent AD hallmarks [10]. Overall, our studies, along with others, suggest that Aβ is likely one of the major mediators causing deficits in axonal transport.

Acknowledgements

This study is supported by the NIH (AG 031852), Alzheimer's Association (IIRG-07-60196, Zen-07-59500) and a pilot grant from Memory and Cognition Center at Case Western Reserve University.

References

1 Smith MA: Alzheimer disease. Int Rev Neurobiol 1998;42:1–54.

2 Reddy PH: Amyloid beta, mitochondrial structural and functional dynamics in Alzheimer's disease. Exp Neurol 2009;218:286–292.

3 Wang X, Su B, Fujioka H, Zhu X: Dynamin-like protein 1 reduction underlies mitochondrial morphology and distribution abnormalities in fibroblasts from sporadic Alzheimer's disease patients. Am J Pathol 2008;173:470–482.

4 Wang X, Su B, Siedlak SL, Moreira PI, Fujioka H, Wang Y, Casadesus G, Zhu X: Amyloid-beta overproduction causes abnormal mitochondrial dynamics via differential modulation of mitochondrial fission/fusion proteins. Proc Natl Acad Sci USA 2008;105:19318–19323.

5 Wang X, Su B, Lee HG, Li X, Perry G, Smith MA, Zhu X: Impaired mitochondrial fission and fusion in Alzheimer's disease. J Neurosci 2009;29:9090–9103.

6 Hollenbeck PJ, Saxton WM: The axonal transport of mitochondria. J Cell Sci 2005;118:5411–5419.

7 Miller KE, Sheetz MP: Axonal mitochondrial transport and potential are correlated. J Cell Sci 2004;117:2791–2804.

8 Rui Y, Tiwari P, Xie Z, Zheng JQ: Acute impairment of mitochondrial trafficking by beta-amyloid peptides in hippocampal neurons. J Neurosci 2006;26:10480–10487.

9 Pigino G, Morfini G, Atagi Y, Deshpande A, Yu C, Jungbauer L, LaDu M, Busciglio J, Brady S: Disruption of fast axonal transport is a pathogenic mechanism for intraneuronal amyloid beta. Proc Natl Acad Sci USA 2009;106:5907–5912.

10 Stokin GB, Lillo C, Falzone TL, Brusch RG, Rockenstein E, Mount SL, Raman R, Davies P, Masliah E, Williams DS, Goldstein LS: Axonopathy and transport deficits early in the pathogenesis of Alzheimer's disease. Science 2005;307:1282–1288.

Biology of Neurodegeneration

Neuro-degenerative Diseases

Neurodegenerative Dis 2010;7:60–63
DOI: 10.1159/000285507

Published online: February 18, 2010

Acetylcholinesterase Variants in Alzheimer's Disease: From Neuroprotection to Programmed Cell Death

David S. Greenberg Debra Toiber Amit Berson Hermona Soreq

Department of Biological Chemistry, The Hebrew University of Jerusalem, Safra Campus – Givat Ram, Jerusalem, Israel

Key Words
Acetylcholinesterase · Alzheimer's disease · Amyloid · Apoptosis · Caspases · Neuroinflammation

Abstract
Background: In Alzheimer's disease (AD), cholinergic neurons are particularly vulnerable for as yet unclear reasons. Here, we report that modified composition, localization and properties of alternative splice variants encoding the acetylcholine-hydrolyzing enzyme acetylcholinesterase (AChE) may be variably involved in disease progression or in systemic efforts to attenuate its progression. ***Objective:*** The purpose of this study was to explore the implications for AD of the cellular and biochemical properties of the various AChE proteins, differing in their N and C termini. ***Methods:*** We have used cell transfection with genetically engineered vectors as well as microinjection to overexpress specific AChE variants and explore the consequences to cellular well-being and survival. Additionally, we employed highly purified recombinant AChE-R and AChE-S to explore putative interactions with the AD β-amyloid peptide. ***Results:*** Our findings demonstrate distinct, and in certain cases inverse cell fate outcome under enforced expression of the human N- and C-terminally modified AChE variants, all of which have similar enzymatic activities. ***Conclusion:*** The N-terminal extension in conjunction with the primary helical C-terminal peptide of 'tailed' AChE-S facilitates, whereas the shorter, naturally unfolded C-terminus of the stress-induced AChE-R variant attenuates Alzheimer's pathology.

Introduction

Alzheimer's disease (AD) has been classified as a cholinergic disorder as early as 1983 [1], when it had been realized that nerve cells producing acetylcholine are the most vulnerable to premature cell death in the AD brain. Cholinergic neurons notably express the acetylcholine-hydrolyzing enzyme acetylcholinesterase (AChE; EC 3.11.7) in about 100-fold higher levels than other neuron types [2], and disease progression is consequently accompanied by a significant, albeit modest decline in hydrolytic AChE activity [3]. Subsequent studies have shown that the AD-associated AChE decline occurs rather late in disease progression [4], which raised the suggestion that it is not likely to be causally involved with the corresponding symptoms.

Intriguingly, the AChE gene can form multiple 3′-alternatively spliced variants [5, 6] as well as alternate 5′-transcripts and N-terminally extended protein products [7–10]. All of these AChE variants share similar hydrolytic activity, but their subcellular localization, cellular

KARGER
Fax +41 61 306 12 34
E-Mail karger@karger.ch
www.karger.com

1660–2854/10/0073–0060$26.00/0

Accessible online at:
www.karger.com/ndd

Hermona Soreq, PhD, Department of Biological Chemistry and
the Interdisciplinary Center of Neural Computation
The Hebrew University of Jerusalem, Safra Campus – Givat Ram
IL–91904 Jerusalem (Israel)
Tel. +972 2658 5109, Fax +972 2652 0258, E-Mail soreq@cc.huji.ac.il

properties and physiological roles were found to be different and sometimes inverse to each other, as is often the case with alternative splicing products of single genes [11]. Realizing that AChE activity reflects a mixture of different variants, it became clear that it is yet unknown the activity of which specific variant(s) of AChE declines in the AD brain and what the potential implication for AD progression of such changes is. Here, we discuss the putative roles of AChE variants with or without an N-terminal extension and two alternative C-terminal choices, S or R, together creating the N-AChE-S, N-AChE-R and the shorter AChE-S and AChE-R variants.

Methods

Expression vectors encoding for the N-terminally extended and the shorter AChE proteins (fig. 1a) were used to test the consequences of enforced expression of each of these variants in cultured cells and microinjected mouse embryos. Brain tissue samples from AD patients and matched nondemented controls as well as transgenic mice overexpressing specific human AChE variants, the doubly mutated amyloid APPswe 'Swedish' gene or both were used in this study. Fluorescence in situ hybridization (FISH) and immunohistochemistry were used to label mRNA and protein products, respectively [10, 11]. siRNA agents were used to suppress AChE expression in cultured cells and in vivo, and highly purified AChE-R produced in transgenic plants [12] enabled both biochemical and cellular loss and gain of function tests of these variants ex vivo and in vivo.

Results

In the entorhinal cortex from AD patients compared to nondemented controls, we found upregulation of an upstream *AChE* promoter which produces the 5′-E1e exon encoding the N-terminally extended N-AChE-S protein. Recombinant N-AChE-S, but none of the other variants, induced programmed cell death, both in microinjected early mouse embryos and in transfected cultured cells of different species and embryonic origins [9, 10] (fig. 1a, b). The apoptotic destiny could be avoided by co-treatment with small molecule anti-AChE agents, an siRNA targeted to the AChE mRNA transcript [Shaltiel et al., in preparation], and inhibitors of GSK and caspase-3, as well as the BCl-2 protein [9] (fig. 1b). Intriguingly, endogenous E1e and N-AChE expression was upregulated in various cultured cells exposed to apoptotic stimuli [9] as well as in the Alzheimer brain (fig. 1c). In our hands, N-AChE-S is the only variant causing cell death [9, 10], suggesting that this variant may be responsible for the

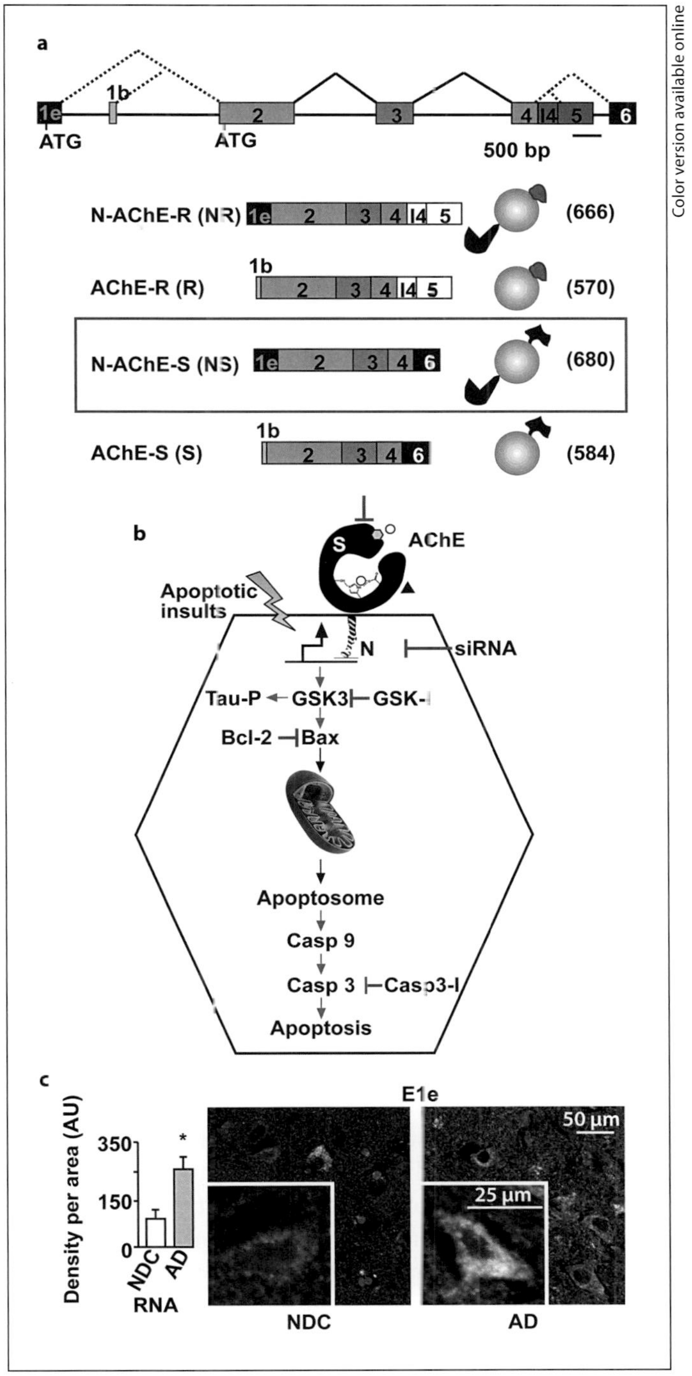

Fig. 1. Different human AChE variants serve for exploring N-AChE-S-related apoptosis. **a** Schematic structure of the human AChE gene (top) and the compositions of AChE variants carrying N-terminal and C-terminal extensions. These were used in transfection experiments for testing their role in AD. **b** N-AChE-S-induced apoptosis may be prevented by various interfering agents. Reproduced from Toiber et al. [9, 10]. **c** FISH tests demonstrating that the 5′-E1e exon is overexpressed in entorhinal cortical neurons from AD patients compared to nondemented controls (NDC).

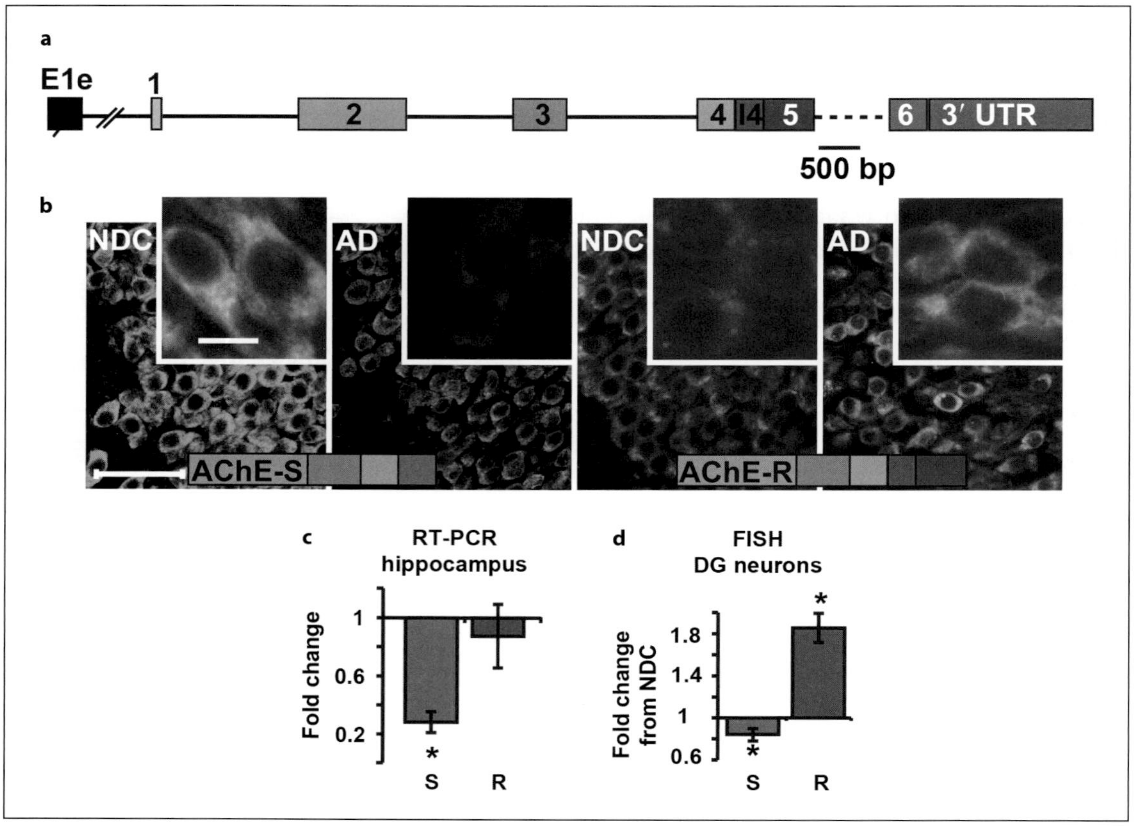

Color version available online

Fig. 2. AChE-R mRNA is overexpressed in the Alzheimer's hippocampus. Reproduced from Berson et al. [15]. **a** Scheme of the primary AChE mRNA transcript. **b** FISH of human hippocampal sections using cRNA probes specific for each variant. **c** Real-time RT-PCR fold change of AChE splice variants from human hippocampal RNA. AChE-S mRNA levels are significantly reduced in AD (n = 10) compared to NDC patients (n = 5; * $p < 0.05$, Mann-Whitney test). **d** Fluorescent signal quantification of **b**. AChE-S mRNA levels are significantly reduced and AChE-R mRNA increased in AD (n = 10) compared to NDC patients (n = 5; * $p < 0.05$, Mann-Whitney test).

apoptosis-related role of AChE reported by others [13, 14]. This corresponds with a positive association between N-AChE- and AChE-S labeling and that of the hyperphosphorylated Tau protein Tau-P in the entorhinal cortex [9]. Additionally, we discovered FISH-validated increases in the 3′ alternatively spliced stress-induced 'readthrough' AChE-R mRNA (fig. 2a, d) in hippocampal dentate gyrus neurons from the AD brain compared to nondemented controls; this was accompanied by RT-PCR-validated decreases in the normally prevalent AChE-S mRNA (also called AChE-T mRNA) [2] (fig. 2b, c). However, intact AChE-R protein levels were drastically reduced in AD [15]. Unlike the N-AChE-S-induced cell death, highly purified recombinant AChE-R produced in engineered plants [16] protected PC12 and neuroblastoma cells from β-amyloid toxicity [15]. Furthermore, in double APP/AChE-R transgenic mice, AChE-R efficiently suppressed β-amyloid fibril formation [15], unlike the AChE-S protein which enhanced the formation of such fibrils in double transgenics [17]. Together, these data suggest that the N-AChE-S, AChE-S and AChE-R variants of AChE play distinct roles in AD.

Discussion

We have found distinct roles for the N-terminally extended N-AChE-S protein which induces cell death, the shorter AChE-S variant which enhances amyloid-associated neurotoxicity and the yet shorter AChE-R protein which may exert neuroprotection by attenuating the formation of β-amyloid fibrils but fails to be produced in the

AD brain. Together, these findings indicate detrimental consequences for alternate AChE promoter usage if unaccompanied by successful production of the AChE-R protein. Changes in AChE gene expression can hence contribute to the AD-associated deterioration in both cortical and hippocampal functioning; and anti-AChEs used as AD drugs should be tested for their capacity to limit the N-AChE-S-induced cell death and delay disease progression.

Acknowledgements

This study was supported by the European Union's Network of Excellence (LSH-2004-1.1.5-3), The German Israel Project (DIP-G 3.2), and The Israel Science Foundation (grants 2007-2011 and 399/07).

References

1 Coyle JT, Price DL, DeLong MR: Alzheimer's disease: a disorder of cortical cholinergic innervation. Science 1983;219:1184–1190.

2 Massoulie J: The origin of the molecular diversity and functional anchoring of cholinesterases. Neurosignals 2002;11:130–143.

3 Darreh-Shori T, Hellstrom-Lindahl E, Flores-Flores C, Guan ZZ, Soreq H, Nordberg A: Long-lasting acetylcholinesterase splice variations in anticholinesterase-treated Alzheimer's disease patients. J Neurochem 2004;88:1102–1113.

4 Davis KL, Mohs RC, Marin D, Purohit DP, Perl DP, Lantz M, Austin G, Haroutunian V: Cholinergic markers in elderly patients with early signs of Alzheimer disease. JAMA 1999;281:1401–1406.

5 Soreq H, Zevin-Sonkin D, Razon N: Expression of cholinesterase gene(s) in human brain tissues: translational evidence for multiple mRNA species. EMBO J 1984;3:1371–1375.

6 Soreq L, Gilboa-Geffen A, Berrih-Aknin S, Lacoste P, Darvasi A, Soreq E, Bergman H, Soreq H: Identifying alternative hyper-splicing signatures in MG-thymoma by exon arrays. PLoS ONE 2008;3:e2392.

7 Meshorer E, Bryk B, Toiber D, Cohen J, Podoly E, Dori A, Soreq H: SC35 promotes sustainable stress-induced alternative splicing of neuronal acetylcholinesterase mRNA. Mol Psychiatry 2005;10:985–997.

8 Meshorer E, Toiber D, Zurel D, Sahly I, Dori A, Cagnano E, Schreiber L, Grisaru D, Tronche F, Soreq H: Combinatorial complexity of 5′ alternative acetylcholinesterase transcripts and protein products. J Biol Chem 2004;279:29740–29751.

9 Toiber D, Berson A, Greenberg D, Melamed-Book N, Diamant S, Soreq H: N-Acetylcholinesterase-induced apoptosis in Alzheimer's disease. PLoS ONE 2008;3:e3108.

10 Toiber D, Greenberg DS, Soreq H: Pro-apoptotic protein-protein interactions of the extended N-AChE terminus. J Neural Transm 2009;116:1435–1442.

11 Shaked I, Soreq H: Studying cholinergic features by transgenic manipulations of AChE gene expression; in Giacobini E, Pepeu G (eds): The Brain Cholinergic System in Health and Disease. London, Informa Healthcare, 2006, pp 125–140.

12 Evron T, Geyer BC, Cherni I, Muralidharan M, Kilbourne J, Fletcher SP, Soreq H, Mor TS: Plant-derived human acetylcholinesterase-R provides protection from lethal organophosphate poisoning and its chronic aftermath. FASEB J 2007;21:2961–2969.

13 Park SE, Kim ND, Yoo YH: Acetylcholinesterase plays a pivotal role in apoptosome formation. Cancer Res 2004;64:2652–2655.

14 Zhang XJ, Yang L, Zhao Q, Caen JP, He HY, Jin QH, Guo LH, Alemany M, Zhang LY, Shi YF: Induction of acetylcholinesterase expression during apoptosis in various cell types. Cell Death Differ 2002;9:790–800.

15 Berson A, Knobloch M, Hanan M, Diamant S, Sharoni M, Schuppli D, Geyer BC, Ravid R, Mor TS, Nitsch RM, Soreq H: Changes in readthrough acetylcholinesterase expression modulate amyloid-beta pathology. Brain 2008;131:109–119.

16 Mor TS, Soreq H: Human cholinesterases from plants for detoxification; in Goodman RM (ed): Encyclopedia of Plant and Crop Science. New York, Marcel Dekker, 2004, pp 564–567.

17 Rees TM, Berson A, Sklan EH, Younkin L, Younkin S, Brimijoin S, Soreq H: Memory deficits correlating with acetylcholinesterase splice shift and amyloid burden in doubly transgenic mice. Curr Alzheimer Res 2005;2:291–300.

Neuro-degenerative Diseases

Neurodegenerative Dis 2010;7:64–67
DOI: 10.1159/000285508

Published online: February 18, 2010

Neuroprotective and Neurotoxic Phenotypes of Activated Microglia in Neonatal Mice with Respective MPTP- and Ethanol-Induced Brain Injury

Hirohide Sawada[a, b] Hiromi Suzuki[c] Toshiharu Nagatsu[b, c] Makoto Sawada[c]

[a]Department of Medical Technology, Kobe Tokiwa University, Kobe, [b]School of Medicine, Fujita Health University, Toyoake, and [c]Research Institute of Environmental Medicine, Nagoya University, Nagoya, Japan

Key Words
Microglia · Neonatal mice · Ethanol · 1-Methyl-4-phenyl-1,2,3,6-tetrahydropyridine

Abstract
Activated microglia play important roles in the inflammatory process and progression in Parkinson's disease. These cells produce various cytokines, nitric oxide, and neurotrophins, which are pleiotropic in their action, i.e., neuroprotective or neurotoxic. In an in vivo study on a mouse model with nigrostriatal lesions produced by the administration of 1-methyl-4-phenyl-1,2,3,6-tetrahydropyridine (MPTP), microglia activated by systemic lipopolysaccharide (LPS) were neurotoxic toward dopamine neurons in aged mice, but unexpectedly, neuroprotective in neonatal mice. In contrast to microglia in the MPTP model, LPS-activated microglia in neonatal mice in a model made by the stereotaxic injection of ethanol into the striatum were neurotoxic, and systemic LPS administration in the ethanol-injury model caused marked increases both in the volume of necrotic lesions and in the number of degenerative neurons in the striatum. Thus, activated microglia in the neonatal mouse brain play either a neuroprotective or neurotoxic role depending on the type of brain injury.

Introduction

Microglia play important roles in inflammatory processes in various neurodegenerative diseases including Parkinson's disease (PD). Activated microglia play either a neuroprotective or neurotoxic role by producing proinflammatory cytokines [e.g., tumor necrosis factor-α (TNF-α), interleukin-1β (IL-1β), nitric oxide (NO), reactive oxygen species (ROS)], or neurotrophic factors [e.g., nerve growth factor (NGF), brain-derived neurotrophic factor (BDNF), glial cell line-derived neurotrophic factor (GDNF)]. Sawada et al. [1] separated two subsets of microglia from mouse brain based on their capacity for intracellular ROS production stimulated by phorbol-12-myristate-13-acetate (PMA): one cell line was neurotoxic when cocultured with neurons and had a high capacity for ROS production, whereas the other cell line was neuroprotective and showed no ROS production. On the other hand, it is well known that neonatal microglia are very proliferative and easily activated under normal circumstances compared with adult microglia [2, 3]. Thus, a question arises as to whether or not activated neonatal microglia are different from those in adult or aged cells in terms of neuroprotective or neurotoxic phenotypes.

KARGER

Fax +41 61 306 12 34
E-Mail karger@karger.ch
www.karger.com

1660–2854/10/0073–0064$26.00/0

Accessible online at:
www.karger.com/ndd

Hirohide Sawada
Department of Medical Technology, Kobe Tokiwa University
2-6-2 Ohtani-cho, Nagata-ku
Kobe, Hyogo 653-0838 (Japan)
Tel. +81 78 611 1821, Fax +81 78 643 4361, E-Mail h-sawada@kobe-tokiwa.ac.jp

Table 1. Effects of LPS-induced activated microglia in mouse models with MPTP- or ethanol-induced neurodegeneration

Model	Toxin administration	Toxin + LPS administration
Neonatal mice (P7) treated with MPTP	Decreased DA neuron numbers in SN Decreased DA and DOPAC levels in midbrain Normal IL-1β and IL-6 levels in midbrain	Normal DA neuron numbers in SN Increased TH activity, DA and DOPAC levels in midbrain Increased IL-1β and IL-6 levels in midbrain
Neonatal mice (P7) treated with ethanol	Moderate decrease in number of striatal neurons in striatum	Severe decrease in number of striatal neurons in striatum
Aged mice (60 weeks) treated with MPTP	Moderate decrease in number of DA neurons in SN	Severe decrease in number of DA neurons in SN

SN = Substantia nigra; TH = tyrosine hydroxylase.

Neuroprotective Phenotype of Microglia Activated by Lipopolysaccharide in Neonatal Mice with MPTP-Induced Injury

Many reports on postmortem PD brains and PD animal models indicate that activated microglia have neurotoxic effects and may play a significant role in progression of the disease. Also aging is thought to be an important factor in idiopathic PD [4]. Aging may promote the toxic change from the protective to the toxic phenotype of activated microglia, as hypothesized by Sawada et al. [1]. This hypothesis of a toxic change in activated microglia had its origin in the in vitro experiments conducted by Vilhardt et al. [5]. Sawada et al. [6] showed in neonatal and aged mice different phenotypes of microglia activated by systemic lipopolysaccharide (LPS) treatment on dopamine (DA) neurons under 1-methyl-4-phenyl-1,2,3,6-tetrahydropyridine (MPTP)-induced injury (table 1). MPTP is a chemical that causes PD-like symptoms in humans and various animals. Although the number of DA neurons in the substantia nigra in aged mice treated with MPTP was significantly decreased, an increase in the number of LPS-activated microglia produced a further decrease in the number of these neurons. By contrast, neonatal (postnatal day 7) mice treated with MPTP showed that the initial decrease in the levels of DA neurons, tyrosine hydroxylase activity, DA, and the metabolite 3,4-dihydroxyphenylacetic acid in the midbrain changed to an increase, along with marked LPS-induced activation of microglia and increased levels of pro-inflammatory cytokines of IL-1β and IL-6. These results suggest that LPS-activated microglia in neonatal mice may have neurotrophic potential. Imai et al. [7] also showed the neuroprotective effects of exogenously administered microglia isolated from neonatal gerbils in an ischemic gerbil model; the exogenous microglia migrated to ischemic hippocampal regions in the host, and enhanced neuroprotection accompanied by the expression of neurotrophic factors BDNF and GDNF.

Neurotoxic Phenotype of Microglia Activated by LPS in Neonatal Mice with Local Ethanol Injury

Sawada et al. [manuscript in preparation] examined whether or not LPS-activated neonatal microglia also show the neuroprotective phenotype in an ethanol-induced brain injury model [8–10] produced by the stereotaxic injection of 100% ethanol (2 μl) into the mouse striatum. This local injection of ethanol produced more severe neuronal damage than seen in the MPTP-induced PD model. This ethanol-induced model produced brain injury without hemorrhage, infection or other unexpected effects that might affect the cytokine networks in the brain. After the ethanol-induced damage, activated microglia accumulated in the boundary area of the necrosis and eliminated damaged neurons by causing delayed neuronal death. A large lesion with a necrotic core was observed in the ethanol-injected striatum, and activated microglia had migrated to the outside of this necrotic mass, where Fluoro-Jade B (FJB)-positive degenerative neurons were observed. By previous treatment with systemic LPS or saline as a control, the volumes of necrotic and degenerative areas in the striatum were further increased along with an increase in the number of activated microglia (table 1). The number of inducible NO-synthesizing enzyme (iNOS)-positive microglia also tended to be increased by the LPS treatment, suggesting NO as a toxic agent. These results suggest that LPS-activated microglia in the neonatal mouse striatum play a neurotoxic role in the ethanol-induced brain injury.

The Mechanisms of Neuroprotective and Neurotoxic Phenotypes of Neonatal Microglia

The mechanisms responsible for the difference in the phenotypes of activated neonatal microglia between the MPTP- and ethanol-injury models remains to be further examined. Neonatal microglia are activated by macrophage colony-stimulating factor (MCSF) from late gestation to 2 weeks, and are very proliferative and easily activated under normal circumstances. As described above, LPS-activated microglia in the neonatal MPTP model showed a neuroprotective phenotype in the substantia nigra, but a neurotoxic phenotype was observed in neonatal mice that received ethanol-induced striatal damage. In the MPTP model, elevated levels of IL-1β and IL-6 in the midbrain were observed, which suggests that these pleiotropic cytokines produced by activated neonatal microglia may have neuroprotective consequences. As a hypothesis, LPS-activated microglia in the ethanol-injury mouse model might be only transiently neuroprotective, rapidly converting to the neurotoxic phenotype that secretes toxic molecules such as NO. Inoue [11] reviewed microglial activation by ATP and ADP released from injured neurons. At low concentrations of ATP, microglia release neurotrophic substances such as plasminogen, TNF-α, and IL-6. Stronger or longer stimulation with ATP induced iNOS synthesis in microglia with high concentrations of NO to cause neuronal death. Thus, a high concentration or long-time exposure to extracellular ATP may change the phenotype from protective to toxic.

Since ethanol itself has been shown to influence microglial activation [12–16], the influence of ethanol on microglial activation by local administration might be different depending on the dose, duration, and timing of exposure. Thus the combined effects of LPS with ethanol on microglial activation may also augment the neurotoxic phenotype. Chronic exposure to ethanol was reported to cause increased production of superoxide anion in cultured neonatal hamster microglia; a similar increase was not seen during acute ethanol exposure [13].

Although the limitations of the local ethanol-injury model should be carefully considered, this model has advantages for examining the protective or toxic mechanisms of activated microglia in a specific brain region at any age. Further studies on the molecules secreted from the LPS-activated microglia around the area injured by ethanol should provide valuable information on mechanisms of neurodegeneration.

Acknowledgements

This work was supported by grants from the Ministry of Health, Labor, and Welfare of Japan (M.S.), the Ministry of Education, Culture, Sports, Science, and Technology of Japan (M.S.), and the Japan Health Sciences Foundation (M.S.).

References

1 Sawada M, Imamura K, Nagatsu T: Role of cytokines in inflammatory process in Parkinson's disease. J Neural Transm 2006; 70(suppl):373–381.
2 Sawada M, Suzumura A, Yamamoto H, Marunouchi T: Activation and proliferation of the isolated microglia by colony stimulating factor-1 and possible involvement of protein kinase C. Brain Res 1990;509:119–124.
3 Thery C, Hetier E, Evrard C, Mallat M: Expression of macrophage colony-stimulating factor gene in the mouse brain during development. J Neurosci Res 1990;26:129–133.
4 Sawada M, Sawada H, Nagatsu T: Effects of aging on neuroprotective and neurotoxic properties of microglia in neurodegenerative diseases. Neurodegenerative Dis 2008;5: 254–256.
5 Vilhardt F, Plastre O, Sawada M, Suzuki K, Wiznerowicz M, Kiyokawa E, Trono D, Krause KH: The HIV-1 Nef protein and phagocyte NADPH oxidase activation. J Biol Chem 2002;277:42136–42143.
6 Sawada H, Hishida R, Hirata Y, Ono K, Suzuki H, Muramatsu S, Nakano I, Nagatsu T, Sawada M: Activated microglia affect the nigro-striatal dopamine neurons differently in neonatal and aged mice treated with 1-methyl-4-phenyl-1,2,3,6-tetrahydropyridine. J Neurosci Res 2007;85:1752–1761.

7 Imai F, Suzuki H, Oda J, Ninomiya T, Ono K, Sano H, Sawada M: Neuroprotective effects of exogenous microglia in global brain ischemia. J Cereb Blood Flow Metab 2007;27:488–500.
8 Takeuchi A, Isobe K, Miyaishi O, Sawada M, Fan ZH, Nakashima I, Kiuchi K: Microglial NO induces delayed neuronal death following acute injury in the striatum. Eur J Neurosci 1998;10:1613–1620.
9 Takeuchi A, Miyaishi O, Kiuchi K, Isobe K: Cu/Zn- and Mn-superoxide dismutases are specifically up-regulated in neurons after focal brain injury. J Neurobiol 2000;45:39–46.
10 Toyama H, Hatano K, Suzuki H, Ichise M, Momosaki M, Kudo G, Ito F, Kato T, Yamaguch H, Katada K, Sawada M, Ito K: In vivo imaging of microglial activation using a peripheral benzodiazepine receptor ligand: [11C]PK-11195 and animal PET following ethanol injury in rat striatum. Ann Nucl Med 2008;22:417–424.
11 Inoue K: Microglial activation by purines and pyrimidines. Glia 2002;40:156–163.
12 Qin L, He J, Hanes RN, Pluzarev O, Hong JS, Crews FT: Increased systemic and brain cytokine production and neuroinflammation by endotoxin following ethanol treatment. J Neuroinflammation 2008;5:10.
13 Colton CA, Snell-Callanan J, Chernyshev ON: Ethanol induced changes in superoxide anion and nitric oxide in cultured microglia. Alcohol Clin Exp Res 1998;22:710–716.
14 Aroor AR, Baker RC: Ethanol inhibition of phagocytosis and superoxide anion production by microglia. Alcohol 1998;15:277–280.
15 Lee H, Jeong J, Son E, Mosa A, Cho GJ, Choi WS, Ha JH, Kim IK, Lee MG, Kim CY, Suk K: Ethanol selectively modulates inflammatory activation signaling of brain microglia. J Neuroimmunol 2004;156:88–95.
16 Suk K: Microglial signal transduction as a target of alcohol action in the brain. Curr Neurovasc Res 2007;4:131–142.

Neuro-degenerative Diseases

Biology of Neurodegeneration

Neurodegenerative Dis 2010;7:68–75
DOI: 10.1159/000285509

Published online: February 18, 2010

LRRK2 and the Stress Response: Interaction with MKKs and JNK-Interacting Proteins

C.H. Hsu[a] D. Chan[a] B. Wolozin[a, b]

Departments of [a]Pharmacology and [b]Neurology, Boston University School of Medicine, Boston, Mass., USA

Key Words

MAP kinase · c-jun NH2-terminal kinase · Scaffold proteins · Parkinson's disease · Immunoprecipitation

Abstract

Increasing evidence supports a putative link between LRRK2 function and the MAP kinase cascades. We recently demonstrated that LRRK2 binds to MKK6, -3, and -7. Previous studies demonstrated that scaffold proteins are essential in the regulation of subcellular localization of stress kinase complexes. The c-jun NH2-terminal kinase (JNK)-interacting proteins (JIPs) are a group of scaffold proteins that play an important role in the regulation of MAP kinase signaling cascades. JIP1–3 are known to regulate the specificity and localization of the JNK pathway, while JIP4 is a specific scaffolding protein for the p38 pathway. We demonstrate that LRRK2 binds to JIP1–4, and is associated with increased levels of total JIP1, -3, -4, oligomeric JIP and ubiquitinated JIP. These results are consistent with a putative role of LRRK2 in regulating the stress kinase cascade.

Introduction

Mutations in leucine-rich repeat kinase 2 (LRRK2) are a common cause of autosomal-dominant Parkinson's disease (PD) and also occur among some sporadic cases of PD [1, 2]. The most prevalent mutation in European populations, G2019S, is associated with approximately 3% of sporadic PD and 30–40% of familial PD cases among Ashkenazi Jews and North African Arabs [3, 4]. Patients with LRRK2 mutation exhibit late disease onset with symptoms indistinguishable from idiopathic PD patients, and are also responsive to L-dopa treatment. The pathology associated with LRRK2 mutations is heterogeneous. Most cases of PD associated with mutations in LRRK2 display Lewy body pathology in the brainstem and substantia nigra – the most common pathological presentation of subjects with mutations in LRRK2 [5, 6]. A small number of cases present with tau-positive neurofibrillary tangle pathology or with no visible inclusion pathology [5, 6].

The biological function of LRRK2 remains unclear. Greatest homology is seen between LRRK2 and the receptor interacting kinase (RIP) family of proteins, which regulate responses to death receptors [7, 8]. In this context, it is notable that LRRK2 binds FADD, a death receptor-mediating protein [9]. LRRK2 is present in the cytoplasm but also associates with numerous membranous organelles, such as the mitochondria, endoplasmic reticulum, trans-Golgi, and plasma membrane [10]. LRRK2 contains several distinct functional domains. Three domains, COR, LRR and WD40, are protein-binding domains. Most attention has focused on the ROC and MKKK domains, which exhibit enzymatic activity. The ROC domain binds GTP and exhibits low

KARGER

Fax +41 61 306 12 34
E-Mail karger@karger.ch
www.karger.com

Accessible online at:
www.karger.com/ndd

Benjamin Wolozin
Departments of Pharmacology and Neurology, Boston University School of Medicine
72 East Concord St., R614
Boston, MA 02118-2526 (USA)
Tel. +1 617 414 2652, Fax +1 617 414 2651, E-Mail bwolozin@bu.edu

level GTPase activity [11, 12]. Studies of LRRK2 ROC protein, produced as recombinant protein, demonstrate that the ROC domain has the capacity to dimerize [13]. Studies of LRRK2 using transfected cells also suggest that the full-length protein also dimerizes [14–17]. The MKKK domain shares homology with mixed lineage kinases, which regulate stress kinase cascades [18]. Multiple studies demonstrate that LRRK2 can autophosphorylate, although the amount of activity generated is low [19–21]. The G2019S LRRK2 mutation increases autophosphorylation activity [19–23]. Many other disease-linked mutations also increase autophosphorylation, but the stimulation is less than for G2019S and does not occur with all disease-linked mutations. A number of putative targets of LRRK2 phosphorylation have been suggested, including E4-BP and moesin, but these results have yet to be confirmed by other groups [24, 25].

Increasing evidence supports a putative link between LRRK2 function and the MAP kinase (MAPK) cascades. LRRK2 was recently shown to phosphorylate MKK3, -4, -6 and -7 [26]. We recently demonstrated that LRRK2 binds to MKK6, -3, and -7, and activates the p38 and c-jun NH2-terminal kinase (JNK) pathway [27]. Association of LRRK2 with MKKs stimulates expression and membrane translocation of these proteins, but does not strongly increase their phosphorylation. Localization of kinases is often facilitated by binding to scaffold proteins, which tether the kinases to particular membrane organelles and bring the kinases together with their substrates. Previous studies demonstrated that scaffold proteins are essential in the regulation of subcellular localization of stress kinase complexes. The JNK-interacting proteins (JIPs) are a group of scaffold proteins that play an important role in the regulation of MAPK signaling cascades [28]. JIP1–3 are known to regulate the specificity and localization of JNK pathway, while JIP4 is a specific scaffolding protein for the p38 pathway [28–30]. Given these data, we hypothesize that the JIP proteins would be integral for the regulation of LRRK2.

Materials and Methods

Constructs

Wild-type (WT) and mutant LRRK2 V5-His tagged and 2xMyc constructs were generated as described in Greggio et al. [20, 21]. Flag-tagged pcDNA3 JIP1–4 plasmids were generous gifts from Dr. Roger Davis (University of Massachusetts).

Cell Culture

HEK293-FT cells were maintained in DEM/10% FBS. Transfections were performed using Lipofectamine 2000 (Invitrogen) as described previously [27, 31].

Coimmunoprecipitation

HEK293-FT cells were transfected with the appropriate constructs for 48 h, and coimmunoprecipitations were performed as described previously [27, 32]. Antibodies were purchased from Sigma (V5, Flag, c-myc, actin). Lysates and immunoprecipitates were loaded and resolved by 3–8% NuPAGE Tris-acetate (for studies of JIPs) or 4–20% Tris-glycine gels (for studies of MKK3) for Western blotting.

Subcellular Fractionation

HEK293-FT cells were transfected with the appropriate constructs for 48 h, and subcellular fractionation was performed as described in Hsu et al. [27] to separate the samples into cytosolic and membrane fractions. Antibody against calnexin (Calbiochem) was used as the membrane marker, and antibody against GAPDH (Biodesign) was used as the cytosolic marker. Lysates were loaded and resolved by 3–8% NuPAGE Tris-acetate (for studies of JIPs) or 4–20% Tris-glycine gels (for studies of calnexin and GAPDH) for Western blotting.

Statistical Analysis

All data were expressed as mean ± SEM and graphed using Prism (GraphPad). One-way ANOVA and Tukey's post-hoc tests were performed to identify statistically significant differences using InStat (GraphPad).

Results

LRRK2 Interacts with MKK3

We have recently shown that LRRK2 binds MKK3, -6 and -7. To confirm these results, we cotransfected HEK-FT 293 cells with WT LRRK2 ± MKK3, and immunoprecipitated the proteins. Figure 1 shows that MKK3 is readily detectable by immunoblot following LRRK2 immunoprecipitation.

LRRK2 Interacts with JIP1–4

The strong association between LRRK2 and MKKs led us to hypothesize that LRRK2 might also interact with the JIPs, and that JIPs might modulate the subcellular translocation of LRRK2 with MKK6. To test this hypothesis, we coexpressed V5His-tagged WT LRRK2 construct with Flag-tagged JIP1–4 constructs in HEK293-FT cells, and performed coimmunoprecipitations to determine whether LRRK2 interacts with the JIPs. Protein complexes containing JIP1–3 (fig. 2a) and JIP4 (fig. 2b) were readily evident upon coimmunoprecipitation of LRRK2 or JIPs. Coexpressing the different proteins also produced a number of additional affects. The expression of LRRK2

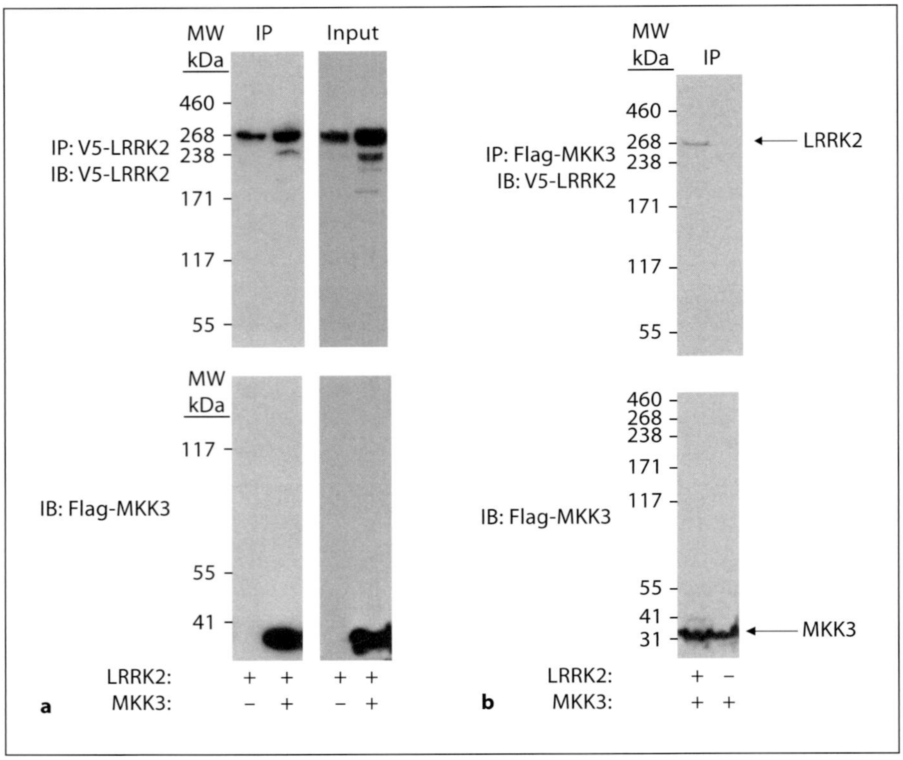

Fig. 1. LRRK2 binds to MKK3. **a** HEK 293 cells were transfected with V5-LRRK2 (WT) ± Flag-MKK3. After 24 h, the lysates were collected and V5-LRRK2 immunoprecipitated. The immunoprecipitates were immunoblotted with either anti-V5 antibody (upper panel, to detect LRRK2) or anti-Flag (lower panel, to detect MKK3). **b** HEK 293 cells were transfected with Flag-MKK3 ± LRRK2 (WT). After 24 h, the lysates were collected and Flag-tagged MKK3 immunoprecipitated. The immunoprecipitates were immunoblotted with either anti-V5 antibody (upper panel, to detect LRRK2) or anti-Flag (lower panel, to detect MKK3). Arrows point to LRRK2 and MKK3. Representative data from three independent experiments.

increase formation of high molecular weight bands in the JIP3 and -4 transfected cells (fig. 2). The appearance of high-molecular-weight bands suggests that LRRK2 might stimulate oligomerization of JIP3 and -4. Coexpressing JIP1–4 with LRRK2 also overall increased levels of JIP expression (fig. 2).

LRRK2 Increases Levels of JIPs

In related work, we showed that the coexpression of MKK6 with LRRK2 induces the expression and translocation of both proteins from the mitochondria to the plasma membrane and the ER, and that this translocation is dependent upon the functionality of MKK6 [27]. We hypothesize that JIPs may be integral components of the complex regulation of the translocation to the plasma membrane. To test this hypothesis, HEK293-FT cells were transfected with or without JIP1–4, and the lysates were fractionated into cytosolic and membrane fractions. The amounts of JIP1–4 were increased in the presence of LRRK2 in both the cytosolic and the membrane fractions (fig. 3). We did not observe that LRRK2 altered the distribution of the JIPs (fig. 3). These results indicate that expressing LRRK2 increases the steady state levels of JIP proteins, but does not alter the gross distribution of JIPs.

LRRK2 Increases JIP4 Ubiquitination

The ability of LRRK2 to increase levels of JIPs suggests the possibility that LRRK2 modulates degradation of JIPs. To investigate whether LRRK2 modulates the catabolism of JIPs, we investigated whether expressing LRRK2 affects ubiquitination of JIP4. LRRK2 was cotransfected with Flag-tagged JIP4 and HA-tagged ubiquitin. JIP4 was immunoprecipitated and probed with anti-HA antibody to determine whether JIP4 ubiquitination is modified by the presence of WT LRRK2 (fig. 4). Coexpressing LRRK2 strongly increased ubiquitination of JIP4 (fig. 4). Immunoblotting for JIP4 also suggested that oligomerization of JIP4 was increased in the presence of LRRK2, although we cannot rule out the possibility that detection of the higher molecular weight species simply reflected elevated levels of JIP4.

JIP4 Oligomerization Is Increased by Disease-Related Mutations in LRRK2

Our previous studies indicate that G2019S and R1441C mutations in LRRK2 exhibit increased binding with MKK6. This observation suggested the possibility that disease-related LRRK2 mutations also enhance binding to JIPs. To explore the effects of disease-related LRRK2 mu-

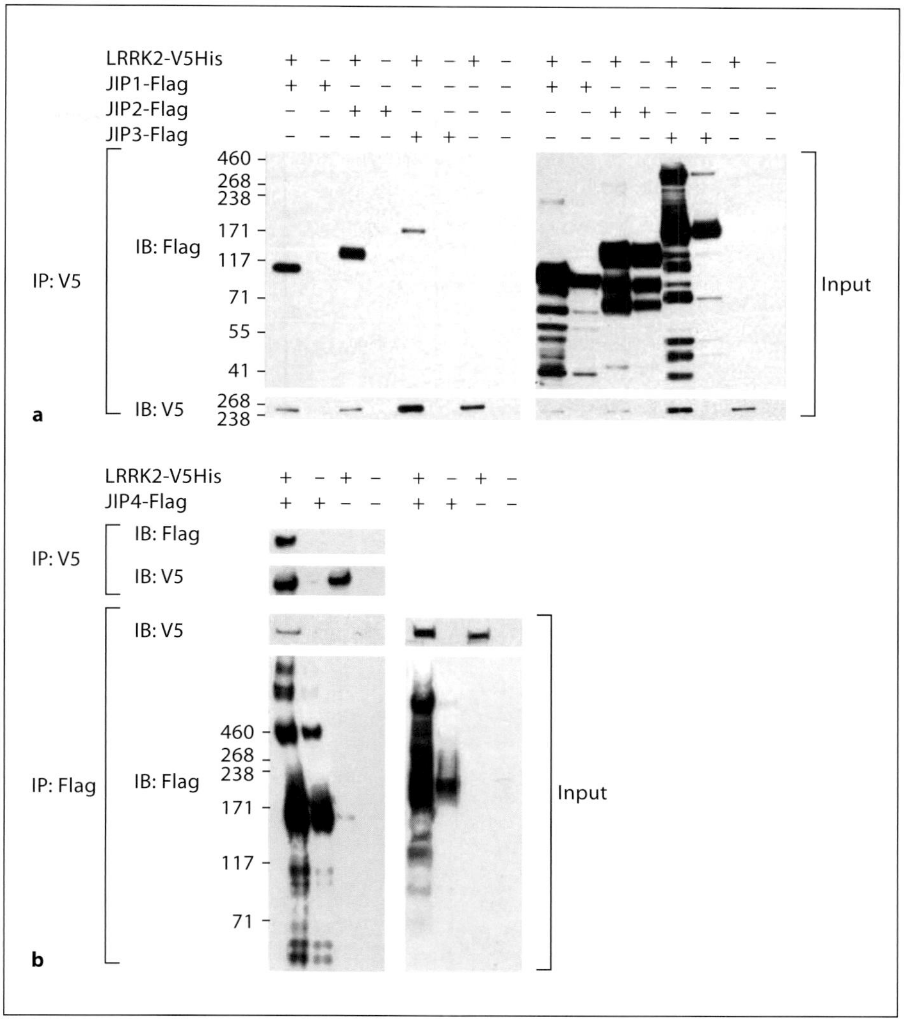

Fig. 2. LRRK2 binds to JIPs. **a** LRRK2 coimmunoprecipitates with JIP1–3. **b** LRRK2 coimmunoprecipitates with JIP4. HEK 293 cells were transfected with Flag-tagged JIP1–3 ± V5-LRRK2 (**a**) or Flag-tagged JIP4 ± V5-LRRK2, and the Flag-JIP complex was immunoprecipitated. Specific association of LRRK2 with each JIP is evident in the complexes shown in the immunoblot in the left panel. Representative data from three independent experiments.

tations on JIP biology, we cotransfected JIP4 with LRRK2 constructs containing mutations linked to disease: G2019S and R1441C, I2020T, Y1699C. The G2019S, R1441C and I2020T mutations were each associated with increased levels of JIP4 and increased levels of oligomerizated complex (fig. 5a). Densitometric quantification indicated that the amount of dimmer was increased for the mutant LRRK2 constructs (fig. 5b), but the apparent increase might also result from the overall increase in total JIP4 levels.

Discussion

Mutations in LRRK2 are among the most common genetic mutations associated with PD. The mechanism by which mutations might contribute to disease is largely unknown, and indeed, the general biology of LRRK2 is poorly understood. In this paper, we set out to understand one aspect of LRRK2 biology evident from its structure. The kinase domain of LRRK2 is homologous to RIP kinases and mixed lineage kinases, which are classes of kinases known to regulate the stress kinase cascades in part through binding to MKKs. We have now shown that LRRK2 also binds to MKKs. We also demonstrate that LRRK2 interacts with a family of scaffold proteins, termed JIPs, which regulate the stress kinase cascades. Cotransfecting LRRK2 increases JIP expression levels, and interaction of LRRK2 with the JIPs might promote their oligomerization, which is thought to be associated with MAPK activation [28]. Most but not all disease-related mutations in LRRK2 that we studied exhibited high-molecular-weight bands indicative of oligomeriza-

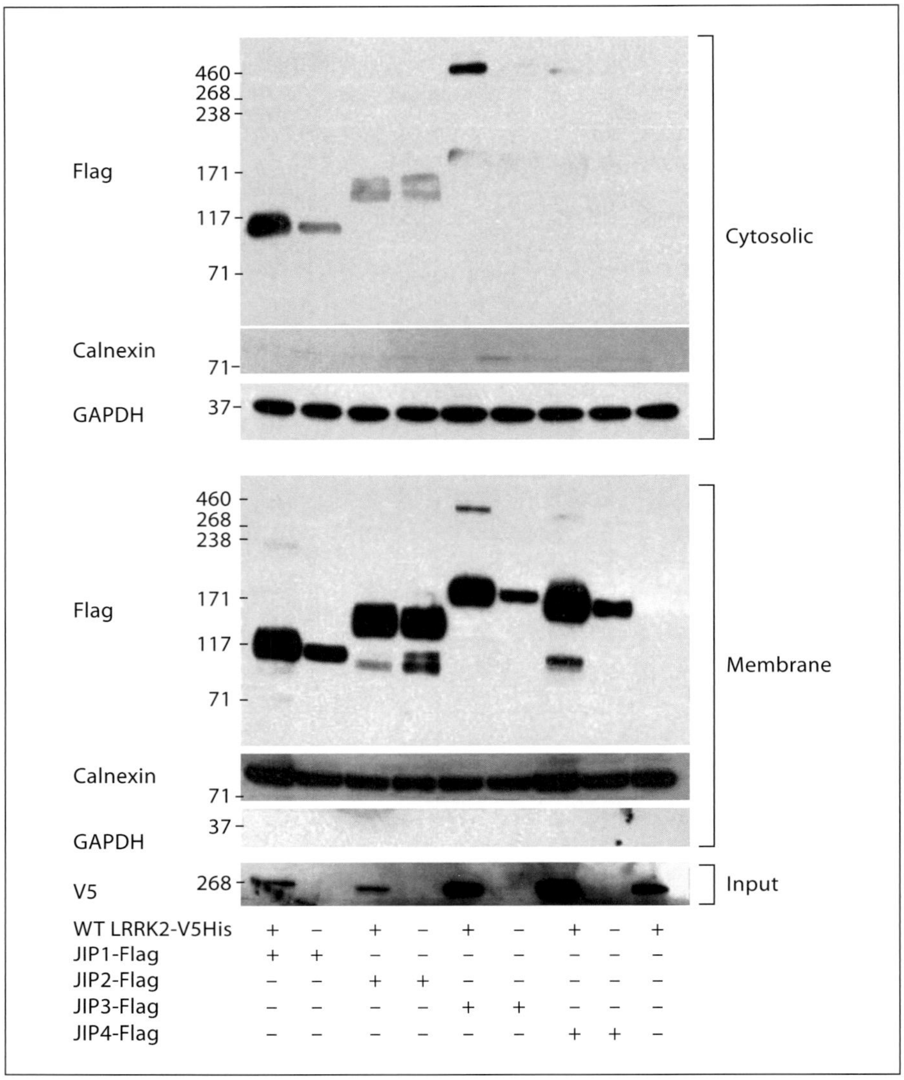

Fig. 3. LRRK2 increases JIP levels but does not induce translocation. HEK 293 cells were transfected with Flag-tagged JIP1–3 ± V5-LRRK2 or Flag-tagged JIP4 ± V5-LRRK2. The resulting lysates were separated into cytoplasmic (upper panel) or membrane (lower panel) components. Cotransfecting LRRK2 increased JIP levels in both the cytoplasmic and membrane fractions equally. Representative data from three independent experiments.

tion. Interestingly, cotransfecting LRRK2 with JIP4, and possibly other JIPs, also increases levels of ubiquitinated JIP4, although the significance of this change is unclear.

Our observation that LRRK2 associates with MKKs and with JIPs is consistent with an increasing body of evidence suggesting that LRRK2 regulates the stress kinase cascade. Studies in *Caenorhabditis elegans* demonstrate that LRRK2 regulates the response to mitochondrial stress (complex I inhibition), and that the response requires the activity of the nematode homologues of MKK6 and p38 [27, 33]. LRRK2 is known to autophosphorylate, although the amount of autophosphorylation is very low. Gloeckner et al. [26] recently demonstrated that LRRK2 can transphosphorylate MKK 3–7 in vitro. The reaction does not appear to be catalytic, though, because levels of MKK phosphorylation were similar to levels of LRRK2 autophosphorylation, despite addition of more than a 10,000-fold excess of MKK. Phosphorylation of MKK by LRRK2 occurs in the amino-domain, which is far from the sites normally associated with MKK activation [26]. The low level of phosphorylation is consistent with a model in which LRRK2 binds the MKKs, phosphorylates the proteins, but then either does not release the MKK or becomes catalytically inactive. Studies from our laboratory demonstrate that LRRK2 binds to MKKs, but interestingly, we find evidence for phosphorylation of MKKs by LRRK2 in vitro, but not in vivo [27]. Our results suggest that binding of LRRK2 to MKK2 increases the

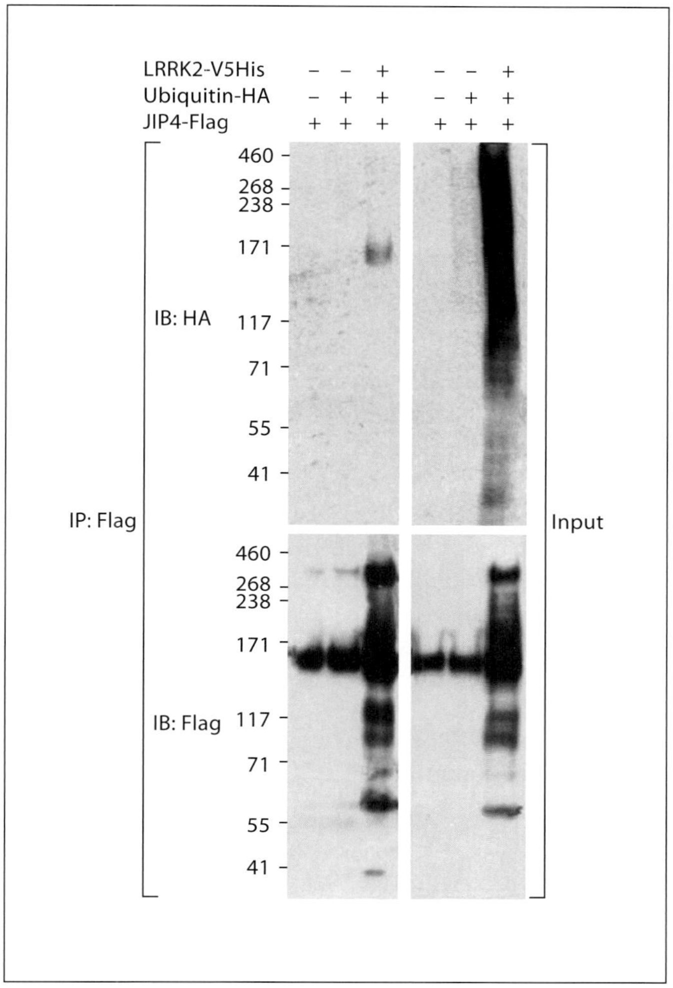

Fig. 4. LRRK2 increases JIP ubiquitination. HEK 293 cells were transfected with Flag-tagged JIP1–3, V5-LRRK2 ± HA ubiquitin. The lysates were subjected to immunoprecipitation with anti-Flag antibody, and probed with antibodies to V5 (for LRRK2), HA (for ubiquitin) or Flag (for JIP4). Cotransfection increased oligomerization of JIP4, and resulted in immunoprecipitation (IP) of ubiquitinated JIP4. Representative data from three independent experiments.

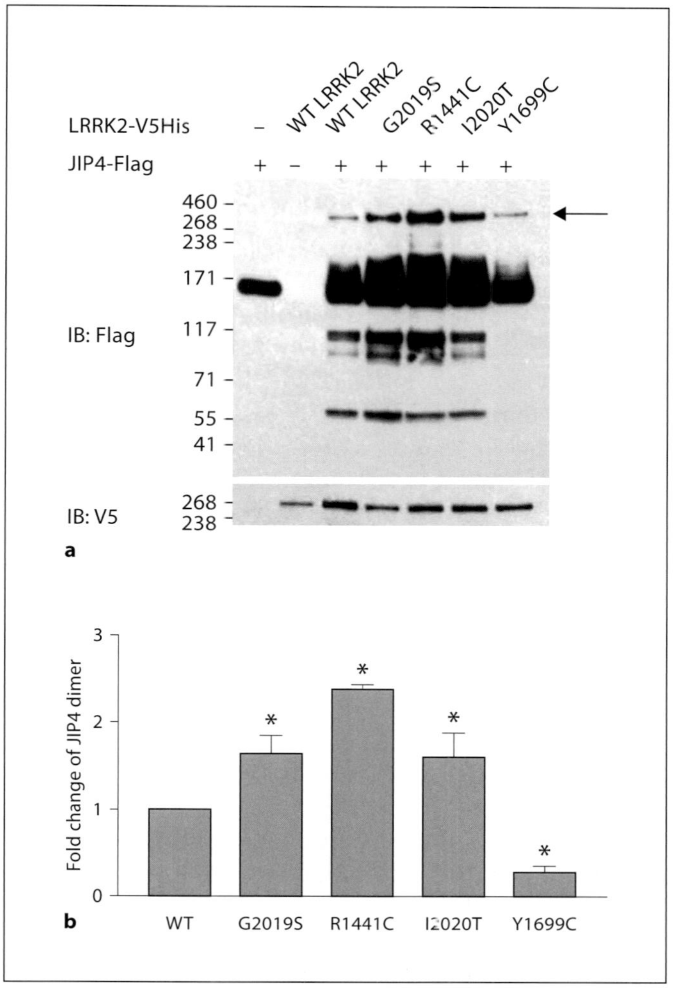

Fig. 5. Disease-linked mutations in LRRK2 increase JIP oligomerization. HEK 293 cells were transfected with Flag-tagged JIP1–3, V5-LRRK2 (WT, G2019S, R1441C, I2020T or Y1699C) ± HA ubiquitin. JIP4 was immunoprecipitated (**a**) and the amount of oligomeric JIP4 quantified (**b**). **a** The arrow points to the oligomer bands used for quantification, and quantification was relative to total JIP4 levels. **b** * $p < 0.05$ (n = 3).

expression and membrane localization of both proteins, as shown by immunocytochemistry and biochemical fractionation.

The interaction of LRRK2 with JIPs is consistent with the observed interaction between LRRK2 and MKKs [27]. JIPs are scaffold proteins for the stress kinase cascade [28]. The ability of LRRK2 to bind JIPs in absence of cotransfected MKKs suggests that LRRK2 binds JIPs directly, or at least through a mechanism that does not require MKKs. Thus, the JIP scaffolding complex appears to contain binding sites for both LRRK2 and MKKs. JIPs function to bring together MKKs with MAPKs (e.g. JNK and p38), and also to direct binding to different sites within the cells. Some JIPs tend to direct binding towards the membrane, such as JIP4, while JIP1–3 are known to bind to microtubules. The interaction of LRRK2 with JIP1–3 suggests that LRRK2 might bind to JIP1–3 as a cargo protein, and that binding might facilitate transport along microtubules. Such transport might be particularly important in neurons where LRRK2 can be found in synaptic fields, such as in the striatum. Other proteins linked to disease also appear to interact with JIPs. α-Synuclein was recently shown to regulate levels of JIP1 [34]. Amyloid precursor protein binds to JIP1 in much the same manner, although the biology of the interaction remains unclear [35].

LRRK2 exhibits a striking ability to increase total levels of JIPs and ubiquitination of JIPs. These two effects in combination suggest that LRRK2 inhibits degradation of JIPs, either through the proteasomal or autophagic systems. Alternatively, LRRK2 might also act to increase JIP translation or transcription. A link between LRRK2 and regulation of protein translation is suggested by the observation that LRRK2 binds and phosphorylates 4E-BP, a regulator of protein translation machinery [24]. A putative role in regulating protein degradation is consistent with the presence of ubiquitin-positive inclusions in most cases of PD that are associated with LRRK2 mutations [5]. Most of these inclusions contain α-synuclein, but some inclusions contain tau protein [5, 36]. The putative ability of LRRK2 to inhibit autophagy or proteasomal function could contribute to increased risk of PD and inclusion formation among subjects with LRRK2 mutations. Several reports also note that LRRK2 overexpression leads to the formation of inclusions containing LRRK2 [20, 37]. Other reports indicate that LRRK2 regulates autophagy [38]. Inhibition of autophagy or proteasomal function could induce inclusion, stimulate inclusion formation as well as increase levels of JIP and JIP oligomers. Further experiments are needed to determine the precise mechanism.

In summary, our data suggest that a strong biological connection exists between LRRK2, the stress kinase cascade and JIPs, a class of scaffold proteins that bind stress kinases. The role of stress kinases in cell death creates a cogent linkage between LRRK2 and cell death. Whether this pathway is the actual pathway linked to the pathophysiology of disease among subjects carrying mutations in LRRK2 remains to be determined. Most of the mutant LRRK2 constructs increased JIP4 levels and oligomerization more than WT with the exception of Y1699C. The incomplete correlation between pathological LRRK2 mutations and enhanced JIP expression/oligomerization suggests that this axis is not the principle mechanism by which LRRK2 causes disease. However, understanding the mechanisms by which LRRK2 modulates the stress kinase cascade could lead to increased understanding of the biology of LRRK2 and potential differences in the pathophysiology of disease among individuals with different LRRK2 mutations.

Acknowledgements

We thank Roger Davis for his generosity in sharing the JIP plasmids. This work was supported by grant awards to B.W. from the Alzheimer Association, the Michael J. Fox Foundation, NIEHS ES15567, and NINDS NS060872.

References

1 Biskup S, Gerlach M, Kupsch A, Reichmann H, Riederer P, Vieregge P, Wullner U, Gasser T: Genes associated with Parkinson syndrome. J Neurol 2008;255(suppl 5):8–17.

2 Taylor JP, Mata IF, Farrer MJ: LRRK2: a common pathway for parkinsonism, pathogenesis and prevention? Trends Mol Med 2006; 12:76–82.

3 Ozelius LJ, Senthil G, Saunders-Pullman R, Ohmann E, Deligtisch A, Tagliati M, Hunt AL, Klein C, Henick B, Hailpern SM, Lipton RB, Soto-Valencia J, Risch N, Bressman SB: LRRK2 G2019S as a cause of Parkinson's disease in Ashkenazi Jews. N Engl J Med 2006; 354:424–425.

4 Lesage S, Durr A, Tazir M, Lohmann E, Leutenegger AL, Janin S, Pollak P, Brice A: LRRK2 G2019S as a cause of Parkinson's disease in North African Arabs. N Engl J Med 2006;354:422–423.

5 Zimprich A, Biskup S, Leitner P, Lichtner P, Farrer M, Lincoln S, Kachergus J, Hulihan M, Uitti RJ, Calne DB, Stoessl AJ, Pfeiffer RF, Patenge N, Carbajal IC, Vieregge P, Asmus F, Muller-Myhsok B, Dickson DW, Meitinger T, Strom TM, Wszolek ZK, Gasser T: Mutations in LRRK2 cause autosomal-dominant parkinsonism with pleomorphic pathology. Neuron 2004;44:601–607.

6 Paisan-Ruiz C, Jain S, Evans EW, Gilks WP, Simon J, van der Brug M, Lopez de Munain A, Aparicio S, Gil AM, Khan N, Johnson J, Martinez JR, Nicholl D, Carrera IM, Pena AS, de Silva R, Lees A, Marti-Masso JF, Perez-Tur J, Wood NW, Singleton AB: Cloning of the gene containing mutations that cause PARK8-linked Parkinson's disease. Neuron 2004;44:595–600.

7 Festjens N, Vanden Berghe T, Cornelis S, Vandenabeele P: RIP1, a kinase on the crossroads of a cell's decision to live or die. Cell Death Differ 2007;14:400–410.

8 Meylan E, Tschopp J: The RIP kinases: crucial integrators of cellular stress. Trends Biochem Sci 2005;30:151–159.

9 Ho CC, Rideout HJ, Ribe E, Troy CM, Dauer WT: The Parkinson disease protein leucine-rich repeat kinase 2 transduces death signals via Fas-associated protein with death domain and caspase-8 in a cellular model of neurodegeneration. J Neurosci 2009;29:1011–1016.

10 Biskup S, Moore DJ, Celsi F, Higashi S, West AB, Andrabi SA, Kurkinen K, Yu SW, Savitt JM, Waldvogel HJ, Faull RL, Emson PC, Torp R, Ottersen OP, Dawson TM, Dawson VL: Localization of LRRK2 to membranous and vesicular structures in mammalian brain. Ann Neurol 2006;60:557–569.

11 West AB, Moore DJ, Choi C, Andrabi SA, Li X, Dikeman D, Biskup S, Zhang Z, Lim KL, Dawson VL, Dawson TM: Parkinson's disease-associated mutations in LRRK2 link enhanced GTP-binding and kinase activities to neuronal toxicity. Hum Mol Genet 2007;16:223–232.

12 Lewis PA, Greggio E, Beilina A, Jain S, Baker A, Cookson MR: The R1441C mutation of LRRK2 disrupts GTP hydrolysis. Biochem Biophys Res Commun 2007;357:668–671.
13 Deng J, Lewis PA, Greggio E, Sluch E, Beilina A, Cookson MR: Structure of the ROC domain from the Parkinson's disease-associated leucine-rich repeat kinase 2 reveals a dimeric GTPase. Proc Natl Acad Sci USA 2008;105:1499–1504.
14 Greggio E, Zambrano I, Kaganovich A, Beilina A, Taymans JM, Daniels V, Lewis P, Jain S, Ding J, Syed A, Thomas KJ, Baekelandt V, Cookson MR: The Parkinson disease-associated leucine-rich repeat kinase 2 (LRRK2) is a dimer that undergoes intramolecular autophosphorylation. J Biol Chem 2008;283: 16906–16914.
15 Klein CL, Rovelli G, Springer W, Schall C, Gasser T, Kahle PJ: Homo- and heterodimerization of ROCO kinases: LRRK2 kinase inhibition by the LRRK2 ROCO fragment. J Neurochem 2009;111:703–715.
16 Sen S, Webber PJ, West AB: Dependence of leucine-rich repeat kinase 2 (LRRK2) kinase activity on dimerization. J Biol Chem 2009; 284:36346–36356.
17 Gotthardt K, Weyand M, Kortholt A, Van Haastert PJ, Wittinghofer A: Structure of the Roc-COR domain tandem of *C. tepidum*, a prokaryotic homologue of the human LRRK2 Parkinson kinase. EMBO J 2008;27: 2239–2249.
18 Wang LH, Besirli CG, Johnson EM Jr: Mixed-lineage kinases: a target for the prevention of neurodegeneration. Annu Rev Pharmacol Toxicol 2004;44:451–474.
19 West AB, Moore DJ, Biskup S, Bugayenko A, Smith WW, Ross CA, Dawson VL, Dawson TM: Parkinson's disease-associated mutations in leucine-rich repeat kinase 2 augment kinase activity. Proc Natl Acad Sci USA 2005;102:16842–16847.
20 Greggio E, Jain S, Kingsbury A, Bandopadhyay R, Lewis P, Kaganovich A, van der Brug MP, Beilina A, Blackinton J, Thomas KJ, Ahmad R, Miller DW, Kesavapany S, Singleton A, Lees A, Harvey RJ, Harvey K, Cookson MR: Kinase activity is required for the toxic effects of mutant LRRK2/dardarin. Neurobiol Dis 2006;23:329–341.
21 Greggio E, Lewis PA, van der Brug MP, Ahmad R, Kaganovich A, Ding J, Beilina A, Baker AK, Cookson MR: Mutations in LRRK2/dardarin associated with Parkinson disease are more toxic than equivalent mutations in the homologous kinase LRRK1. J Neurochem 2007;102:93–102.
22 Biskup S, West AB: Zeroing in on LRRK2-linked pathogenic mechanisms in Parkinson's disease. Biochim Biophys Acta 2009; 1792:625–633.
23 Greggio E, Cookson MR: Leucine-rich repeat kinase 2 mutations and Parkinson's disease: three questions. ASN Neuro 2009;1: e00002.
24 Imai Y, Gehrke S, Wang HQ, Takahashi R, Hasegawa K, Oota E, Lu B: Phosphorylation of 4E-BP by LRRK2 affects the maintenance of dopaminergic neurons in Drosophila. EMBO J 2008;27:2432–2443.
25 Jaleel M, Nichols RJ, Deak M, Campbell DG, Gillardon F, Knebel A, Alessi DR: LRRK2 phosphorylates moesin at threonine-558: characterization of how Parkinson's disease mutants affect kinase activity. Biochem J 2007;405:307–317.
26 Gloeckner CJ, Schumacher A, Boldt K, Ueffing M: The Parkinson disease-associated protein kinase LRRK2 exhibits MAPKKK activity and phosphorylates MKK3/6 and MKK4/7, in vitro. J Neurochem 2009;109: 959–968.
27 Hsu CH, Chan D, Greggio E, Guillily MD, Segal L, Saha S, Cookson MR, Wolozin B: Association of Parkinson's disease-related protein LRRK2 with MKK6 stimulates their mutual membrane translocation. J Neurochem 2010; Jan 7, Epub ahead of print.
28 Whitmarsh AJ: The JIP family of MAPK scaffold proteins. Biochem Soc Trans 2006; 34:828–832.
29 Kelkar N, Standen CL, Davis RJ: Role of the JIP4 scaffold protein in the regulation of mitogen-activated protein kinase signaling pathways. Mol Cell Biol 2005;25:2733–2743.
30 Verhey KJ, Meyer D, Deehan R, Blenis J, Schnapp BJ, Rapoport TA, Margolis B: Cargo of kinesin identified as JIP scaffolding proteins and associated signaling molecules. J Cell Biol 2001;152 959–970.
31 Zerbinatti CV, Cordy JM, Chen CD, Guillily M, Suon S, Ray WJ, Seabrook GR, Abraham CR, Wolozin B: Oxysterol-binding protein-1 (OSBP1) modulates processing and trafficking of the amyloid precursor protein. Mol Neurodegener 2008;3:5.
32 Ostrerova N, Petrucelli L, Farrer M, Mehta N, Alexander P, Choi P, Palacino J, Hardy J, Wolozin B: α-Synuclein shares physical and functional homology with 14-3-3 proteins. J Neurosci 1999;19:5782–5791.
33 Saha S, Guillily MD, Ferree A, Lanceta J, Chan D, Ghosh J, Hsu CH, Segal L, Raghavan K, Matsumoto K, Hisamoto N, Kuwahara T, Iwatsubo T, Moore L, Goldstein L, Cookson M, Wolozin B: LRRK2 modulates vulnerability to mitochondrial dysfunction in *Caenorhabditis elegans*. J Neurosci 2009;29: 9210–9218.
34 Hashimoto M, Hsu LJ, Rockenstein E, Takenouchi T, Mallory M, Masliah E: alpha-Synuclein protects against oxidative stress via inactivation of the c-Jun N-terminal kinase stress-signaling pathway in neuronal cells. J Biol Chem 2002;277:11465–11472.
35 Scheinfeld MH, Ghersi E, Davies P, D'Adamio L: Amyloid beta protein precursor is phosphorylated by JNK-1 independent of, yet facilitated by, JNK-interacting protein (JIP)-1. J Biol Chem 2003;278:42058–42063.
36 Rajput A, Dickson DW, Robinson CA, Ross OA, Dachsel JC, Lincoln SJ, Cobb SA, Rajput ML, Farrer MJ: Parkinsonism, Lrrk2 G2019S, and tau neuropathology. Neurology 2006;67: 1506–1508.
37 Smith WW, Pei Z, Jiang H, Moore DJ, Liang Y, West AB, Dawson VL, Dawson TM, Ross CA: Leucine-rich repeat kinase 2 (LRRK2) interacts with parkin and mutant LRRK2 induces neuronal degeneration. Proc Natl Acad Sci USA 2005;102:18676–18681.
38 Plowey ED, Cherra SJ 3rd, Liu YJ, Chu CT: Role of autophagy in G2019S-LRRK2-associated neurite shortening in differentiated SH-SY5Y cells. J Neurochem 2008;105:1048–1056.

Biology of Neurodegeneration

Neuro-degenerative Diseases

Neurodegenerative Dis 2010;7:76–79
DOI: 10.1159/000285510

Published online: February 18, 2010

Misframed Proteins and Neurodegeneration: A Novel View on Alzheimer's and Parkinson's Diseases

F.J.A. Dennissen N. Kholod H.W.M. Steinbusch F.W. Van Leeuwen

Department of Neuroscience, Faculty of Health, Medicine and Life Sciences, Maastricht University, Maastricht, The Netherlands

Key Words

Ubiquitin · Amyloid precursor protein · Ubiquitin-proteasome system · Protein quality control · Molecular misreading

Abstract

Sporadic forms of Alzheimer's and Parkinson's diseases are the most frequent forms of their kind. Together with Huntington's disease, they belong to the so called 'conformational diseases' as they share a common feature in the accumulation of insoluble protein deposits. In this review, we focus on the significance of the ubiquitin-proteasome system in conformational diseases and the possible consequences due to the accumulation of aberrant proteins. In all forms of Alzheimer's and Huntington's diseases, but not in Parkinson's disease, we have shown the presence of misframed proteins such as misframed ubiquitin (UBB^{+1}) of which we have determined the functional relevance in vitro and in vivo. Misframed proteins are the result of the inaccurate transcription of monotonic sequences in the genome and their subsequent translation. This process has been called 'molecular misreading'. In the present review, we will discuss the present state of the art with regard to UBB^{+1} and amyloid precursor protein APP^{+1}.

Introduction

For the majority of Alzheimer's disease (AD) and Parkinson's disease (PD) cases (i.e. the sporadic forms), no suitable explanations are available. For AD, the amyloid cascade hypothesis has received the most attention, but it appears that other hypotheses are necessary to explain a multifactorial disease such as AD; especially as it has turned out that immunization against Aβ42 resulted in the disappearance of Aβ plaques without relieving cognitive functions [1, 2]. Therefore, attention is focused now on other functions of the amyloid precursor protein (APP) in other parts of the molecule as well [3]. A decade ago, we reported on the occurrence of molecular misreading in APP and ubiquitin B (UBB) and found the resulting misframed APP^{+1} and misframed UBB^{+1} to accumulate in the hallmarks of AD, suggesting a function.

Molecular Misreading

Molecular misreading is the result of a dinucleotide deletion (e.g. ΔGA, ΔGU) in simple monotonic base sequences at the RNA level resulting in '+1 proteins' (e.g. UBB^{+1} and APP^{+1} [4]). The mechanism of molecular misreading is unknown, but it has been suggested that the RNA polymerase may stutter or show slippage on homopolymeric runs in the DNA template [5].

KARGER

Fax +41 61 306 12 34
E-Mail karger@karger.ch
www.karger.com

1660–2854/10/0073–0076$26.00/0

Accessible online at:
www.karger.com/ndd

F.W. Van Leeuwen
Department of Neuroscience
Universiteitsingel 50
NL–6229 ER Maastricht (The Netherlands)
Tel. +31 43 3881044, Fax +31 43 3671096, E-Mail f.vanleeuwen@np.unimaas.nl

Misframed Ubiquitin B

UBB^{+1} accumulates in the hallmarks of all forms of tauopathies and polyglutamine diseases but not in synucleinopathies [6] (fig. 1), suggesting that –1 proteins may be involved in these neurodegenerative diseases.

Ubiquitin is tagged to a degron within a target protein with its C-terminal glycine via multiple enzymatic steps (E1, E2, E3, and E4) [7] (fig. 2, left panel). The resulting polyubiquitin chains are an efficient trigger for subsequent 26S proteasomal degradation. UBB^{+1} lacks the C-terminal glycine residue and has 20 amino acids added to its C-terminus instead. Consequently, UBB^{+1} cannot ubiquitinate, is ubiquitinated, inhibits the ubiquitin proteasome system (UPS) dose dependently and impairs mitochondrial trafficking [8, 9]. Moreover, polyubiquitinated UBB^{+1} is refractory to deubiquitination. UBB^{+1} has been claimed to be the first naturally occurring identified

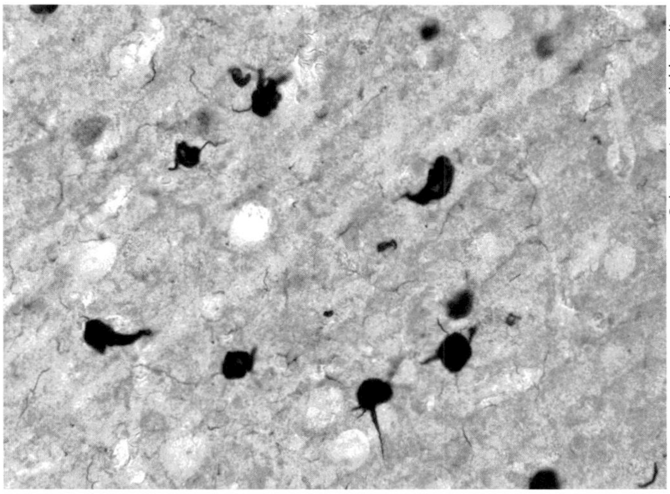

Fig. 1. UBB^{+1} staining in 50-μm Vibratome in the temporal cortex (layers 2 and 5) of a 92-year-old patient suffering from AD; intense immunoreactivity can be seen in neurofibrillary tangles.

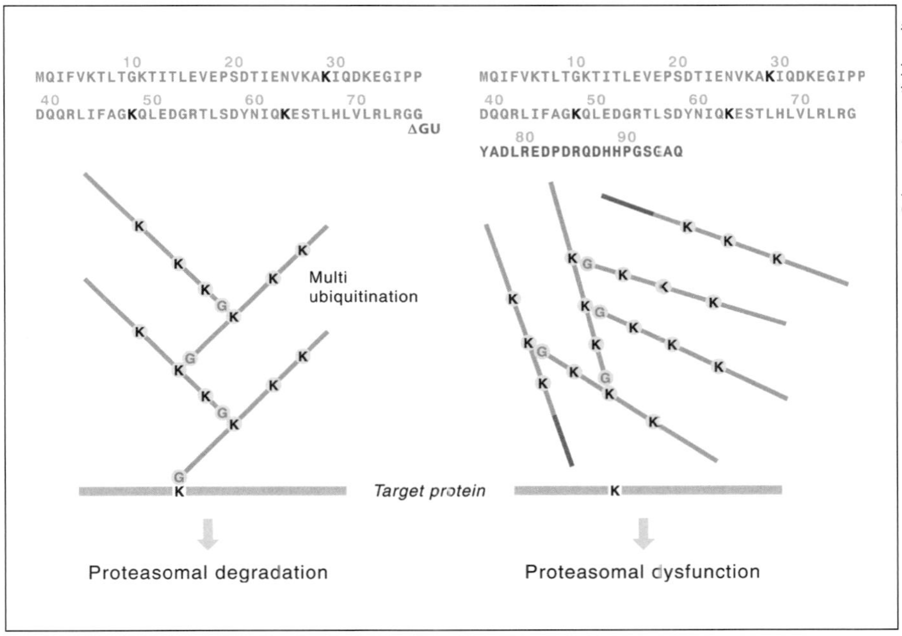

Fig. 2. Multiubiquitination of proteasome substrates. Simplified and schematic representation of how ubiquitin acts via multiubiquitination through a number of enzymatic steps (E_1, E_2 and E_3; left panel; for details see [7]). The lysine moieties (K) at positions 29, 48 and 63 are involved in the multiubiquitination and degradation. At the C-terminus of UBB, a GAGAG motif is present. It was shown that adjacent to this motif a dinucleotide deletion (ΔGU) occurs, resulting in an extension of 20 amino acids (right panel). Due to the dinucleotide deletion, the G_{76} moiety at the C-terminus, essential for binding to a target protein, is not synthetized. Consequently, this molecule cannot ubiquitinate. In fact, UBB^{+1} is the first naturally occurring identified UFD substrate [10]. Of much interest is that it was recently suggested that E3 enzymes form a 'forked' polyubiquitin chain in which two ubiquitin chains are linked to adjacent lysines on a preceding ubiquitin moiety (e.g. K29, K48) and K63 [13]. The forked polyubiquitin chains appeared to be relatively resistant to disassembly or degradation by the 26S proteasomes [15]. It is thus possible that ubiquitinated UBB^{+1} is an inhibitor of the proteasome [6].

ubiquitin fusion degradation (UFD) substrate [10]. Very recently, it was shown that the TRIP12-HECT domain can act as the E3 enzyme for the UFD pathway [11]. Evidence was also presented that the UBB^{+1} extension is just a few amino acids too short to be efficiently degraded by the proteasome. A possible mechanism how UBB^{+1} may cause proteasomal dysfunction is shown in figure 2, right panel [12–15].

Furthermore, in HD we showed in vitro that UBB^{+1} is an aggravating factor in polyglutamine-induced neurodegeneration [16]. The UPS in younger human controls (<53 years, [17]) is apparently able to degrade this problematic substrate. However, the suboptimal functioning UPS in elderly people and AD patients causes accumulation of UBB^{+1}. Therefore, the presence of UBB^{+1} can be regarded as a reporter for proteasomal dysfunction [6].

In order to study the effect of UBB^{+1} in vivo, we generated transgenic mouse lines expressing UBB^{+1} in neurons of the cortex, striatum and hippocampus. These mice showed moderate proteasomal inhibition, proteomic changes and a behavioral phenotype (impaired contextual memory) [18]. To determine whether the impaired contextual memory of the UBB^{+1} transgenic mice is reflected as reduced synaptic plasticity, we currently measure long-term potentiation in both the CA1 region and the dentate gyrus of the hippocampus. As AD is a multifactorial disease, we have crossed line 3413 with a model for AD ($APP_{Swe}/PSEN1\Delta_{exon9}$). Currently, we are studying the effect of UBB^{+1} on Aβ load during aging in the triple-transgenic line ($UBB^{+1}/APP_{Swe}/PSEN1\Delta_{exon9}$).

Misframed amyloid precursor protein ΔGA deletions in GAGAG motifs in APP in the N-terminal growth-promoting domain (exons 9 and 10, RERMS motif, 328–332, [19]) give rise to APP^{+1}(329–348). APP^{+1} accumulates in the neurofibrillary tangles and neuropil threads of AD and Down syndrome patients [4]. In cerebrospinal fluid, APP^{+1} correlated negatively with increasing Braak stages [20]. This means that APP^{+1} is an additional biomarker for the early diagnosis of AD. In vitro and in vivo studies showed that APP^{+1} was readily released and that it promotes the synthesis of Aβ40 [21, 22]. This negative correlation may be explained by the accumulation of UBB^{+1}, reducing the axonal flow [8] in patients older than 53 years. Interestingly, we observed beaded APP^{+1} fibers in all human postmortem brain hippocampi and cortices [17, 21]. This fact was not really appreciated until recently when the N-terminus of APP (1–286) was found to bind DR6 to trigger axon pruning [3].

Acknowledgements

The authors are greatly indebted to the International Foundation of Alzheimer's disease (04507/04830/06502), the Jan Dekker en Ludgardine Bouwman Stichting (04-22), the Matty Brand Stichting, Hersenstichting Nederland (15F07(2).48 and 2008(1).17), Van Leersum Foundation KNAW (2008), the Society Progressive Supranuclear Palsy (440-4) and the International Parkinson Foundation (2008).

References

1 Holmes C, Boche D, Wilkinson D, Yadegarfar G, Hopkins V, Bayer A, Jones RW, Bullock R, Love S, Neal JW, Zotova E, Nicoll JA: Long-term effects of Abeta42 immunisation in Alzheimer's disease: follow-up of a randomised, placebo-controlled phase I trial. Lancet 2008;372:216–223.

2 Schnabel J: Alzheimer's theory makes a splash. Nature 2009;459:310.

3 Nikolaev A, McLaughlin T, O'Leary DD, Tessier-Lavigne M: APP binds DR6 to trigger axon pruning and neuron death via distinct caspases. Nature 2009;457:981–989.

4 van Leeuwen FW, de Kleijn DP, van den Hurk HH, Neubauer A, Sonnemans MA, Sluijs JA, Koycu S, Ramdjielal RD, Salehi A, Martens GJ, Grosveld FG, Peter J, Burbach H, Hol EM: Frameshift mutants of beta amyloid precursor protein and ubiquitin-B in Alzheimer's and Down patients. Science 1998;279:242–247.

5 Gerez L, de Haan A, Hol EM, Fischer DF, van Leeuwen FW, van Steeg H, Benne R: Molecular misreading: the frequency of dinucleotide deletions in neuronal mRNAs for beta-amyloid precursor protein and ubiquitin B. Neurobiol Aging 2005;26:145–155.

6 Fischer DF, De Vos RA, Van Dijk R, De Vrij FM, Proper EA, Sonnemans MA, Verhage MC, Sluijs JA, Hobo B, Zouambia M, Steur EN, Kamphorst W, Hol EM, Van Leeuwen FW: Disease-specific accumulation of mutant ubiquitin as a marker for proteasomal dysfunction in the brain. FASEB J 2003;17:2014–2024.

7 Schwartz AL, Ciechanover A: Targeting proteins for destruction by the ubiquitin system: implications for human pathobiology. Annu Rev Pharmacol Toxicol 2009;49:73–96.

8 Tan Z, Sun X, Hou FS, Oh HW, Hilgenberg LG, Hol EM, van Leeuwen FW, Smith MA, O'Dowd DK, Schreiber SS: Mutant ubiquitin found in Alzheimer's disease causes neuritic beading of mitochondria in association with neuronal degeneration. Cell Death Differ 2007;14:1721–1732.

9 van Tijn P, de Vrij FM, Schuurman KG, Dantuma NP, Fischer DF, van Leeuwen FW, Hol EM: Dose-dependent inhibition of proteasome activity by a mutant ubiquitin associated with neurodegenerative disease. J Cell Sci 2007;120:1615–1623.

10 Lindsten K, de Vrij FM, Verhoef LG, Fischer DF, van Leeuwen FW, Hol EM, Masucci MG, Dantuma NP: Mutant ubiquitin found in neurodegenerative disorders is a ubiquitin fusion degradation substrate that blocks proteasomal degradation. J Cell Biol 2002;157:417–427.

11 Park Y, Yoon SK, Yoon JB: The HECT domain of TRIP12 ubiquitinates substrates of the ubiquitin fusion degradation pathway. J Biol Chem 2009;284:1540–1549.
12 Verhoef LG, Heinen C, Selivanova A, Halff EF, Salomons FA, Dantuma NP: Minimal length requirement for proteasomal degradation of ubiquitin-dependent substrates. FASEB J 2009;23:123–133.
13 Paine S, Bedford L, Thorpe JR, Mayer RJ, Cavey JR, Bajaj N, Sheppard PW, Lowe J, Layfield R: Immunoreactivity to Lys63-linked polyubiquitin is a feature of neurodegeneration. Neurosci Lett 2009;460:205–208.
14 Shabek N, Herman-Bachinsky Y, Ciechanover A: Ubiquitin degradation with its substrate, or as a monomer in a ubiquitination-independent mode, provides clues to proteasome regulation. Proc Natl Acad Sci USA 2009;106:11907–11912.
15 Kim HT, Kim KP, Uchiki T, Gygi SP, Goldberg AL: S5a promotes protein degradation by blocking synthesis of nondegradable forked ubiquitin chains. EMBO J 2009;28:1867–1877.
16 de Pril R, Fischer DF, Maat-Schieman ML, Hobo B, de Vos RA, Brunt ER, Hol EM, Roos RA, van Leeuwen FW: Accumulation of aberrant ubiquitin induces aggregate formation and cell death in polyglutamine diseases. Hum Mol Genet 2004;13:1803–1813.
17 van Leeuwen FW, van Tijn P, Sonnemans MA, Hobo B, Mann DM, Van Broeckhoven C, Kumar-Singh S, Cras P, Leuba G, Savioz A, Maat-Schieman ML, Yamaguchi H, Kros JM, Kamphorst W, Hol EM, de Vos RA, Fischer DF: Frameshift proteins in autosomal dominant forms of Alzheimer disease and other tauopathies. Neurology 2006;66:S86–S92.
18 Fischer DF, van Dijk R, van Tijn P, Hobo B, Verhage MC, van der Schors RC, Li KW, van Minnen J, Hol EM, van Leeuwen FW: Long-term proteasome dysfunction in the mouse brain by expression of aberrant ubiquitin. Neurobiol Aging 2009;30:847–863.
19 Pawlik M, Otero DA, Park M, Fischer WH, Levy E, Saitoh T: Proteins that bind to the RERMS region of beta amyloid precursor protein. Biochem Biophys Res Commun 2007;355:907–912
20 Hol EM, van Dijk R, Gerez L, Sluijs JA, Hobo B, Tonk MT, de Haan A, Kamphorst W, Fischer DF, Benne R, van Leeuwen FW: Frameshifted beta-amyloid precursor protein (APP+1) is a secretory protein, and the level of APP+1 in cerebrospinal fluid is linked to Alzheimer pathology. J Biol Chem 2003;278:39637–39643.
21 van Dijk R, Fischer DF, Sluijs JA, Sonnemans MA, Hobo B, Mercken L, Mann DM, Hol EM, van Leeuwen FW: Frame-shifted amyloid precursor protein found in Alzheimer's disease and Down's syndrome increases levels of secreted amyloid beta40. J Neurochem 2004;90:712–723.
22 Fischer DF, Hol EM, Hobo B, van Leeuwen FW: Alzheimer-associated APP+1 transgenic mice: frameshift beta-amyloid precursor protein is secreted in cerebrospinal fluid without inducing neuropathology. Neurobiol Aging 2006;27:1445–1450.

Biology of Neurodegeneration

Neuro-degenerative Diseases

Neurodegenerative Dis 2010;7:80–83
DOI: 10.1159/000285511

Published online: February 18, 2010

Impaired Neurotransmitter Release in Alzheimer's and Parkinson's Diseases

Jie Shen

Center for Neurologic Diseases, Brigham and Women's Hospital, Program in Neuroscience, Harvard Medical School, Boston, Mass., USA

Key Words

Synapse · Age-related neurodegeneration · Presenilin · Parkin · Nicastrin

Abstract

Mutations in several causative genes have been linked to monogenic forms of Alzheimer's disease (AD) or Parkinson's disease (PD). To look for possible common pathogenic mechanisms underlying age-related neurodegeneration in AD and PD, we employed genetic approaches to investigate systematically the roles of these gene products (e.g. presenilins (PS) for AD; Parkin, DJ-1, PINK1 and LRRK2 for PD) in the mouse brain, especially in neural circuits that are particularly vulnerable in AD or PD. Our series of genetic studies revealed that PS play cell type-specific roles in the developing brain with the most prominent function in the maintenance of neural progenitor cells. In the adult cerebral cortex, where the pathogenesis of AD occurs, loss of PS results in progressive memory impairment and age-related neurodegeneration. Specifically, PS are involved in the regulation of long-term potentiation and NMDA receptor functions. Interestingly, our further genetic dissection in the hippocampal Schaeffer collateral pathway highlighted the importance of presynaptic PS in the activity-dependent regulation of glutamate release and long-term potentiation induction via modulation of calcium release from intracellular stores. Intriguingly, our independent genetic analysis of Parkin, DJ-1, PINK1 and LRRK2 showed a common defect in activity-dependent dopamine release caused by PD-linked mutations in these genes. Together, our genetic studies suggest that presynaptic dysfunction might be a converging early pathogenic event before neurodegeneration in AD and PD.

Alzheimer's disease (AD) is the most common form of dementia and neurodegenerative disorder. AD is characterized clinically by progressive memory loss and deterioration of cognitive functions, and neuropathologically by extracellular amyloid plaques, intracellular neurofibrillary tangles, and synaptic and neuronal loss. Presenilins (PS1 and PS2) are the major causative genes of early-onset (<65 years of age) familial AD and harbor ~90% of FAD mutations identified to date. PS are essential components of γ-secretase, a multi-subunit protease complex that catalyzes the intramembranous cleavage of a number of type I transmembrane proteins, including Notch and the amyloid precursor protein. Notch is a key physiological substrate of γ-secretase, as evidenced by similar developmental phenotypes exhibited by PS and Notch mutant mice [reviewed in 1], and the dependence of Notch

KARGER

Fax +41 61 306 12 34
E-Mail karger@karger.ch
www.karger.com

Accessible online at:
www.karger.com/ndd

Jie Shen
New Research Building
Rm 636E, 77 Avenue Louis Pasteur
Boston, MA 02115 (USA)
Tel. +1 617 525 5561, Fax +1 617 525 5522, E-Mail jshen@rics.bwh.harvard.edu

signaling on the γ-secretase-mediated release of its intracellular domain [2, 3].

PS play important roles during embryonic development. *PS1*$^{-/-}$ mice exhibit perinatal lethality and somitogenesis defects [4, 5], while mice deficient for both PS1 and PS2 die before embryonic day 9.5 and display early patterning defects [6]. Our investigations of PS function in neural development revealed essential roles for PS in maintenance of neural progenitor cells, differentiation and migration of postmitotic neurons and generation of radial glia [1, 4, 7–9]. PS1 also regulates neuronal migration in a non-cell-autonomous manner by controlling proliferation of meningeal fibroblasts, which in turn affects the survival of Cajal Rezius neurons, pioneer neurons that are important for proper neuronal migration [8]. PS regulate these processes primarily through the Notch signaling pathway [1–3, 7, 10]. However, it is unclear whether Notch is the key functional mediator of PS in the adult brain.

To investigate the role of PS in synaptic function in the adult cerebral cortex, which is the most relevant experimental system for the investigation of the pathogenesis of AD, we generated a viable *PS1* conditional knockout, in which expression of PS1 is selectively eliminated in excitatory pyramidal neurons of the forebrain beginning at postnatal day ~18 [11]. PS is normally expressed highly in pyramidal neurons of the cerebral cortex. This hypomorphic *PS* mutant mouse exhibits a specific but mild deficit in spatial memory [11]. Synaptic transmission and plasticity in the hippocampal CA3-CA1 synapse, however, are normal [11]. Analysis of conditional *PS*-null mice lacking both PS1 and PS2 in the postnatal forebrain revealed impairments in hippocampal memory and long-term potentiation (LTP) prior to any neuropathological changes, demonstrating a requirement for PS in normal synaptic plasticity and memory [12]. More specifically, we found a selective reduction in NMDA receptor-mediated responses and synaptic levels of NMDA receptors and αCaMKII in mutant mice. Furthermore, in the absence of PS, levels of CBP and transcription of CREB/CBP target genes are reduced [12, 13], even though subsequently we found that CREB-mediated transcription is regulated indirectly by PS [14]. Strikingly, *PS* cDKO mice develop in an age-dependent manner synaptic, dendritic and neuronal degeneration with accompanying astrogliosis and hyperphosphorylation of tau, demonstrating an essential role for PS in neuronal survival [12, 15]. Furthermore, PS promote memory and neuronal survival in a γ-secretase-dependent manner, as conditional inactivation of nicastrin, another component of the γ-secretase complex, in the adult cerebral cortex similarly resulted in progressive memory impairment and neurodegeneration [16]. Based on these in vivo findings and a large number of reports on the effects of FAD-linked mutations in culture and in vitro systems as well as in *C. elegans*, we proposed that PS mutations may cause dementia and neurodegeneration in AD via a partial loss-of-function mechanism [17]. The fact that synaptic impairments precede progressive neurodegeneration suggests that synaptic dysfunction caused by loss of PS function promotes subsequent neuronal degeneration.

To determine the precise synaptic site of PS function, we performed a systematic genetic analysis through the restriction of PS inactivation to hippocampal CA1 or CA3 neurons [18]. This strategy permitted analysis of the effects of PS inactivation in either presynaptic or postsynaptic neurons of the Schaeffer collateral pathway. We found that LTP induced by theta burst stimulation is decreased after presynaptic but not postsynaptic deletion of PS. Moreover, presynaptic but not postsynaptic inactivation of PS impairs short-term plasticity and synaptic facilitation. The probability of evoked glutamate release, measured with the open-channel NMDA receptor antagonist MK-801, is reduced by presynaptic inactivation of PS. Strikingly, depletion of calcium internal stores by thapsigargin or inhibition of calcium release from these stores by ryanodine receptor inhibitors mimics and occludes the effects of presynaptic PS inactivation. Collectively, our genetic and electrophysiological studies demonstrate that loss of PS function impairs LTP induction and glutamatergic neurotransmitter release by a presynaptic mechanism. These findings, which distinguish unequivocally between presynaptic and postsynaptic functions of PS, raise the possibility that presynaptic mechanisms may play a primary role in AD pathophysiology. In support of this hypothesis, PS are localized to presynaptic terminals [18], and amyloid precursor protein C-terminal fragments, precursors of Aβ, accumulate in presynaptic terminals of *PS1* conditional knockout mice [19].

Parkinson's disease (PD) is the most common movement disorder characterized by resting tremor, rigidity and bradykinesia. These clinical features are thought to result from reduced dopaminergic input to the striatum, which is caused by the loss of dopaminergic neurons in the substantia nigra. The occurrence of PD is largely sporadic, but clinical syndromes resembling sporadic PD have been linked to mutations in at least 5 distinct genes (*α-synuclein, parkin, DJ-1, PINK1* and *LRRK2*). The recessive inheritance mode of the mutations and the existence of large deletions in the *parkin*, *DJ-1* and *PINK1* genes indicate a loss-of-function pathogenic mechanism. Parkin can function as an E3 ubiquitin ligase [20–23] or as a transcription regulator [24]. DJ-1 itself can be oxidized, thus protecting cells from oxidative damage [25, 26]. PINK1 is a protein kinase localized in the mitochondrion and other subcellular compartments [27–30]. Our previous generation and multidisciplinary analysis of *parkin*$^{-/-}$, *DJ-1*$^{-/-}$ and *PINK1*$^{-/-}$ mice have demonstrated that each of these gene products is required for normal dopaminergic function and evoked dopamine release in nigrostriatal terminals [31–34]. Furthermore, inactivation of each or all three of these recessive PD genes does not cause dopaminergic neurodegeneration [31, 33–35]. In addition, our studies have further shown that loss of PINK1 or Parkin impairs mitochondrial function [36, 37]. A role for PINK1 and Parkin in mitochondria is also supported by genetic studies in *Drosophila* [38–42]. Thus, two converging cellular pathogenic mechanisms have emerged from genetic studies of recessive parkinsonism [43]. Specifically, presynaptic dopaminergic dysfunction in evoked release may be a central pathogenic precursor before leading to frank dopaminergic neuron loss in PD.

In summary, our genetic approaches to the studies of AD and PD [44] have uncovered a novel pathogenic mechanism, suggesting that defects in presynaptic neurotransmitter release may represent a convergent mechanism leading to neurodegeneration in affected circuits in AD and PD. Therapeutic strategies directed toward restoring normal neurotransmitter release may be effective in combating circuit dysfunction and neurodegeneration in these disorders.

Acknowledgements

The author would like to thank Adair Swain for assistance. This work was supported by grants from the NINDS.

References

1 Wines-Samuelson M, Shen J: Presenilins in the developing, adult, and aging cerebral cortex. Neuroscientist 2005;11:441–451.
2 De Strooper B, Annaert W, Cupers P, Saftig P, Craessaerts K, Mumm JS, Schroeter EH, Schrijvers V, Wolfe MS, Ray WJ, Goate A, Kopan R: A presenilin-1-dependent gamma-secretase-like protease mediates release of Notch intracellular domain. Nature 1999; 398:518–522.
3 Song W, Nadeau P, Yuan M, Yang X, Shen J, Yankner BA: Proteolytic release and nuclear translocation of Notch-1 are induced by presenilin-1 and impaired by pathogenic presenilin-1 mutations. Proc Natl Acad Sci USA 1999;96:6959–6963.
4 Shen J, Bronson RT, Chen DF, Xia W, Selkoe DJ, Tonegawa S: Skeletal and CNS defects in Presenilin-1-deficient mice. Cell 1997;89: 629–639.
5 Wong PC, Zheng H, Chen H, Becher MW, Sirinathsinghji DJ, Trumbauer ME, Chen HY, Price DL, Van der Ploeg LH, Sisodia SS: Presenilin 1 is required for Notch1 and DII1 expression in the paraxial mesoderm. Nature 1997;387:288–292.
6 Donoviel DB, Hadjantonakis AK, Ikeda M, Zheng H, Hyslop PS, Bernstein A: Mice lacking both presenilin genes exhibit early embryonic patterning defects. Genes Dev 1999; 13:2801–2810.
7 Handler M, Yang X, Shen J: Presenilin-1 regulates neuronal differentiation during neurogenesis. Development 2000;127:2593–2606.
8 Wines-Samuelson M, Handler M, Shen J: Role of presenilin-1 in cortical lamination and survival of Cajal-Retzius neurons. Dev Biol 2005;277:332–346.
9 Kim WY, Shen J: Presenilins are required for maintenance of neural stem cells in the developing brain. Mol Neurodegener 2008;3: 2.
10 Yang X, Klein R, Tian X, Cheng HT, Kopan R, Shen J: Notch activation induces apoptosis in neural progenitor cells through a p53-dependent pathway. Dev Biol 2004;269:81–94.
11 Yu H, Saura CA, Choi SY, Sun LD, Yang X, Handler M, Kawarabayashi T, Younkin L, Fedeles B, Wilson MA, Younkin S, Kandel ER, Kirkwood A, Shen J: APP processing and synaptic plasticity in presenilin-1 conditional knockout mice. Neuron 2001;31:713–726.
12 Saura CA, Choi SY, Beglopoulos V, Malkani S, Zhang D, Shankaranarayana Rao BS, Chattarji S, Kelleher RJ 3rd, Kandel ER, Duff K, Kirkwood A, Shen J: Loss of presenilin function causes impairments of memory and synaptic plasticity followed by age-dependent neurodegeneration. Neuron 2004; 42:23–36.
13 Beglopoulos V, Shen J: Regulation of CRE-dependent transcription by presenilins: prospects for therapy of Alzheimer's disease. Trends Pharmacol Sci 2006;27:33–40.
14 Watanabe H, Smith MJ, Heilig E, Beglopoulos V, Kelleher RJ 3rd, Shen J: Indirect regulation of presenilins in CREB-mediated transcription. J Biol Chem 2009;284:13705–13713.
15 Beglopoulos V, Sun X, Saura CA, Lemere CA, Kim RD, Shen J: Reduced beta-amyloid production and increased inflammatory responses in presenilin conditional knock-out mice. J Biol Chem 2004;279:46907–46914.
16 Tabuchi K, Chen G, Sudhof TC, Shen J: Conditional forebrain inactivation of nicastrin causes progressive memory impairment and age-related neurodegeneration. J Neurosci 2009;29:7290–7301.
17 Shen J, Kelleher RJ 3rd: The presenilin hypothesis of Alzheimer's disease: evidence for a loss-of-function pathogenic mechanism. Proc Natl Acad Sci USA 2007;104:403–409.
18 Zhang C, Wu B, Beglopoulos V, Wines-Samuelson M, Zhang D, Dragatsis I, Sudhof TC, Shen J: Presenilins are essential for regulating neurotransmitter release. Nature 2009; 460:632–636.
19 Saura CA, Chen G, Malkani S, Choi SY, Takahashi RH, Zhang D, Gouras GK, Kirkwood A, Morris RG, Shen J: Conditional inactivation of presenilin 1 prevents amyloid accumulation and temporarily rescues contextual and spatial working memory impairments in amyloid precursor protein transgenic mice. J Neurosci 2005;25:6755–6764.
20 Imai Y, Soda M, Takahashi R: Parkin suppresses unfolded protein stress-induced cell death through its E3 ubiquitin-protein ligase activity. J Biol Chem 2000;275:35661–35664.

21 Shimura H, Hattori N, Kubo S, Mizuno Y, Asakawa S, Minoshima S, Shimizu N, Iwai K, Chiba T, Tanaka K, Suzuki T: Familial Parkinson disease gene product, parkin, is a ubiquitin-protein ligase. Nat Genet 2000;25:302–305.
22 Shimura H, Schlossmacher MG, Hattori N, Frosch MP, Trockenbacher A, Schneider R, Mizuno Y, Kosik KS, Selkoe DJ: Ubiquitination of a new form of alpha-synuclein by parkin from human brain: implications for Parkinson's disease. Science 2001;293:263–269.
23 Zhang Y, Gao J, Chung KK, Huang H, Dawson VL, Dawson TM: Parkin functions as an E2-dependent ubiquitin- protein ligase and promotes the degradation of the synaptic vesicle-associated protein, CDCrel-1. Proc Natl Acad Sci USA 2000;97:13354–13359.
24 Alves da Costa C, Sunyach C, Giaime E, West A, Corti O, Brice A, Abou-Sleiman PM, Wood NW, Takahashi H, Goldberg MS, Shen J, Checler F: Transcriptional repression of p53 by parkin and impairment by autosomal recessive juvenile Parkinson's disease-associated mutations. Nat Cell Biol 2009;11:1370–1375.
25 Kahle PJ, Waak J, Gasser T: DJ-1 and prevention of oxidative stress in Parkinson's disease and other age-related disorders. Free Radic Biol Med 2009;47:1354–13561.
26 Mitsumoto A, Nakagawa Y, Takeuchi A, Okawa K, Iwamatsu A, Takanezawa Y: Oxidized forms of peroxiredoxins and DJ-1 on two-dimensional gels increased in response to sublethal levels of paraquat. Free Radic Res 2001;35:301–310.
27 Gandhi S, Muqit MM, Stanyer L, Healy DG, Abou-Sleiman PM, Hargreaves I, Heales S, Ganguly M, Parsons L, Lees AJ, Latchman DS, Holton JL, Wood NW, Revesz T: PINK1 protein in normal human brain and Parkinson's disease. Brain 2006;129:1720–1731.
28 Pridgeon JW, Olzmann JA, Chin LS, Li L: PINK1 protects against oxidative stress by phosphorylating mitochondrial chaperone TRAP1. PLoS Biol 2007;5:e172.
29 Lin W, Kang UJ: Characterization of PINK1 processing, stability, and subcellular localization. J Neurochem 2008;106:464–474.
30 Weihofen A, Ostaszewski B, Minami Y, Selkoe DJ: Pink1 Parkinson mutations, the Cdc37/Hsp90 chaperones and Parkin all influence the maturation or subcellular distribution of Pink1. Hum Mol Genet 2008;17:602–616.
31 Goldberg MS, Fleming SM, Palacino JJ, Cepeda C, Lam HA, Bhatnagar A, Meloni EG, Wu N, Ackerson LC, Klapstein GJ, Gajendiran M, Roth BL, Chesselet MF, Maidment NT, Levine MS, Shen J: Parkin-deficient mice exhibit nigrostriatal deficits but not loss of dopaminergic neurons. J Biol Chem 2003;278:43628–43635.
32 Goldberg MS, Pisani A, Haburcak M, Vortherms TA, Kitada T, Costa C, Tong Y, Martella G, Tscherter A, Martins A, Bernardi G, Roth BL, Pothos EN, Calabresi P, Shen J: Nigrostriatal dopaminergic deficits and hypokinesia caused by inactivation of the familial Parkinsonism-linked gene DJ-1. Neuron 2005;45:489–496.
33 Kitada T, Pisani A, Karouani M, Haburcak M, Martella G, Tscherter A, Platania P, Wu B, Pothos EN, Shen J: Impaired dopamine release and synaptic plasticity in the striatum of parkin$^{-/-}$ mice. J Neurochem 2009;110:613–621.
34 Kitada T, Pisani A, Porter DR, Yamaguchi H, Tscherter A, Martella G, Bonsi P, Zhang C, Pothos EN, Shen J: Impaired dopamine release and synaptic plasticity in the striatum of PINK1-deficient mice. Proc Natl Acad Sci USA 2007;104:11441–11446.
35 Yamaguchi H, Shen J: Absence of dopaminergic neuronal degeneration and oxidative damage in aged DJ-1-deficient mice. Mol Neurodegener 2007;2:10.
36 Gautier CA, Kitada T, Shen J: Loss of PINK1 causes mitochondrial functional defects and increased sensitivity to oxidative stress. Proc Natl Acad Sci USA 2008;105:11364–11369.
37 Palacino JJ, Sagi D, Goldberg MS, Krauss S, Motz C, Wacker M, Klose J, Shen J: Mitochondrial dysfunction and oxidative damage in parkin-deficient mice. J Biol Chem 2004;279:18614–18622.
38 Clark IE, Dodson MW, Jiang C, Cao JH, Huh JR, Seol JH, Yoo SJ, Hay BA, Guo M: *Drosophila* pink1 is required for mitochondrial function and interacts genetically with parkin. Nature 2006;441:1162–1166.
39 Greene JC, Whitworth AJ, Kuo I, Andrews LA, Feany MB, Pallanck LJ: Mitochondrial pathology and apoptotic muscle degeneration in *Drosophila* parkin mutants. Proc Natl Acad Sci USA 2003;100:4078–4083.
40 Park J, Lee SB, Lee S, Kim Y, Song S, Kim S, Bae E, Kim J, Shong M, Kim JM, Chung J: Mitochondrial dysfunction in *Drosophila* PINK1 mutants is complemented by parkin. Nature 2006;441:1157–1161.
41 Pesah Y, Pham T, Burgess H, Middlebrooks B, Verstreken P, Zhou Y, Harding M, Bellen H, Mardon G: *Drosophila* parkin mutants have decreased mass and cell size and increased sensitivity to oxygen radical stress. Development 2004;131:2183–2194.
42 Yang Y, Gehrke S, Imai Y, Huang Z, Ouyang Y, Wang JW, Yang L, Beal MF, Vogel H, Lu B: Mitochondrial pathology and muscle and dopaminergic neuron degeneration caused by inactivation of *Drosophila* Pink1 is rescued by Parkin. Proc Natl Acad Sci USA 2006;103:10793–10798.
43 Shen J, Cookson MR: Mitochondria and dopamine: new insights into recessive parkinsonism. Neuron 2004;43:301–304.
44 Beglopoulos V, Shen J: Gene-targeting technologies for the study of neurological disorders. Neuromolecular Med 2004;6:13–30.

Biology of Neurodegeneration

Neuro-degenerative Diseases

Neurodegenerative Dis 2010;7:84–87
DOI: 10.1159/000285512

Published online: February 18, 2010

Stem Cell Biology in the Study of Pathological Conditions

K. Sugaya

College of Medicine, University of Central Florida, Orlando, Fla., USA

Key Words
Neural stem cell · Amyloid precursor protein · Reelin

Abstract
The current focus of researchers is to create certain types of cells in vitro as transplantation materials. The problem of this approach is that terminally differentiated cells may not integrate into the host. To overcome this problem, we may want to transplant premature cells, which can migrate and differentiate due to environmental cues received from the host, allowing for intrinsic proper functioning of the cells. Thus, we have to consider the effects that the pathological environment might have on the transplanted cells. Here, we show the effects of amyloid precursor protein and reelin on neural stem cell (NSC) differentiation, and demonstrate how we have regulated this effect to produce desirable cells under pathological conditions. We found that amyloid precursor protein increases glial differentiation via the notch and cytokine-signaling pathway, while reelin induces radial glial differentiation followed by neuronal differentiation via increasing phosphorylation of adapter protein disabled-1. Since amyloid and reelin are found in plaques within Alzheimer's disease, these findings may closely associate with NSC biology in the context of its pathology. By regulating these factors in Alzheimer's disease, we may be able to not only guide differentiation of transplanted NSCs, but also to modify progression of disease by guiding differentiation of endogenous NSCs.

Introduction

Advances in stem cell technology may bring a cure for neurodegenerative diseases. We have shown that neural stem cell (NSC) transplantation improved cognitive function in aged animals [1]. More recently, we successfully produced embryonic stem cell-like cells from adult stem cells by overexpression of nanog, an embryonic stem cell gene [2]. Now it is time to consider how Alzheimer's disease (AD) pathology affects NSC biology, since successful neuroregeneration is dependent on the effective production of neurons from NSC in the patient's brain. In the current study, we investigated two factors, amyloid precursor protein (APP) and reelin, which are found in amyloid plaques of AD.

Although amyloid-β (Aβ) deposition has been a hallmark of AD, the physiological function of APP is not clear. Our previous study suggested that high concentration of APP induces glial differentiation while physiological level of APP promotes migration and differentiation of NSC [3]. Reelin, which is also a component of plaques, has been shown to be an important signal for neuronal migration and proper positioning of neurons [4]. Reelin signal is transmitted into the cells after reelin binds its receptors, apolipoprotein receptor 2 (ApoER2) and the very low density lipoprotein receptor (VLDLR). Reelin binding initiates disabled-1 (Dab-1) binding to the internalization (NPXY) motif of ApoER2 and VLDLR, leading to the induction of Dab1 tyrosine phosphor-

KARGER

Fax +41 61 306 12 34
E-Mail karger@karger.ch
www.karger.com

1660–2854/10/0073–0084$26.00/0

Accessible online at:
www.karger.com/ndd

Kiminobu Sugaya
6900 Lake Nona Blvd.
BMS room 412
Orlando, FL 32827-7407 (USA)
Tel. +1 407 266 7045, Fax +1 407 266 7017, E-Mail ksugaya@mail.ucf.edu

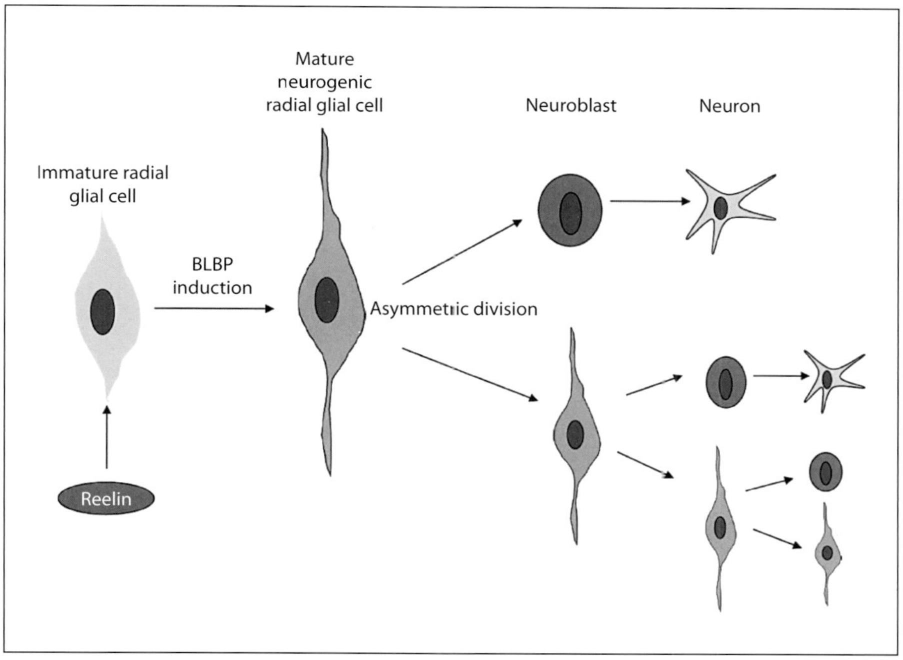

Fig. 1. Schematic diagram that illustrates the proposed role for reelin in neurogenesis. Reelin binding to the surface of an immature radial glial cell induces BLBP expression in this cell and drives its maturation. The maturation includes morphological changes and a shift from a proliferative phase (symmetric division) to a neurogenic phase (asymmetric division) that will result in the generation of neurons.

Color version available online

ylation [5]. Mice deficient in this type of signaling generate a phenotype characterized by inversion of the cortical layers, and abnormalities in laminated brain structures [6].

APP Induces Glial Differentiation by Notch and the IL-6 Signaling Pathway

In the later stage of neural differentiation, glial differentiation is induced by various factors. To date, IL-6 cytokine families, bone morphogenic factors, basic fibroblast growth factor (bFGF), and Notch signaling have been known for an important mechanism that is involved in the glial differentiation process [7]. IL-6-induced Janus kinase/signal transducer and activator of transcription (JAK/STAT) signaling pathway is a central part of the glial differentiation process [8]. Once the IL-6 cytokine families interact with their cognate receptors (e.g. IL-6 receptor-α), the resultant complexes are then associated with gp130, a crucial signal-transducing component of IL-6 receptor [9]. Formation of these receptor heterodimers stimulates a downstream transcription factor, STAT proteins, by activating JAKs, especially JAK1 and JAK2. Predominantly, STAT3 molecules are phosphorylated, and then the phosphorylated STAT3s form dimerization and undergo translocation into the nucleus. Finally, STAT3 dimers bind to the putative STAT3 binding element of GFAP promoter, a typical astrocytic marker for glial differentiation [10].

APP promotes dose-dependent phosphorylation of STAT3-p-Tyr705 residues in NSCs [11]. The siRNA silencing expression of JAK1 and STAT3 abolish GFAP expression induced by APP, suggesting that APP-induced glial differentiation is mediated by JAK/STAT in the IL-6/gp130 signaling pathway. Also, inhibition of JAKs using selective inhibitors (AG490; Tyrphostin B42) suppressed phosphorylation of STAT3 and GFAP expression. Thus, these results indicate that sAPP-induced glio-genesis is mediated by the IL-6/gp130 signaling pathway through gp130, and by downstream-signaling molecules, JAKs and STAT3.

We observed a higher intracellular domain of notch (NICD) generation in APP23 mice brain compared to WT, indicating that APP increases Notch proteolysis and involvement of notch signaling in APP-induced glial differentiation. We found that APP increased NICD generation and GFAP expression in vitro and in vivo, while application of an antibody recognizing APP (22C11) dependently suppressed the generation of NICDs. These results suggest that sAPP-induced glial differentiation is mediated through the Notch signaling pathway. Recently, cross-talk between Notch and JAK/STAT pathways through physical interaction between Hes1 and JAK2

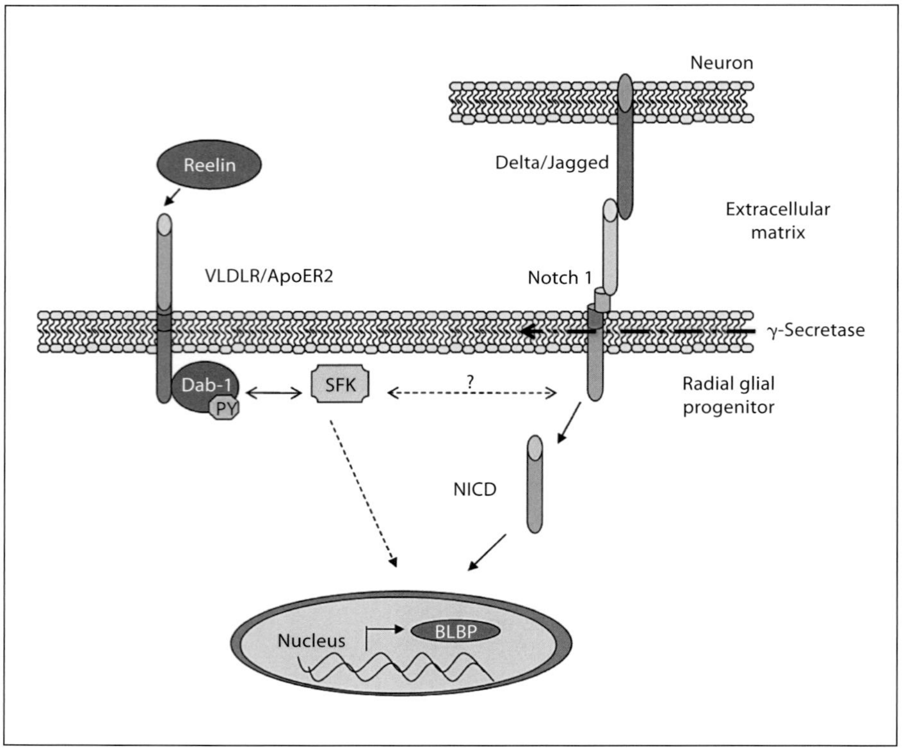

Color version available online

Fig. 2. Schematic diagram that demonstrates the proposed cross-talk between reelin and Notch-1 signaling pathways. Upon Notch-1 activation, the released NICD translocates to the nucleus and induces BLBP expression. Reelin signaling is also known to induce BLBP expression. We propose a cross-talk between the two pathways and suggest that reelin signaling increases NICD levels leading to BLBP expression.

was reported [12]. In our study, APP upregulated Hes1, and treatment with γ-secretase inhibitor (L-685, 458) significantly inhibited Hes1 and GFAP expression. Treatment with L-685, 458 also suppressed phosphorylation of STAT3-Tyr 705 induced by APP. These results suggest that APP potentiates glial differentiation of NSCs by cross-talk between Notch and gp130/IL-6 signaling pathways.

Reelin Induces Radial Glial Differentiation of NSC

We found that reelin treatment increases neuronal differentiation of HNCs, while it activates Notch signaling. Since Notch activation can induce both the radial glial phenotype and its transformation into astrocytes [13, 14], we hypothesized that reelin signaling may act to fine-tune Notch activation, favoring the induction of the radial glial phenotype prenatally. This in turn can explain how the degeneration of the cells that produce reelin in the cortex coincides with transformation of the radial glial cells into astrocytes postnatally [15, 16]. Recently, brain lipid-binding protein (BLBP) expression in cortical radial glia as well as its role in radial process extension was found to be dependent on reelin expression [17]. A recent study showed that Notch signaling could also regulate the molecular and the morphological differentiation of radial glia through the transcriptional activation of BLBP [18]. In our study, in vitro addition of reelin to NSCs, isolated from the cortex of a 14-week-old human fetus, induced BLBP expression and a radial glial phenotype similar to that induced by Notch activation. The inhibition of Notch activation by inhibiting the activity of γ-secretase abolished reelin's effect, suggesting the dependency of reelin signaling on Notch activation. Furthermore, reelin treatment increased the level of NICD, indicating that reelin can directly activate Notch. Finally, Dab-1 was observed to bind to Notch, thus providing evidence of the physical interaction between these two pathways. FGF and epidermal growth factor (EGF) deprivation transform NSCs into a transient phenotype that is between radial glial cells and immature astrocytes [19], while FGF and EGF pathways are known to promote the formation of radial glia [20, 21].

Reelin treatment reinduces the formation of radial glia from HNSs that have been deprived of FGF and EGF. The newly formed radial glia were characterized by increased process extension with BLBP expression. The induction of neurogenic radial glia was determined by finding the percentage of BLBP-positive-expressing cells and a bipolar morphology with at least one thin process longer than 50 μm [22, 23]. We found that the percentage of neurogenic radial glial cells significantly increased from 3.4% in the control-treated cells to 9.5% in the reelin-treated cells.

Conclusions

Since amyloid and reelin are found in plaques, a major hallmark of AD, these results indicate the close association of AD pathology with NSC biology. By regulating these factors in AD, we may be able to not only efficiently produce neurons from transplanted NSCs but also to reduce gliosis, along with minimizing the reduction of the neuronal population found in AD, by guiding differentiation of endogenous NSCs.

References

1 Qu T, Brannen CL, Kim HM, Sugaya K: Human neural stem cells improve cognitive function of aged brain. Neuroreport 2001;12:1127–1132.
2 Sugaya K, Alvarez A, Marutle A, Kwak YD, Choumkina E: Stem cell strategies for Alzheimer's disease therapy. Panminerva Med 2006;48:87–96.
3 Kwak YD, Brannen CL, Qu T, Kim HM, Dong X, Soba P, Majumdar A, Kaplan A, Beyreuther K, Sugaya K: Amyloid precursor protein regulates differentiation of human neural stem cells. Stem Cells Dev 2006;15:381–389.
4 D'Arcangelo G, Miao GG, Chen SC, Scares HD, Morgan JI, Curran T: A protein related to extracellular matrix proteins deleted in the mouse mutant reeler. Nature 1995;374:719–723.
5 Forster E, Jossin Y, Zhao S, Chai X, Frotscher M, Goffinet AM: Recent progress in understanding the role of Reelin in radial neuronal migration, with specific emphasis on the dentate gyrus. Eur J Neurosci 2006;23:901–909.
6 Trommsdorff M, Gortthardt M, Hiesberger T, Shelton J, Stockinger W, Nimpf J, Hammer RE, Richardson JA, Herz J: Reeler/disabled-like disruption of neuronal migration in knockout mice lacking the VLDL receptor and ApoE receptor 2. Cell 1999;97:689–701.
7 Nakashima K, Taga T: Mechanisms underlying cytokine-mediated cell-fate regulation in the nervous system. Mol Neurobiol 2002;25:233–244.
8 He F, Ge W, Martinowich K, Becker-Catania S, Coskun V, Zhu W, Wu H, Castro D, Guillemot F, Fan G, de Vellis J, Sun YE: A positive autoregulatory loop of Jak- STAT signaling controls the onset of astrogliogenesis. Nat Neurosci 2005;8:616–625.
9 Hibi M, Murakami M, Saito M, Hirano T, Taga T, Kishimoto T: Molecular cloning and expression of an IL-6 signal transducer, gp130. Cell 1990;63:1149–1157.
10 Bonni A, Sun Y, Nadal-Vicens M, Bhatt A, Frank DA, Rozovsky I, Stahl N, Yancopoulos GD, Greenberg ME: Regulation of gliogenesis in the central nervous system by the JAK-STAT signaling pathway. Science 1997;278:477–483.
11 Wang Y, Fuller GM: Phosphorylation and internalization of gp130 occur after IL-6 activation of Jak2 kinase in hepatocytes. Mol Biol Cell 1994;5:819–828.
12 Kamakura S, Oishi K, Yoshimatsu T, Nakafuku M, Masuyama N, Gotoh Y: Hes binding to STAT3 mediates crosstalk between Notch and JAK-STAT signalling. Nat Cell Biol 2004;6:547–554.
13 Gaiano N, Nye JS, Fishell G: Radial glial identity is promoted by Notch1 signaling in the murine forebrain. Neuron 2000;26:395–404.
14 Chambers CB, Peng Y, Nguyen H, Gaiano N, Fishell G, Nye JS: Spatiotemporal selectivity of response to Notch1 signals in mammalian forebrain precursors. Development 2001;128:689–702.
15 Super H, Uylings HB: The early differentiation of the neocortex: a hypothesis on neocortical evolution. Cereb Cortex 2001;11:1101–1109.
16 Martin R, Gutierrez A, Penafiel A, Marin-Padilla M, de la Calle A: Persistence of Cajal-Retzius cells in the adult human cerebral cortex. An immunohistochemical study. Histol Histopathol 1999;14:487–490.
17 Hartfuss E, Forster E, Bock HH, Hack MA, Leprince P, Luque JM, Herz J, Frotscher M, Götz M: Reelin signaling directly affects radial glia morphology and biochemical maturation. Development 2003;130:4597–4609.
18 Patten BA, Peyrin JM, Weinmaster G, Corfas G: Sequential signaling through Notch1 and erbB receptors mediates radial glia differentiation. J Neurosci 2003;23:6132–6140.
19 Liu X, Bolteus AJ, Balkin DM, Henschel O, Bordey A: GFAP-expressing cells in the postnatal subventricular zone display a unique glial phenotype intermediate between radial glia and astrocytes. Glia 2006;54:394–410.
20 Kabos P, Kabosova A, Neuman T: Blocking HES1 expression initiates GABAergic differentiation and induces the expression of p21(CIP1/WAF1) in human neural stem cells. J Biol Chem 2002;277:8763–8766.
21 Kamakura S, Oishi K, Yoshimatsu T, Nakafuku M, Masuyama N, Gotoh Y: Hes binding to STAT3 mediates crosstalk between Notch and JAK-STAT signalling. Nat Cell Biol 2004;6:547–554.
22 Gregg C, Weiss S: Generation of functional radial glial cells by embryonic and adult forebrain neural stem cells. J Neurosci 2003;23:11587–11601.
23 Yoon K, Nery S, Rutlin ML, Radtke F, Fishell G, Gaiano N: Fibroblast growth factor receptor signaling promotes radial glial identity and interacts with Notch signaling in telencephalic progenitors. J Neurosci 2004;24:9497–9506.

Disease Models

Neuro-degenerative Diseases

Neurodegenerative Dis 2010;7:88–95
DOI: 10.1159/000285513

Published online: February 18, 2010

Possible Involvement of Transthyretin in Hippocampal β-Amyloid Burden and Learning Behaviors in a Mouse Model of Alzheimer's Disease (TgCRND8)

Sihem Doggui   Jonathan Brouillette   Jean-Guy Chabot   Mark Farso
Rémi Quirion

Douglas Mental Health University Institute and Department of Psychiatry, McGill University, Montreal, Que., Canada

Key Words
Transthyretin · Alzheimer's disease · TgCRND8 mouse · Human amyloid precursor protein transgenic mouse · Deposition of β-amyloid · Morris water maze · Spatial learning

Abstract
Background: Alzheimer's disease (AD) is a neurodegenerative disease characterized by progressive memory loss, possibly triggered by the accumulation of β-amyloid (Aβ) peptides and the hyperphosphorylation of Tau neurofilament protein. Recent findings have shown that transthyretin (TTR) is a potent scavenger of Aβ peptide deposits, suggesting a possible neuroprotective role for TTR in neurodegenerative processes associated with amyloidogenesis, such as AD. ***Methods:*** To investigate the relationship between TTR and Aβ deposition, we crossed mouse carrying a deletion of TTR ($TTR^{-/-}$) with a transgenic mouse model of AD (TgCRND8), and Aβ burden and spatial learning capacities were evaluated at 4 and 6 months of age (exclusion of the 6 month-old TgCRND8/$TTR^{-/-}$ group due to low survival rate). ***Results:*** Rather surprisingly, Aβ plaque burden was significantly reduced in the hippocampus of 4-month-old TgCRND8/$TTR^{+/-}$, and to a lesser extent in TgCRND8/$TTR^{-/-}$, as compared to age-matched TgCRND8/$TTR^{+/+}$. No difference in plaque burden was found between any groups in 6-month-old animals. At 4 and 6 months of age, all populations of these hybrid transgenic mice displayed similar magnitude of spatial memory deficits in the Morris water maze task. ***Conclusion:*** Since TgCRND8 mice represent an aggressive model of Aβ deposition with plaques developing as early as 3 months of age, along with spatial learning deficits, it may be already too late at 4 and 6 months of age to observe significant changes due to the deletion of the TTR gene.

Introduction

Alzheimer's disease (AD) is among the most common forms of dementia, affecting 20 million people worldwide [1]. This neurodegenerative disease is primarily characterized by progressive memory impairments and other cognitive deficits including disorientation and deficits in executive functions [2–4]. Neuropathological hallmarks of AD include increase in the levels of β-amyloid (Aβ)-enriched senile plaques and hyperphosphorylated Tau

S.D. and J.B. contributed equally to the study.

KARGER
Fax +41 61 306 12 34
E-Mail karger@karger.ch
www.karger.com

1660–2854/10/0073–0088$26.00/0

Accessible online at:
www.karger.com/ndd

Rémi Quirion, OC, PhD, FRSC, CQ
Douglas Mental Health University Institute, Institute of Neuroscience, Mental Health and Addiction, 6875 LaSalle Boulevard, Montréal, QC H4H 1R3 (Canada)
Tel. +1 514 761 6131, ext. 2934, Fax +1 514 762 3034
E-Mail remi.quirion@douglas.mcgill.ca

neurofibrillary tangles in various brain regions (e.g. hippocampus, cortex) implicated in cognitive functions [5].

Aβ peptides are soluble serum and cerebrospinal fluid (CSF) components normally produced from proteolytic cleavage of the transmembrane amyloid precursor protein (APP) by β- and γ-secretases [6]. In AD, the amyloid cascade hypothesis suggests that neurotoxic Aβ peptides accumulate as extracellular insoluble fibrils in plaques as well as within neurons or as soluble extracellular oligomers that bind to neuronal surfaces [5, 7]. Genetic studies of familial cases of AD have revealed autosomal dominant mutations in three distinct genes: APP [8], presenilin1 [9] and presenilin 2 [10]. These mutations most likely can accelerate the development of AD-related pathology.

Using a high-density microarray approach, we have recently identified various genes, including transthyretin (TTR), that are differentially expressed in the hippocampi of aged memory-impaired (AI) versus aged memory-unimpaired rats [11]. Decreased TTR gene expression was associated with memory deficits in AI rats [11], while aged mice lacking TTR displayed accelerated spatial memory impairments [11, 12]. TTR is a well-known transporter of retinol and thyroxine from the periphery to the brain [13, 14]. TTR has also been identified as the major Aβ-binding protein in CSF enabling to sequester Aβ peptides [15–20]. Buxbaum et al. [21] have reported that the ability of TTR to bind to Aβ may protect against the neurotoxic effects of 'free' amyloid peptides. Other studies using AD mouse models have demonstrated the important relationship between TTR and amyloid clearance. For instance, increased hippocampal Aβ levels have been reported following a local treatment with anti-TTR antibody in a mouse model of AD [22], while an upregulation of TTR gene expression with a concomitant reduction in Aβ levels was observed in APPSwe/PS1ΔE9 transgenic (Tg) mice exposed to an enriched environment [23]. More than 80 different TTR variants have been reported in humans [24]. While a TTR point mutation appeared to be associated with dementia [25], TTR polymorphisms have not been identified with risk of AD [26, 27]. But a significant association between few TTR single nucleotide polymorphisms and hippocampal atrophy has recently been observed [27]. However, the finding of lower TTR levels in the CSF of AD patients has led to the suggestion of the possible use of CSF TTR as a biomarker of AD [28–34]. Taking into consideration the important relationship between TTR and Aβ peptides, we hypothesized that decreases in the level of TTR gene expression could accelerate AD-like pathologies in a Tg mouse model of AD. In the present study, we have thus examined Aβ plaque burden and spatial learning abilities in TTR knockout mice overexpressing an APP gene containing the Swedish (K670N and M671L) and the Indiana (V717F) familial AD mutations (TgCRND8 [35]) at 4 and 6 months of age.

Materials and Methods

Animals

Animal care was according to protocols and guidelines of the McGill University Animal Care Committee and the Canadian Council for Animal Care.

APP TgCRND8 Mice

These Tg hemizygous mice were kindly provided by David Westaway (Centre for Research in Neurodegenerative Diseases, University of Toronto, now at the University of Alberta, Edmonton, Alta., Canada). These mice harbor a double APP 695 mutation (Swedish KM670/671NL and Indiana V717F APP) under control of the Syrian hamster prion gene promoter. Three month-old TgCRND8 mice have been reported to display increased brain levels of human Aβ peptides and concomitant impairment in acquisition and learning reversal, as revealed by the reference memory version of the Morris water maze (MWM) [35]. All animals were bred in our animal facility and maintained on an outbred C3H/C57BL6 background [35].

TTR Knockout ($TTR^{-/-}$) Mice

$TTR^{-/-}$ mice were purchased from Jackson Laboratory (Bar Harbor, Me., USA) and maintained on a mixed C57BL/6 × 129S background. These mice were bred (F2 generation) in our animal facility.

Hybrid TgCRND8/TTR Mouse

Hybrid Tg+/TTR mice were obtained by mating male TgCRND8 with $TTR^{-/-}$ female mice. The heterozygous $TTR^{+/-}$ F1 male mice carrying the mutant APP cDNA were mated with heterozygous $TTR^{+/-}$ F1 female mice. Four- and six-month-old $TTR^{+/+}$, $TTR^{+/-}$ and $TTR^{-/-}$ F2 progenies carrying the mutant APP cDNA (TgCRND8/$TTR^{+/+}$, TgCRND8/$TTR^{+/-}$ and TgCRND8/$TTR^{-/-}$) on the hybrid C3H × C57BL/6 × 129S were used in the present study. However, results from the 6-month-old TgCRND8/$TTR^{-/-}$ group were excluded from the present study because only one mouse survived.

All mice were housed (5 animals per cage) under 12 h light/dark cycles (lights on at 08:00 a.m.) with constant humidity and temperature and food and tap water ad libitum. After weaning, Tg (TgCRND8), TTR-KO and hybrid (TgCRND8/TTR) mice were identified by PCR amplification of ear genomic DNA using specific primer pairs as previously described [36, 37].

MWM Task

Spatial memory was determined using the reference memory version of the MWM task, where the hidden escape platform remained in the centre of the same quadrant throughout all training days [38]. In a 1.4-meter diameter pool, mice were required to find a submerged platform (15 cm in diameter) located 1 cm below the surface of water (24°C), rendered opaque by the addition of skim milk powder. Animals were pseudo-randomly started from a different position at each trial and used distal visuospatial cues to find the hidden platform [38]. Each animal was given three trials of 90 s per day with a 40-min intertrial interval over 5 consecutive days. If the platform was not located within 90 s, animals were guided to it and remained there for 10 s before removal. After the acquisition phase on day 5, mice were given one probe trial of 60 s in which the platform was removed from the pool to evaluate the number of times the animal crossed the previous location of the platform, time spent in the target quadrant, and swimming speed. This trial was followed by one cued trial of 60 s in which the platform was visible to assess visual, sensorimotor or motivational deficits to escape from water. The experimenter was blind to the genotype and treatment performed on mice. Data derived from the MWM task were recorded on a computer using a video tracking system (HVS, Buckingham, UK). To control for possible effects due to circadian cycles, all trials were performed at approximately the same time of the day, between 11 and 15 h. Statistical significance of each test was assessed using the appropriate ANOVA design and simple main effects were analyzed with the F test when the interaction was significant. Tukey's honestly significant difference test was used as post-hoc pairwise comparison test.

Tissue Preparation and Immunofluorescence

Mice were anesthetized and transcardially perfused with saline. Brains were removed and bisected in the mid-sagittal plane. The right hemispheres were snap frozen, and the left ones for immunohistochemistry were immersion-fixed in 4% paraformaldehyde and embedded in paraffin. Eight-micrometer-thick coronal sections were prepared for immunofluorescence staining.

The Aβ immunofluorescence staining was performed by pretreating the sections with formic concentrated (98%) formic acid for 5 min, followed by incubation in Tris-buffered saline (TBS; pH 7.6) containing normal goat serum (10% v/v) and 0.05% Tween 20 (0.05%). Sections were then incubated with the primary mouse monoclonal antibody (6E10, 1:1,000; Covance Research Products Inc., Denver, Pa., USA; 6F/3D, 1:100; Dako Canada Inc., Mississauga, Ont., Canada) in TBS containing 1% NGS (overnight; 4°C) followed by a biotinylated goat anti-mouse IgG (1:200 in TBS containing 2% NGS; Vector Laboratories, Burlingame, Calif., USA) for 1 h. After TBS washes, the slides were incubated with streptavidin conjugated to Alexa Fluor 488 (1:200; Invitrogen Canada, Burlington, Ont., Canada,) for 2 h and mounted in Vectashield containing DAPI (Vector Laboratories).

Hippocampal Aβ Burden

Amyloid plaque burden was estimated by directly measuring plaque area on twelve 8-μm-thick coronal sections that were evenly spaced (40 μm apart) throughout the region of interest. Each section from the 'systematic-uniform-random' set was immunostained by using either 6E10 (compact and diffuse Aβ plaques) or 6F/3D (compact Aβ plaques) antibody. Quantification of hippocampal amyloid plaque area was done under the Nikon Eclipse E800 microscope (×10; Nikon Canada Inc., Mississauga, Ont., Canada) fitted with a SPOT 741 RT digital camera (Diagnostic Instruments, Sterling Heights, Mich., USA). Digital images were analyzed using MCID version 6 Elite imaging software (Imaging Research Inc., St. Catharines, Ont., Canada). The plaque size distribution was also determined. Plaques were categorized as being either <500, 500–1,000, 1,000–2,000, 2,000–3,000, or >3,000 μm^2 in size. One-way ANOVA followed by the Dunnett multiple comparison test was used to compare different groups with $p < 0.05$ being considered significant (GraphPad Software, San Diego, Calif., USA).

Results

TTR Deficiency Does Not Increase the Deposition of Aβ in the Hippocampus

To evaluate whether or not TTR affected the deposition of Aβ, we measured the area occupied by Aβ plaques and the Aβ plaque size distribution in the hippocampus of 4- and 6-month-old mice expressing the double-mutated form of the APP 695 in the presence (TgCRND8/$TTR^{+/+}$), hemizygous deletion (TgCRND8/$TTR^{+/-}$) or absence (TgCRND8/$TTR^{-/-}$) of murine TTR. As already pointed out in the 'Materials and Methods' section, since only one mouse survived, results from the 6-month-old TgCRND8/$TTR^{-/-}$ group were excluded. As previously reported [35], the Aβ deposition was increased with age since the Aβ plaque area was bigger at 6 months compared to 4-month-old Tg mice (fig. 1a, b). When the Aβ plaques were stained using the 6E10 antibody, which labels both compact and diffuse senile plaques, Aβ burden did not significantly differ between groups (fig. 1a). Interestingly, a significant reduction in total hippocampal Aβ burden was observed in 4-month-old TgCRND8/$TTR^{+/-}$ compared to age-matched TgCRND8/$TTR^{+/+}$ (fig. 1b) when compact Aβ plaques were immunostained using the 6F3D antibody. To determine whether TTR can affect the formation of new plaques and/or plaque growth, we examined the distribution of plaque size. There was no significant difference in plaque size and distribution between the Tg mice studied here at either 4 or 6 months of age (fig. 1c).

TTR Expression Does Not Affect Spatial Memory Deficits in TgCRND8 Mice

To determine whether the absence of endogenous murine TTR gene expression has an effect on cognitive memory parameters in TgCRND8, we carried out the reference memory version of the MWM task, a hippocampus-dependent behavioral task [38], on 4- and 6-month-old mice expressing the double-mutated form of the APP 695 in the presence (TgCRND8/$TTR^{+/+}$), hemizygous deletion (TgCRND8/$TTR^{+/-}$) or absence (TgCRND8/$TTR^{-/-}$) of murine TTR. Results from the 6-month-old

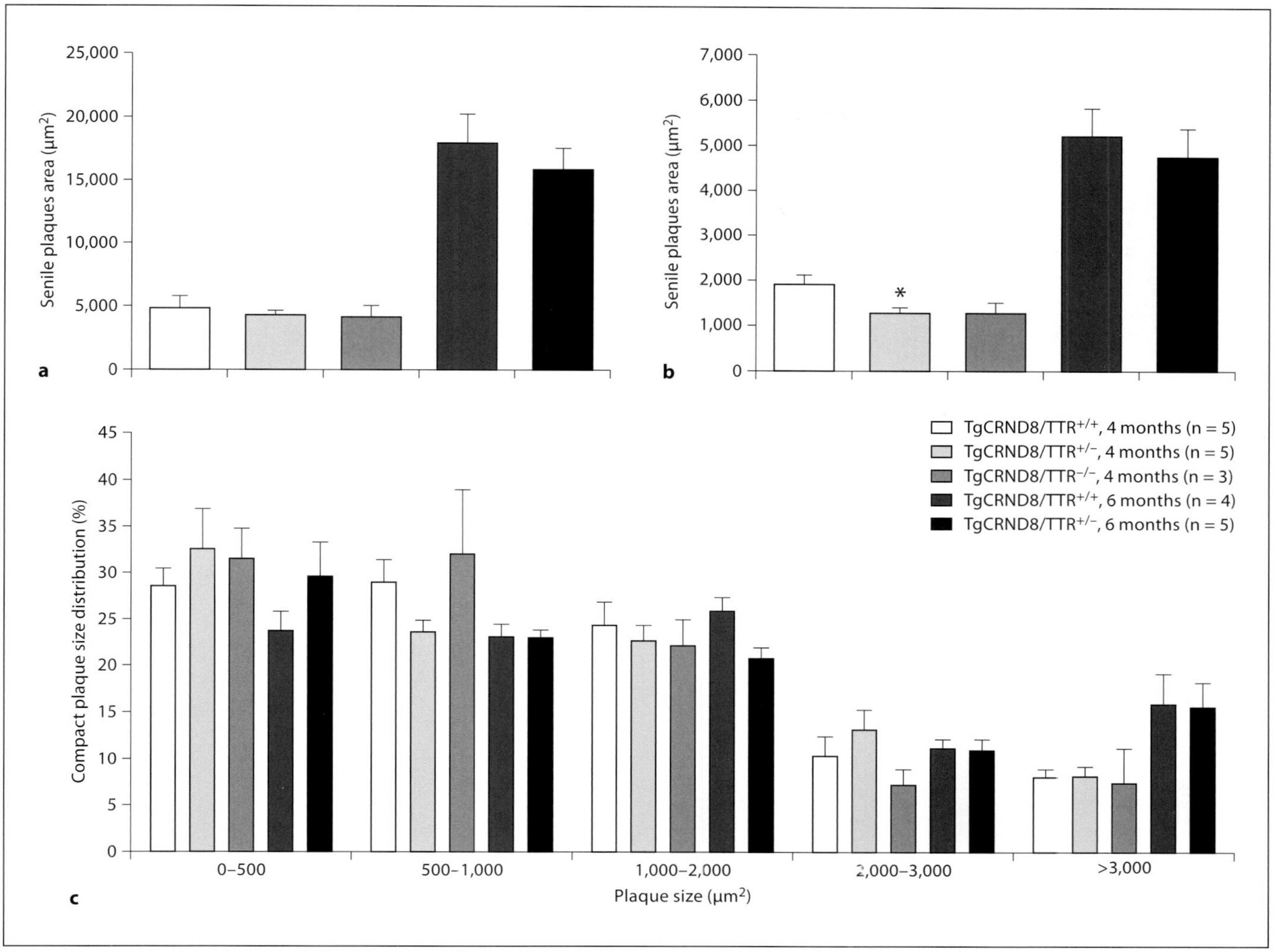

Fig. 1. Quantitative analysis of Aβ burden in the hippocampus of TgCRND8/TTR$^{+/+}$, TgCRND8/TTR$^{+/-}$ and TgCRND8/TTR$^{-/-}$ mice using the 6E10 antibody labeling both compact and diffuse senile plaques (**a**) and 6F3D antibody recognizing only the compact Aβ plaques (**b**). A significant decrease in the area covered by Aβ plaques was observed in 4-month-old TgCRND8/TTR$^{+/-}$ animals using the 6F3D antibody. **c** The level of TTR gene expression did not affect the plaque size distribution. All results are mean ± SEM.

TgCRND8/TTR$^{-/-}$ group were excluded given that only one mouse survived.

There were no significant learning differences between 4- and 6-month-old non-Tg mice (fig. 2a, b). As previously reported [35, 39, 40], TgCRND8 mice at both ages took longer than non-Tg mice to locate the hidden escape platform (fig. 2a, b). Tg APP 695 mice showing hemizygous or homozygous deletion of TTR also displayed a longer escape latency than the wild type on days 3–5 (fig. 2a, b). However, there were no significant differences in learning deficits between the various Tg animals tested here at both ages (fig. 2a, b). Learning deficits were confirmed immediately after the end of training by performing a probe trial of 60 s in which the platform was removed. Tg mice showed no preference for the quadrant that previously contained the platform (fig. 2c) and had fewer platform crossings (fig. 2d). Performance of the various groups during the MWM task could not be attributed to the difference in the swimming speed (fig. 2e) or to visual, sensorimotor or motivational deficits (fig. 2f), as no significant differences were observed in the speed and escape latency to a visible platform.

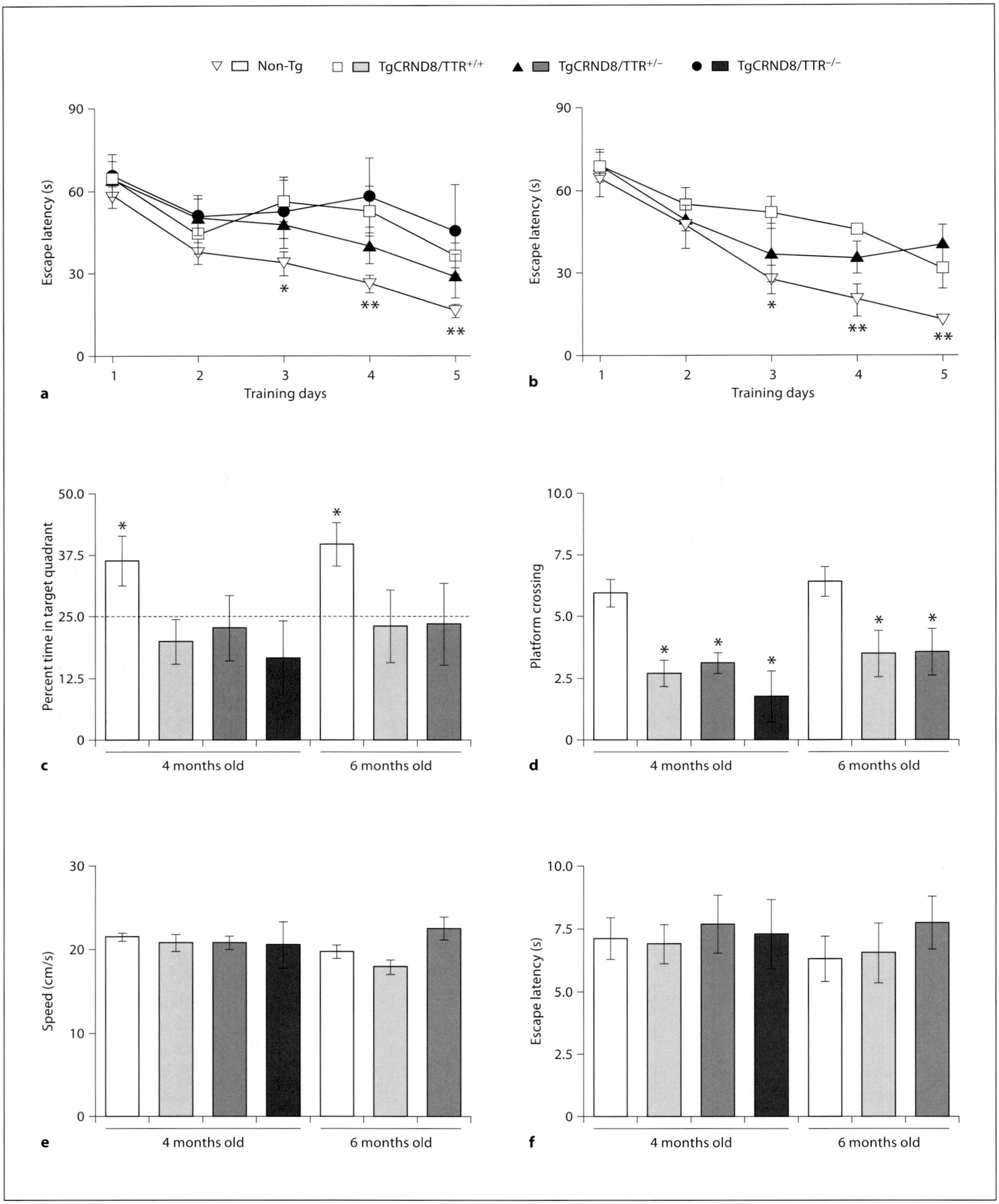

Non-Tg
TgCRND8/TTR+/+
TgCRND8/TTR+/−
TgCRND8/TTR−/−
Escape latency (s)
Training days
a
b
Percent time in target quadrant
Platform crossing
4 months old
6 months old
c
d
Speed (cm/s)
Escape latency (s)
e
f

Discussion

The main result of the present study is the apparent lack of effect of the deletion of the TTR gene on amyloid burden and amyloid plaque size in the hippocampus of 4- and 6-month-old TgCRND8 mice. Similar amyloid plaque deposition was detected among the 3 hybrid Tg mice at each time-point studied. Moreover, all three TgCRND8/TTR genotypes studied here displayed similar spatial memory deficits at both 4 and 6 months of age compared to their non-Tg littermates. Indeed, learning deficits observed in both 4- and 6-month-old TgCRND8 mice expressing TTR were of the same magnitude as those of mice partially (TgCRND8/TTR$^{+/-}$) or fully devoid (TgCRND8/TTR$^{-/-}$) of TTR expression. A very early onset of Aβ deposition, both as compact and diffuse plaques, accompanied by astrogliosis/microgliosis, along with spatial learning deficits has been observed in TgCRND8 mice [35]. For example, at 3 months of age, this Tg AD mouse model displayed amyloid pathology roughly comparable to that of 10-month-old Tg2576 mice [35]. Thus, we can assume that it was too late to observe significant alterations by TTR gene deletion in Aβ plaque burden and memory deficits at 4 and 6 months of age in our rapidly progressing AD hybrid mouse model.

TTR is a homotetrameric protein synthesized by the liver, spleen and choroid plexus [41]. It plays an essential role in the transport of retinol and thyroxine [13, 14]. Our group has recently shown that TTR gene expression is significantly decreased in the hippocampus of memory-impaired versus memory-unimpaired aged rats [11]. Moreover, memory deficits are also observed in aging mice that lack TTR [11, 12]. In addition, we have also reported that retinoic acid treatment reverses cognitive deficits in these knockout mice as well as in aged rats, suggesting that TTR is a critical component of the retinoid pathway for the maintenance of memory capacities during aging [11].

Our initial hypothesis was based on our results from memory-impaired aged rats and TTR KO mice [11], and other studies that proposed a role of TTR as an Aβ scavenger [15–20]. Other previous in vivo and in vitro work has also suggested that TTR plays a role in modulating Aβ fibril formation, aggregation and clearance. For instance, lower levels of brain TTR have been noted in AD patients compared to age-matched controls and were negatively correlated with the number of senile plaques [33, 34]. While the lack of neurodegeneration was associated with increased levels of TTR in the hippocampus of preplaque Tg2576 mice, a Tg AD mouse model [42], a lower TTR transcript expression concomitant with higher Aβ levels has been recently reported in older animals [43]. In other studies, neutralization of TTR by a chronic infusion of a TTR antibody into the hippocampus led to increased levels of Aβ in a mouse model of AD [22], and in Aβ Tg *Caenorhabditis elegans* expressing TTR Aβ aggregation was reduced [44]. Under in vitro conditions, CSF TTR was shown to bind Aβ and to prevent Aβ fibril formation [18], and in cell culture TTR has been shown to inhibit Aβ aggregation and toxicity [45].

Various studies have reported on the existence of a link between amyloid deposition and TTR expression using different Tg mouse models of AD. An increase in brain levels of Aβ and a higher Aβ burden were observed in 7-month-old CeAPPswe/PS1ΔE9 mice with hemizygous deletion of TTR [46]. Similarly, another group found that chronic infusion of an antibody against TTR into the hippocampus of mice overexpressing APP with the Swedish mutation increased the incidence of neuropathological changes including Aβ plaque density [22]. Most recently, Buxbaum et al. [21] examined the role of both murine (mTTR) and human (hTTR) TTR in APP23 mice carrying a Swedish autosomal dominant APP mutation. These mice were crossed with those overexpressing the wild-type hTTR gene (APP23/hTTR), whilst others lacked mTTR (APP23/mTTR$^{-/-}$). Cognitive function was markedly improved in APP23 mice overexpressing hTTR

Fig. 2. TTR gene expression did not alter spatial memory deficits of APP 695 Tg (TgCRND8) mice in the MWM task. Escape latencies before finding the hidden platform (three trials of 90 s per day with a 40-min intertrial interval) were longer in APP Tg animals at 4 (**a**; TgCRND8/TTR$^{+/+}$, n = 7; TgCRND8/TTR$^{+/-}$, n = 9; TgCRND8/TTR$^{-/-}$, n = 4) and 6 (**b**; TgCRND8/TTR$^{+/+}$, n = 6; TgCRND8/TTR$^{+/-}$, n = 7) months compared to age-matched non-Tg littermates (4 months, n = 20; 6 months, n = 7). * $p < 0.05$; ** $p < 0.01$. Escape latencies were not significantly different in TTR-deficient mice harboring APP 695 mutation at both ages. **c** The time spent in the target quadrant during the probe trial by the various Tg animals was around 25% chance level. **d** All APP695 Tg mice harboring various TTR gene expression crossed the previous site of the platform less frequently than non-Tg age-matched littermates (* $p < 0.05$) during the probe trial. No significant difference in swimming speed during the probe trial and a similar escape latency to a visible platform were observed among all the groups. All results are mean ± SEM.

compared to age-matched APP23 mice. Interestingly, amyloid burden was also decreased in APP23 mice carrying hTTR, suggesting that TTR could reduce the formation of Aβ aggregates and plaques [21]. In contrast to these earlier studies, our results suggest that the degree of Aβ plaque burden is not significantly affected by the level of expression of TTR in 4- and 6-month-old TgCRND8 mice. However, our findings are in agreement with a most recent study showing a significant reduction in total and vascular Aβ burden in Tg2576/$TTR^{-/-}$ mice [47]. The dramatic differences between our study and recently published data [21, 46] on the role of TTR deletion in the Aβ deposition in vivo may be due in part to the cDNA construct used and the onset of amyloid pathogenesis. Compared to other APP Tg mice used in similar studies (CeAPPswe/PS1ΔE9, APP23, Tg2576) [21, 46, 47], TgCRND8 mice inherit a highly aggressive amyloidopathy (onset at 3 months of age) accompanied by cognitive deficits [35]. For example, in CeAPPswe/PS1ΔE9 and APP23 mice the first Aβ deposits are found at about 6 months of age [48, 49], while Aβ plaque onset is observed at 9 months of age in Tg2576 mice [35].

Since the effect of TTR deletion may be critical before the onset of Aβ deposition, further studies are underway to examine brain Aβ levels, Aβ plaque burden and spatial learning abilities in TTR-deficient TgCRND8 mice at earlier stage (as early as 4–6 weeks of age) than the current time-points studied, expecting to obtain similar results as those reported in previous studies [21, 46].

Acknowledgements

This work was supported by grants from the Canadian Institutes of Health Research (CIHR) to R.Q. and a student scholarship from CIHR to J.B. The authors also thank Mira Thakur for correcting the manuscript and Dr. Stéphane Bastianetto for useful discussion.

References

1 Goedert M, Spillantini MG: A century of Alzheimer's disease. Science 2006;314:777–781.
2 Artero S, Tierney MC, Touchon J, Ritchie K: Prediction of transition from cognitive impairment to senile dementia: a prospective, longitudinal study. Acta Psychiatr Scand 2003;107:390–393.
3 Perry RJ, Hodges JR: Attention and executive deficits in Alzheimer's disease. A critical review. Brain 1999;122:383–404.
4 Lambon Ralph MA, Patterson K, Graham N, Dawson K, Hodges JR: Homogeneity and heterogeneity in mild cognitive impairment and Alzheimer's disease: a cross-sectional and longitudinal study of 55 cases. Brain 2003;126:2350–2362.
5 Hardy J, Selkoe DJ: The amyloid hypothesis of Alzheimer's disease: progress and problems on the road to therapeutics. Science 2002;297:353–356.
6 Haass C: Take five-BACE and the γ-secretase quartet conduct Alzheimer's amyloid β-peptide generation. EMBO J 2004;23:483–488.
7 Walsh DM, Selkoe DJ: Aβ oligomer – a decade of discovery. J Neurochem 2007;101:1172–1184.
8 Goate A, Chartier-Harlin MC, Mullan M, Brown J, Crawford F, Fidani L, Giuffra L, Haynes A, Irving N, James L, Mant R, Newton P, Rooke K, Roques P, Talbot C, Pericak-Vance M, Roses A, Williamson R, Rossor M, Owen M, Hardy J: Segregation of a missense mutation in the amyloid precursor protein gene with familial Alzheimer's disease. Nature 349;1991:704–706.
9 Campion D, Flaman JM, Brice A, Hannequin D, Dubois B, Martin C, Moreau V, Charbonnier F, Didierjean O, Tardieu S, Penet C, Puel M, Pasquier F, Le Doze F, Bellis G, Calenda A, Heilig R, Martinez M, Mallet J, Bellis M, Clerget-Darpoux F, Agid Y, Frebourg T: Mutations of the presenilin I gene in families with early-onset Alzheimer's disease. Hum Mol Genet 1995;4:2373–2377.
10 Sherrington R, Rogaev EL, Liang Y, Rogaeva EA, Levesque G, Ikeda M, Chi H, Lin C, Li G, Holman K, Tsuda T, Mar L, Foncin J-F, Bruni AC, Montesi MP, Sorbi S, Rainero I Pinessi L, Nee L, Chumakov I, Pollen D, Brookes A, Sanseau P, Polinsky RJ, Wasco W, Da Silva HAR, Haines JL, Pericak-Vance MA, Tanzi RE, Roses AD, Fraser PE, Rommens JM, St George-Hyslop PH: Cloning of the gene bearing missense mutations in early-onset familial Alzheimer's disease. Nature 1995;375:754–760.
11 Brouillette J, Quirion R: Transthyretin: a key gene involved in the maintenance of memory capacities during aging. Neurobiol Aging 2008;29:1721–1732.
12 Sousa JC, Marques, F, Dias-Ferreira E, Cerqueira JJ, Sousa N, Palha JA: Transthyretin influences spatial reference memory. Neurobiol Learn Mem 2007;88:381–385.
13 Chanoine JP, Alex S, Fang SL, Stone S, Leonard JL, Körhle J, Braverman LE: Role of transthyretin in the transport of thyroxine from the blood to the choroid plexus, the cerebrospinal fluid, and the brain. Endocrinology 1992;130:933–938.
14 Monaco HL: The transthyretin-retinol-binding protein complex. Biochim Biophys Acta 2000;1482:65–72.
15 Carro E, Trejo JL, Gomez-Isla T, LeRoith D, Torres-Aleman I: Serum insulin-like growth factor I regulates brain amyloid-β levels. Nat Med 2002;8:1390–1397.
16 Carro E, Trejo JL, Spuch C, Bohl D, Heard JM, Torres-Aleman I: Blockade of the insulin-like growth factor I receptor in the choroid plexus originates Alzheimer's-like neuropathology in rodents: new cues into the human disease? Neurobiol Aging 2006;27:1618–1631.
17 Costa R, Gonçalves A, Saraiva MJ, Cardoso I: Transthyretin binding to Aβ peptide impact on Aβ fibrillogenesis and toxicity. FEBS Lett 2008;582:936–942.
18 Schwarzman AL, Gregori L, Vitek MP, Lyubski S, Strittmatter WJ, Enghilde JJ, Bhasin R, Silverman J, Weisgraber KH, Coyle PK, Zagorski MG, Talafous J, Eseinberg M, Saunders AM, Roses AD, Goldgaber D: Transthyretin sequesters amyloid β protein and prevents amyloid formation. Proc Natl Acad Sci USA 1994;91:8368–8372.
19 Schwarzman AL, Tsiper M, Wente H, Wang A, Vitek MP, Vasiliev V, Goldgaber D: Amyloidogenic and anti-amyloidogenic properties of recombinant transthyretin variants. Amyloid 2004;11:1–9.
20 Sousa JC, Cardoso I, Marques F, Saraiva MJ, Palha JA: Transthyretin and Alzheimer's disease: where in the brain? Neurobiol Aging 2007;28:713–718.

21 Buxbaum JN, Ye Z, Reixach N, Friske L, Levy C, Das P, Golde T, Masliah E, Roberts AR, Bartfai T: Transthyretin protects Alzheimer's mice from the behavioral and biochemical effects of Aβ toxicity. Proc Natl Acad Sci USA 2008;105:2681–2686.
22 Stein TD, Anders NJ, DeCarli C, Chan SL, Mattson MP, Johnson JA: Neutralization of transthyretin reverses the neuroprotective effects of secreted amyloid precursor protein (APP) in APP_{SW} mice resulting in tau phosphorylation and loss of hippocampal neurons: support for the amyloid hypothesis. J Neurosci 2004;24:7707–7717.
23 Lazarov O, Robinson J, Tang Y-P, Hairston IS, Korade-Mirnics Z, Lee V M-Y, Hersh LB, Sapolsky RM, Mirnics K, Sisodia SS: Environmental enrichment reduces Aβ levels and amyloid deposition in transgenic mice. Cell 2005;120:701–713.
24 Connors LH, Lim A, Prokaeva T, Roskens VA, Costello CE: Tabulation of human transthyretin (TTR) variants. Amyloid 2003;10: 160–184.
25 Remes AM, Finnilä S, Mononen H, Tuominen H, Takalo R, Herva R, Majamaa K: Hereditary dementia with intracerebral hemorrhages and cerebral amyloid angiopathy. Neurology 2004;63:234–240.
26 Palha JA, Moreira P, Wisniewshi T, Frangione B, Saraiva MJ: Transthyretin gene in Alzheimer's disease patients. Neurosci Lett 1996;204:212–214.
27 Cuenco KT, Friedland R, Baldwin CT, Guo J, Vardarajan B, Lunetta KL, Cupples LA, Green RC, DeCarli C, Farrer LA: Association of *TTR* polymorphisms with hippocampal atrophy in Alzheimer disease families. Neurobiol Aging DOI:10.1016/j.neurobiolaging.2009.02.014.
28 Castano EM, Roher AE, Esh CL, Kokjohn TA, Beach T: Comparative proteomics of cerebrospinal fluid in neuropathologically-confirmed Alzheimer's disease and non-demented elderly subjects. Neurol Res 2006;28: 155–163.
29 Davidsson P, Sjogren M: Proteome studies of CSF in AD patients. Mech Ageing Dev 2006; 127:133–137.
30 Finehout EJ, Franck Z, Choe LH, Relkin N, Lee KH: Cerebrospinal fluid proteomic biomarkers for Alzheimer's disease. Ann Neurol 2007;61:120–129.
31 Gloeckner SF, Meyne F, Wagner F, Heinemann U, Krasnianski A, Meissner B, Zerr I: Quantitative analysis of transthyretin, tau and amyloid-beta in patients with dementia. J Alzheimers Dis 2008;14:17–25.
32 Lovell MA, Lynn BC, Xiong S, Quinn JF, Kaye J, Markesbery WR: An aberrant protein complex in CSF as a biomarker of Alzheimer disease. Neurology 2008;70:2212–2218.
33 Merched A, Serot JM, Visvikis S, Aguillon D, Faure G, Siest G: Apolipoprotein E, transthyretin and actin in the CSF of Alzheimer's patients: relation with the senile plaques and cytoskeleton biochemistry. FEBS Lett 1998; 425:225–228.
34 Serot J-M, Christmann D, Dubost T, Couturier M: Cerebrospinal fluid transthyretin: aging and late onset Alzheimer's disease. J Neurol Neurosurg Psychiatry 1997;63:506–508.
35 Chishti, MA, Yang DS, Janus C, Phinney AL, Horne P, Pearson J, Strome R, Zuker, N, Loukides J, French J, Turner S, Lozza G, Grilli M, Kunicki S, Morissette C, Paquette J, Gervais F, Bergeron C, Fraser PE, Carlson GA, St George-Hyslop P, Westaway D: Early-onset amyloid deposition and cognitive deficits in transgenic mice expressing a double mutant form of amyloid precursor protein 695. J Biol Chem 2001;276:21562–21570.
36 Dudal S, Morissette C, Lacombe D, Tremblay P, Gervais F: Differences in the amyloid-beta induced inflammatory response in microglia from C57BL/6 and A/J strains of mice. J Neuroimmunol 2004;153:26–35.
37 Episkopou V, Maeda S, Nishiguchi S, Shimada K, Gaitanaris GA, Gottesman ME, Robertson EJ: Disruption of the transthyretin gene results in mice with depressed levels of plasma retinol and thyroid hormone. Proc Natl Acad Sci USA 1993;90:2375–2379.
38 Morris R: Developments of a water-maze procedure for studying spatial learning in the rat. J Neurosci Methods 1984;11:47–60.
39 Hyde LA, Kazdoba TM, Grilli M, Lozza G, Brusa R, Zhang Q, Wong GT, McCool MF, Zhang L, Parker EM, Higgins GA: Age-progressing cognitive impairments and neuropathology in transgenic CRND8 mice. Behav Brain Res 2005;160:344–355.
40 Janus C, Pearson J, McLaurin J, Mathews PM, Jiang Y, Schmidt SD, Chishti MA, Horne P, Heslin D, French J, Mount HTJ, Nixon RA, Mercken M, Bergeron C, Fraser PE, St George-Hyslop P, Westaway D: Aβ peptide immunization reduces behavioural impairment and plaques in a model of Alzheimer's disease. Nature 2000;408:979–982.
41 Hamilton JA, Benson MD: Transthyretin: a review from a structural perspective. Cell Mol Life Sci 2001;58:1491–1521.
42 Stein TD, Johnson JA: Lack of neurodegeneration in transgenic mice overexpressing mutant amyloid precursor protein is associated with increased levels of transthyretin and the activation of cell survival pathways. J Neurosci 2002;22:7380–7388.
43 Tsai KJ, Yang CH, Lee PC, Wang WT, Chiu MJ, Shem CKJ: Asymmetric expression patterns of brain transthyretin in normal mice and a transgenic mouse model of Alzheimer's disease. Neuroscience 2009;159:638–646.
44 Link CD: Expression of human beta-amyloid peptide in transgenic *Caenorhabditis elegans*. Proc Natl Acad Sci USA 1995;92:9368–9372.
45 Giunta S, Valli MB, Galeazzi R, Fattoretti P, Corder EH, Galeazzi L: Transthyretin inhibition of amyloid beta aggregation and toxicity. Clin Biochem 2005;38:1112–1119.
46 Choi SH, Leight SN, Lee VM-Y, Li T, Wong PC, Johnson JA, Saraiva MJ, Sisodia, SS: Accelerated Aβ deposition in APPswe/PS1ΔE9 mice with hemizygous deletions of TTR (transthyretin). J Neurosci 2007;27:7006–7010.
47 Wati H, Kawarabayashi T, Matsubara E, Kasai A, Hirasawa T, Kubota T, Harigaya Y, Shoji M, Maeda S: Transthyretin accelerates vascular Aβ deposition in a mouse model of Alzheimer's disease. Brain Pathol 2009;19: 48–57.
48 Jankowsky JL, Fadale DJ, Anderson J, Xu GM, Gonzales V, Jenkins NA, Copeland NG, Lee MK, Younkin LH, Wagner SL, Youkin SG, Borchelt DR: Mutant presenilins specifically elevate the levels of the 42 residue β-amyloid peptide in vivo; evidence for augmentation of a 42-specific γ secretase. Hum Mol Genet 2004;13:159–170.
49 Sturchler-Pierrat C, Abramowski D, Duke M, Wiederhold K-H, Mistl C, Rothacher S, Ledermann B, Bürki K, Frey P, Paganetti PA, Waridel C, Calhoun ME, Jucker M, Probst A, Staufenbiel M, Sommer B: Two amyloid precursor protein transgenic mouse models with Alzheimer disease-like pathology. Proc Natl Acad Sci USA 1997;94:13287–13292.

Disease Models

Neuro-degenerative Diseases

Neurodegenerative Dis 2010;7:96–98
DOI: 10.1159/000285514

Published online: February 18, 2010

Early-Stage Inflammation and Experimental Therapy in Transgenic Models of the Alzheimer-Like Amyloid Pathology

A.C. Cuello M.T. Ferretti W.C. Leon M.F. Iulita T. Melis A. Ducatenzeiler M.A. Bruno F. Canneva

Department of Pharmacology and Therapeutics, McGill University, Montreal, Que., Canada

Key Words

Alzheimer's disease · Central nervous system · Inflammation · Intracellular Aβ · Aβ oligomers and minocycline

Abstract

Background: Intracellular accumulation of β-amyloid (Aβ) is one of the early features in the neuropathology of Alzheimer's disease (AD) and Down's syndrome. This can be reproduced in cell and transgenic animal models of the AD-like amyloid pathology. In a transgenic rat model, our lab has previously shown that the intracellular accumulation of Aβ is sufficient to provoke cognitive impairments and biochemical alterations in the cerebral cortex and hippocampus in the absence of amyloid plaques. ***Objective:*** To investigate an early, pre-plaque inflammatory process in AD-like transgenic models and establish whether the neurotoxic effects of Aβ oligomers and proinflammatory responses can be arrested with minocycline. ***Methods:*** For these studies, we used naïve mice and transgenic animal models of the AD-like amyloid pathology and applied neurochemical, immunohistochemical and behavioral experimental approaches. ***Results:*** In the early stages of the AD-like amyloid pathology, intracellular Aβ oligomers accumulate within neurons of the cerebral cortex and hippocampus. Coincidental with this, behavioral impairments occur prior to the appearance of amyloid plaques, together with an upregulation of MHC-II, i-NOS and COX-2, well-known proinflammatory markers. Treatment with minocycline corrected behavioral impairments, lowered inflammatory markers and levels of Aβ trimers. ***Conclusion:*** A pharmacological approach targeting the early neuroinflammatory effects of Aβ might be a promising strategy to prevent or delay the onset of AD.

In view of the increasing evidence supporting a pathological role for intracellular neuronal accumulation of β-amyloid (Aβ) in Alzheimer's disease (AD), we generated transgenic animal models overexpressing the human amyloid precursor protein – APP751 – bearing the Swedish (K670N, M671L) and Indiana (V717F) mutations under the control of the murine Thy1.2 promoter. These mono-transgenic animals, coded McGill-Thy1-APP, display the AD-like amyloid pathology in the presence of intracellular Aβ immunoreactive material, prior to the deposition of amyloid plaques.

Immunohistochemical analysis and Western blotting revealed that intracellular accumulation of Aβ oligomers

KARGER

Fax +41 61 306 12 34
E-Mail karger@karger.ch
www.karger.com

1660–2854/10/0073–0096$26.00/0

Accessible online at:
www.karger.com/ndd

A.C. Cuello
Department of Pharmacology and Therapeutics
3655 Promenade Sir-William-Osler, Room 1210
Montreal, QC H3G 1Y6 (Canada)
Tel. +1 514 398 3618, Fax +1 514 398 8317, E-Mail claudio.cuello@mcgill.ca

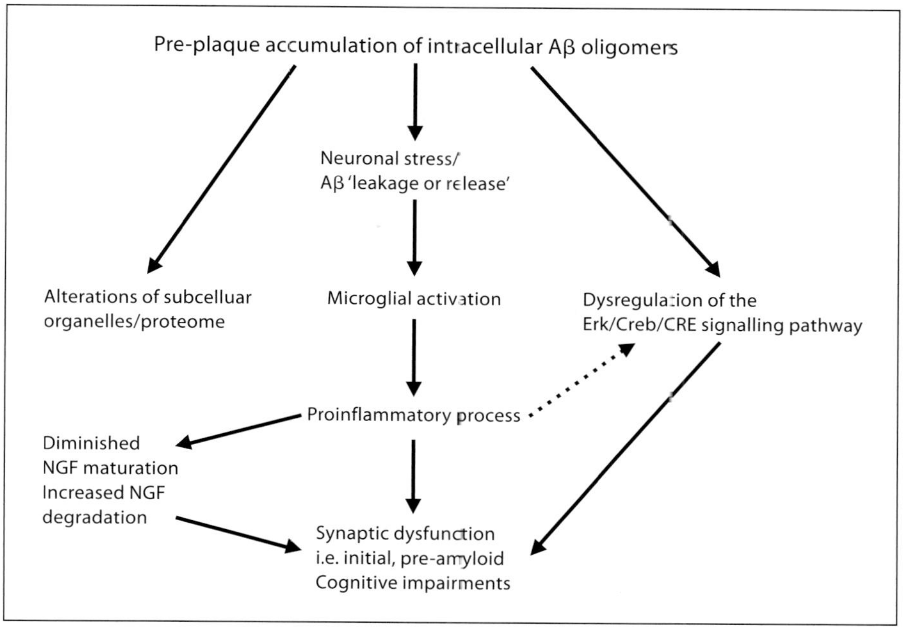

Fig. 1. Schematic representation of the early, pre-plaque components of the AD-like amyloid pathology leading to synaptic dysfunction and cognitive impairments.

Table 1. Effects of early, pre-plaque treatment of McGill-Thy1-APP mice with minocycline on neurochemical and behavioral parameters

Untreated Tg mice	Minocycline-treated Tg mice
i-NOS ↑↑ MHC-II ↑↑ COX-2 ↑↑	Normalized i-NOS, MHC-II and COX-2
Behavioral impairments	Correction of behavioral impairments
Aβ trimers ↑↑↑	Aβ trimers ↑

occurs as early as at 1 week in mice, while amyloid plaque deposition was detected after 3 months of age. The oligomeric nature of the Aβ peptides was confirmed by dot blot and immunohistochemistry of unfixed frozen sections to rule out the possibility that immunoreactivity of fixed tissue was due to artificial aggregates.

Our model also displayed early behavioral impairments in the performance of the Morris Water Maze task. Interestingly, learning and memory deficits occurred when the amyloid pathology was limited to intracellular Aβ oligomerization within pyramidal neurons of the cerebral cortex and hippocampus, prior to the deposition of plaques. Learning and memory were progressively impaired with age and with increasing Aβ load.

In addition, upregulation of specific proinflammatory markers followed the early intracellular accumulation of Aβ oligomers. In particular, Western blotting of hippocampal homogenates revealed an increase in the levels of i-NOS, MHC-II and neuronal COX-2 in Tg animals compared with age-matched non-Tg littermates. COX-2 immunoreactivity was detected in areas associated with Aβ-bearing neurons.

We further stained brain sections from Tg animals with Iba-1, a structural marker for microglia, and morphologically distinguished an early activation of these cells prior to plaque deposition. In contrast, stained sections from control animals revealed resting microglial cells, with a small flattened soma and long, thin, highly ramified processes as opposed to activated cells with larger soma and retraction and thickening of the processes. Immunohistochemical analysis further revealed a recruitment of activated microglial cells around neurons with intracellular accumulation of Aβ oligomers.

The appearance of an early inflammatory response coincidental with the intracellular accumulation of Aβ suggested that inflammation is at least one of the earliest neurotoxic effects of the peptide. Therefore, targeting this early phenomenon with minocycline, which is well known for its anti-inflammatory actions in the central nervous system, which crosses the blood brain barrier and displays limited toxicity of the gastrointestinal tract [for review, see 1], might delay or prevent the AD-like amyloid pathology. As proof of principle, we treated Tg animals with 50 mg/kg of minocycline for a month prior to the appearance of extracellular amyloid plaques, sacrificed them at 3 months of age and observed a decrease in the levels of inflammatory markers. Behavioral deficits were also corrected. Unexpectedly, early treatment also lowered the levels of Aβ trimers (table 1).

In these studies, we have shown that intracellular Aβ oligomerization in transgenic models of the AD-like amyloid pathology is an early phenomenon and prominent in pyramidal neurons of the cerebral cortex and hippocampus. The accumulation of intracellular Aβ oligomers is coincidental with behavioral impairments and proinflammatory responses observed in AD-like transgenic models prior the appearance of amyloid plaques. Furthermore, it is likely that Aβ oligomers unleash the proinflammatory responses as injections of synthetic Aβ oligomer preparations into the hippocampus of naïve rats can elicit a similar inflammatory process, as well as a dysregulation of the nerve growth factor (NGF) metabolism [2]. The NGF dysmetabolism appears very early in the AD-like amyloid pathology and an indication of this can be observed in the brains of MCI sufferers [3].

These Aβ-induced inflammatory changes and behavioral deficits can be arrested with minocycline treatment in both naïve rats (injected with Aβ oligomers in the hippocampus) and in the McGill-Thy1-APP transgenic models. Our lab has previously shown that the pathological intracellular accumulation of Aβ also disrupts the CREB-CRE gene regulation pathway [4–6], which is essential to synaptic plasticity. It is therefore likely that all the above factors affect synaptic function and collectively explain the early cognitive impairments detected prior to the appearance of amyloid plaques, as schematically represented in figure 1.

Acknowledgements

This work was supported by the CIHR grant MOP-62735 and by the US Alzheimer's Association grant IIRG-06-25861. A.C.C. is the holder of a Frosst-Merk endowed chair in Pharmacology. M.T.F is the recipient of a fellowship from Regione Autonoma della Sardegna, Italy. W.C.L. is the recipient of a fellowship from Universidad de Los Andes, Venezuela. M.F.I. is the recipient of the McGill University Provost's Graduate Fellowship. F.C. is a Frosst-Merk Postdoctoral Fellow.

References

1 Yong VW, Wells J, Giuliani F, Casha S, Power C, Metz LM: The promise of minocycline in neurology. Lancet Neurol 2004;3:744–751.

2 Bruno MA, Leon WC, Fragoso G, Mushynski WG, Almazan G, Cuello AC: Aβ-induced NGF dysmetabolism in Alzheimer's disease. J Neuropathol Exp Neurol 2009;68:857–869.

3 Bruno MA, Mufson EJ, Cuello AC: Increased MMP-9 cortical level and activity in subjects with mild cognitive impairment (abstract 2007-A-101716-SFN). 37th Annu Meet Soc Neurosci Annu Meet, San Diego, November 2007.

4 Echeverria V, et al: Altered mitogen-activated protein kinase signaling, tau hyperphosphorylation and mild spatial learning dysfunction in transgenic rats expressing the beta-amyloid peptide intracellularly in hippocampal and cortical neurons. Neuroscience 2004;129:583–592.

5 Echeverria V, Ducatenzeiler A, Chen CH, Cuello AC: Endogenous beta-amyloid peptide synthesis modulates cAMP response element-regulated gene expression in PC12 cells. Neuroscience 2005;135:1193–1202.

6 Arvanitis DN, Ducatenzeiler A, Ou JN, Grodstein E, Andrews SD, Tendulkar SR, Ribeiro-da-Silva A, Szyf M, Cuello AC: High intracellular concentrations of amyloid-beta block nuclear translocation of phosphorylated CREB. J Neurochem 2007;103:216–228.

Disease Models

Neuro-degenerative Diseases

Neurodegenerative Dis 2010;7:99–102
DOI: 10.1159/000285515

Published online: February 18, 2010

Transgenic Zebrafish as a Novel Animal Model to Study Tauopathies and Other Neurodegenerative Disorders in vivo

Dominik Paquet Bettina Schmid Christian Haass

Deutsches Zentrum für Neurodegenerative Erkrankungen – Standort München and Adolf-Butenandt-Institute, Department of Biochemistry, Ludwig-Maximilians University, Munich, Germany

Key Words
Zebrafish · Gal4-UAS · Tau · Alzheimer's disease · Frontotemporal dementia · Drug screening

Abstract
Our ageing society is confronted with a dramatic increase in patients suffering from tauopathies such as Alzheimer's disease, frontotemporal dementia and others. Typical neuropathological lesions including tangles composed of hyperphosphorylated tau protein as well as severe neuronal cell death characterize these disorders. No mechanism-based cures are available at present. Genetically modified animals are invaluable models to understand the molecular disease mechanisms and to screen for modifying compounds. We recently introduced tau-transgenic zebrafish as a novel model for tauopathies. Our model allows recapitulating key pathological features of tauopathies within an extremely short time. Moreover, life imaging of tau-dependent neuronal cell death was performed for the very first time. This demonstrated tau-dependent neuronal cell loss independent of tangle formation. Finally, we exemplified that the zebrafish frontotemporal dementia model can be used to screen for drugs that prevent abnormal tau phosphorylation and neuronal cell death.

Neurodegenerative diseases including Alzheimer's disease (AD) and frontotemporal dementia (FTD) are the most frequent cause of dementia in our ageing society. These disorders are characterized by posttranslationally modified amyloidogenic proteins, such as amyloid β-peptide (Aβ) in AD and tau in AD and FTD, which form neurotoxic oligomers and are finally deposited as insoluble amyloid fibers in senile plaques or tangles [1–3].

Neurodegenerative diseases with deposition of insoluble tau protein are now commonly termed tauopathies. The tau protein is an important target for drug development, since its pathological alterations correlate with disease progression and memory loss in AD and other tauopathies [4]. Moreover, tau suppression improves memory function in transgenic FTD models [5]. Furthermore, mutations in the tau gene, such as the Tau-P301L mutation, have been identified in patients with a genetically inherited form of autosomal dominant FTD [6]. Among the first pathological alterations of tau is its pathologic phosphorylation at multiple residues [2]. Subsequently, the hyperphosphorylated tau species become insoluble and form paired helical filaments, which are finally deposited in the cell bodies of neurons as neurofibrillary tangles (NFT). The biochemical and pathological properties of tau have been extensively studied both in vitro and in vivo. Over the last decade, several tau trans-

KARGER

Fax +41 61 306 12 34
E-Mail karger@karger.ch
www.karger.com

1660–2854/10/0073–0099$26.00/0

Accessible online at:
www.karger.com/ndd

Christian Haass, PhD
Deutsches Zentrum für Neurodegenerative Erkrankungen, Standort München
Adolf-Butenandt-Institute, Department of Biochemistry
Ludwig-Maximilians University, Schillerstrasse 44, DE–80336 Munich (Germany)
Tel. +49 89 2180 75472, Fax +49 89 2180 415, E-Mail chaass@med.uni-muenchen.de

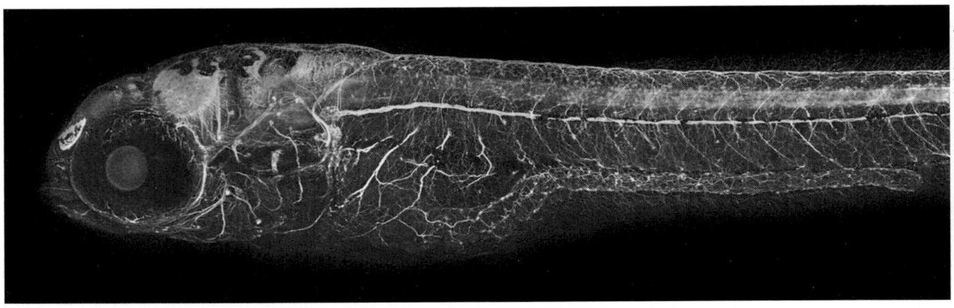

Fig. 1. The translucent body of zebrafish larvae allows imaging of cellular and subcellular processes in high detail. Triple immunostaining of a 5-day-old tau-transgenic zebrafish, using antibodies against acetylated tubulin, showing neuronal projections in green, total tau in red and AT8-phosphorylated tau in blue.

genic animal models have been developed. Invertebrates such as worms and flies and vertebrates like mice have been used to understand pathogenic mechanisms [for detailed reviews, see 7, 8]. In addition, chemical modifiers of the disease which could be further explored to develop novel treatment approaches have been investigated in these animals. Invertebrate systems offer experimental advantages, including low costs, small size, excellent genetic tractability, a simple and rapidly developing nervous system and a short life span. However, the evolutionary and morphological distance between invertebrates and humans makes the direct translation of experimental results rather difficult and unreliable. Therefore, neurotoxic mechanisms evoked by amyloidogenic proteins may be more faithfully reproduced in vertebrate brains. For this reason, transgenic mice have been the major species used for modeling AD and FTD.

The generation of these mouse models began with the expression of wild-type tau, which led to its pathologic phosphorylation, but not filament formation. This key feature of tauopathies was only reproduced upon expressing tau with familial FTD-associated tau mutations. Subsequently, the FTD-like phenotypes could be further enhanced by the addition of Aβ, indicating cross-talk between Aβ and tau aggregation. Finally, coexpression of mutant tau with the Swedish mutation of the β-amyloid precursor protein as well as the familial AD-associated presenilin 1 M146V mutation, led to the enhanced formation of NFTs, again supporting the amyloid cascade hypothesis. However, tau seems to be the primary mediator of toxicity and memory loss, since inhibition of tau expression in such triple transgenic mice allowed recovery of memory and a reduction in neuronal cell loss. Interestingly, under these conditions NFTs continued to accumulate, suggesting that soluble tau oligomers but not tangles may be the primary neurotoxic species [1, 7, 8].

The abovementioned models greatly expanded our knowledge on the formation of the typical neuropathology of AD and FTD and the pathologic misfunction of disease-associated genes. However, the initial steps leading to tau phosphorylation and synaptic dysfunction, which in humans may occur presymptomatically are still poorly understood in vivo. It is extremely difficult to investigate early subtle changes and disease propagation in living mice, since their brain is not readily accessible for imaging and they need a rather long time to develop disease symptoms. In addition, large-scale screening for anti-aggregation drugs, or neurotoxicity-ameliorating compounds, is not feasible in mice. Transgenic zebrafish larvae combine many of the advantages of invertebrate and vertebrate models. Their translucent body allows whole-body imaging of cellular and subcellular processes in high detail (fig. 1) both in fixed animals and in vivo [9]. In addition, large-scale compound screens, which are feasible due to the small size of the fish larvae, have already been performed [10]. Two zebrafish models of tauopathies have already been described. Tomasiewicz et al. [11] injected cDNA constructs encoding human Tau-GFP fusion proteins into zebrafish eggs to study tau pathology. While this approach led to tau phosphorylation at a pathologically relevant epitope in a small number of neurons expressing the injected DNA, it failed to generate transgenic lines with stable and reproducible expression. In addition, tangle formation, disease progression as well as neuronal loss were not described. The generation of stable transgenic lines was first achieved by Bai et al. [12], who described a human tau-transgenic fish using the zebrafish Enolase2 promoter. This promoter allowed expressing tau specifically in the nervous system; however, no signs of tau pathology were observed at larval stages of development. This might be due to insufficient tau protein levels, since high expression levels have been shown to be essential for a concentration-dependent amyloid aggregation mechanism in model systems [13]. We have therefore developed a Gal4-UAS-based expression system to efficiently generate transgenic zebrafish overexpressing high levels of human Tau-P301L or other disease-associated proteins under control of the neuronal zebrafish HuC promoter. The Gal4-UAS system amplifies gene expression by both the strong herpes simplex virus VP16 transcriptional activator, which is fused to Gal4, and the use of 14 UAS sites, to which the Gal4-VP16 binds [14]. The tau-transgenic fish rapidly reproduced pathological signatures of tauopathies already in early developmental stages in a time-dependent manner [15]. Pathological misfolding of tau and hyperphosphorylation at several well-studied epitopes occurred within a few hours of development, and expression of late-stage pathological markers, such as AT8, rapidly progressed over time. Furthermore, NFTs with typical neuropathological features developed after 5 weeks. In addition, the fish displayed abnormal motoneuron function, leading to a retarded escape response. After a few days, they also developed significant neurodegeneration in the nervous system, and the new model allowed for the first time to image the degeneration of neurons live in an animal model by in vivo time-lapse microscopy. Strikingly, tau-dependent neuronal cell loss was observed well before tangles formed. Thus, our findings may suggest that in contrast to the common opinion, tangles themselves are not neurotoxic but rather soluble tau oligomers. Alternatively, elevated levels of tau monomers might also be toxic, as they may trap cellular proteins and prevent them from executing their physiological functions.

We also used the fish to identify and validate newly developed drugs, which may modify the pathologic hyperphosphorylation of tau. Hyperphosphorylation is believed to be a key initiator of detachment of normal tau from microtubules and subsequent oligomerization and aggregation. Preventing hyperphosphorylation by kinase inhibitors could slow further progression of pathology and thus be an efficient treatment option for AD and FTD [16]. These inhibitors can be developed on a large scale by structure-based design [17], but this approach requires in vivo validation in cell culture and animal models. We validated two newly identified inhibitors of GSK3, a major kinase in tau phosphorylation [18]. Interestingly, one compound was highly active in preventing abnormal tau phosphorylation, while the other was completely inactive in fish, though equally potent in cell culture. The inactivity of one of the inhibitors could be due to low penetration through the developing blood-brain barrier or rapid degradation or metabolism of the compound. This result illustrates the usefulness of the fish model as an effective in vivo screening tool to quickly and directly identify promising compounds and eliminate substances without reasonable in vivo activity early in the screening process. In addition, the tauopathy-like phenotypes of the transgenic zebrafish may also allow performing unbiased large-scale compound screens to identify new drug targets and new compounds capable not only of reducing tau hyperphosphorylation, but also of restoring axonal transport deficits and preventing synapse dysfunction as well as neuronal cell death.

Since the versatility of the Gal4/UAS-based vector system also allows to quickly subclone and express other proteins associated with neurodegenerative disease, the advantages of the fish system may now also be used to study related disease, such as Parkinson disease or the tau-negative cases of FTD.

Taken together, transgenic zebrafish could be a promising tool to further elucidate the early pathological processes leading synaptic dysfunction in neurodegenerative diseases and also to streamline pharmacological screening for new and effective drugs.

Acknowledgements

This work was supported by grants from the Deutsche Forschungsgemeinschaft (SFB 596 to B.S. and C.H.; the Center for Integrated Protein Science, to C.H. and B.S., and the Leibniz Award, to C.H.), Elitenetzwerk Bayern and Universität Bayern (to D.P.), and from the European Community's Seventh Framework Programme (FP7/2007-2013) under grant agreement No. 200611 (MEMOSAD, to C.H., B.S., and D.P.). C.H. is supported by a 'Research Professorship' of the LMU.

References

1 Haass C, Selkoe DJ: Soluble protein oligomers in neurodegeneration: lessons from the Alzheimer's amyloid beta-peptide. Nat Rev Mol Cell Biol 2007;8:101–112.
2 Grundke-Iqbal I, Iqbal K, Tung YC, Quinlan M, Wisniewski HM, Binder LI: Abnormal phosphorylation of the microtubule-associated protein tau (tau) in Alzheimer cytoskeletal pathology. Proc Natl Acad Sci USA 1986; 83:4913–4917.
3 Kosik KS, Joachim CL, Selkoe DJ: Microtubule-associated protein tau (tau) is a major antigenic component of paired helical filaments in Alzheimer disease. Proc Natl Acad Sci USA 1986;83:4044–4048.
4 Braak H, Braak E: Neuropathological stageing of Alzheimer-related changes. Acta Neuropathol 1991;82:239–259.

5 Santacruz K, Lewis J, Spires T, Paulson J, Kotilinek L, Ingelsson M, Guimaraes A, DeTure M, Ramsden M, McGowan E, Forster C, Yue M, Orne J, Janus C, Mariash A, Kuskowski M, Hyman B, Hutton M, Ashe KH: Tau suppression in a neurodegenerative mouse model improves memory function. Science 2005; 309:476–481.

6 Hutton M, Lendon CL, Rizzu P, Baker M, Froelich S, Houlden H, Pickering-Brown S, Chakraverty S, Isaacs A, Grover A, Hackett J, Adamson J, Lincoln S, Dickson D, Davies P, Petersen RC, Stevens M, de Graaff E, Wauters E, van Baren J, Hillebrand M, Joosse M, Kwon JM, Nowotny P, Che LK, Norton J, Morris JC, Reed LA, Trojanowski J, Basun H, Lannfelt L, Neystat M, Fahn S, Dark F, Tannenberg T, Dodd PR, Hayward N, Kwok JB, Schofield PR, Andreadis A, Snowden J, Craufurd D, Neary D, Owen F, Oostra BA, Hardy J, Goate A, van Swieten J, Mann D, Lynch T, Heutink P: Association of missense and 5′-splice-site mutations in tau with the inherited dementia FTDP-17. Nature 1998;393: 702–705.

7 Götz J, Deters N, Doldissen A, Bokhari L, Ke Y, Wiesner A, Schonrock N, Ittner L: A decade of tau transgenic animal models and beyond. Brain Pathol 2007;17:91–103.

8 Götz J, Ittner L: Animal models of Alzheimer's disease and frontotemporal dementia. Nat Rev Neurosci 2008;9:532–544.

9 Rubinstein AL: Zebrafish: from disease modeling to drug discovery. Curr Opin Drug Discov Devel 2003;6:218–223.

10 Zon LI, Peterson RT: In vivo drug discovery in the zebrafish. Nat Rev Drug Discov 2005; 4:35–44.

11 Tomasiewicz HG, Flaherty DB, Soria JP, Wood JG: Transgenic zebrafish model of neurodegeneration. J Neurosci Res 2002;70: 734–745.

12 Bai Q, Garver JA, Hukriede NA, Burton EA: Generation of a transgenic zebrafish model of tauopathy using a novel promoter element derived from the zebrafish eno2 gene. Nucleic Acids Res 2007;35:6501–6516.

13 Price DL, Sisodia SS, Borchelt DR: Genetic neurodegenerative diseases: the human illness and transgenic models. Science 1998; 282:1079–1083.

14 Koster RW, Fraser SE: Tracing transgene expression in living zebrafish embryos. Dev Biol 2001;233:329–346.

15 Paquet D, Bhat R, Sydow A, Mandelkow E, Berg S, Hellberg S, Fälting J, Distel M, Köster RW, Schmid B, Haass C: A zebrafish model of tauopathy allows in vivo imaging of neuronal cell death and drug evaluation. J Clin Invest 2009;119:1382–1395.

16 Mazanetz MP, Fischer PM: Untangling tau hyperphosphorylation in drug design for neurodegenerative diseases. Nat Rev Drug Discov 2007;6:464–479.

17 Bhat R, Xue Y, Berg S, Hellberg S, Ormo M, Nilsson Y, Radesater AC, Jerning E, Markgren PO, Borgegard T, Nylof M, Gimenez-Cassina A, Hernandez F, Lucas JJ, Diaz-Nido J, Avila J: Structural insights and biological effects of glycogen synthase kinase 3-specific inhibitor ar-a014418. J Biol Chem 2003;278:45937–45945.

18 Doble BW, Woodgett JR: Gsk-3: tricks of the trade for a multi-tasking kinase. J Cell Sci 2003;116:1175–1186.

Disease Models

Neuro-degenerative Diseases

Neurodegenerative Dis 2010;7:103–107
DOI: 10.1159/000285516

Published online: February 18, 2010

Generation of Tau Aggregates and Clearance by Autophagy in an Inducible Cell Model of Tauopathy

Y. Wang U. Krüger E. Mandelkow E.-M. Mandelkow

Max-Planck Unit for Structural Molecular Biology, Hamburg, Germany

Key Words
Alzheimer's disease · Autophagy · Paired helical filaments · Tau protein · Protein aggregation · Proteolysis

Abstract
We have studied the mechanism of aggregation in an inducible cell model of Tau pathology. When the repeat domain of human Tau (Tau_{RD}) carrying the FTDP-17 mutation ΔK280 is expressed, the cells develop aggregates, as seen by thioflavin S fluorescence, electron microscopy, and sarkosyl extraction methods. By contrast, mutants of Tau_{RD} that are unable to generate β-structure do not aggregate. Enhanced aggregation leads to enhanced toxicity, visible by live cell microscopy and LDH release assay. The aggregation process is initiated by the sequential cleavage of Tau_{RD} which yields highly amyloidogenic fragments. This cleavage occurs only with proaggregant Tau_{RD}, and not with the nonaggregating mutants, indicating that β-structure makes Tau_{RD} vulnerable to both proteolytic degradation and aggregation. Aggregation is reversed by switching off the expression of Tau_{RD}, by inhibitor compounds, and by certain protease inhibitors. In all cases, the enhanced toxicity is rescued. The clearance of the aggregates involves autophagy, whereas proteasomal degradation plays only a minor role.

Introduction

Tau, a microtubule-associated protein which occurs mainly in the central nervous system, is upregulated during neuronal differentiation, and localizes mainly to neuronal axons [1, 2]. Tau is highly soluble due to its large fraction of hydrophilic amino acids [3]; nevertheless, Tau forms insoluble aggregates in Alzheimer's disease and other neurodegenerative diseases termed tauopathies [for reviews see 4, 5]. Therefore, it is one of the prime objectives of AD research to understand the mechanism of Tau aggregation and to develop strategies for preventing or reversing the aggregation [6].

Because of the unusual solubility of Tau protein, it has been difficult to develop cell or animal models that mimic the aggregation. In the case of transgenic mice, robust aggregation was achieved only with the enhanced expression of Tau proteins that harbor one of the FTDP-17 mutations [7]. In the case of cell models, the difficulties are compounded by the short lifetimes of cells that are normally not sufficient for the aggregation process to occur [8]. To overcome these problems we made use of the mutation ΔK280 because this shows a particularly high tendency to aggregate in vitro [9]. This can be explained by the high propensity for β-structure in the repeat domain which forms the core of Alzheimer paired helical filaments (PHFs) [10, 11].

KARGER

Fax +41 61 306 12 34
E-Mail karger@karger.ch
www.karger.com

1660–2854/10/0073–0103$26.00/0

Accessible online at:
www.karger.com/ndd

E.-M. Mandelkow
Max-Planck Unit for Structural Molecular Biology
Notkestrasse 85
DE–22607 Hamburg (Germany)
Tel. +49 40 8998 2810, Fax +49 40 8971 6822, E-Mail mand@mpasmb.desy.de

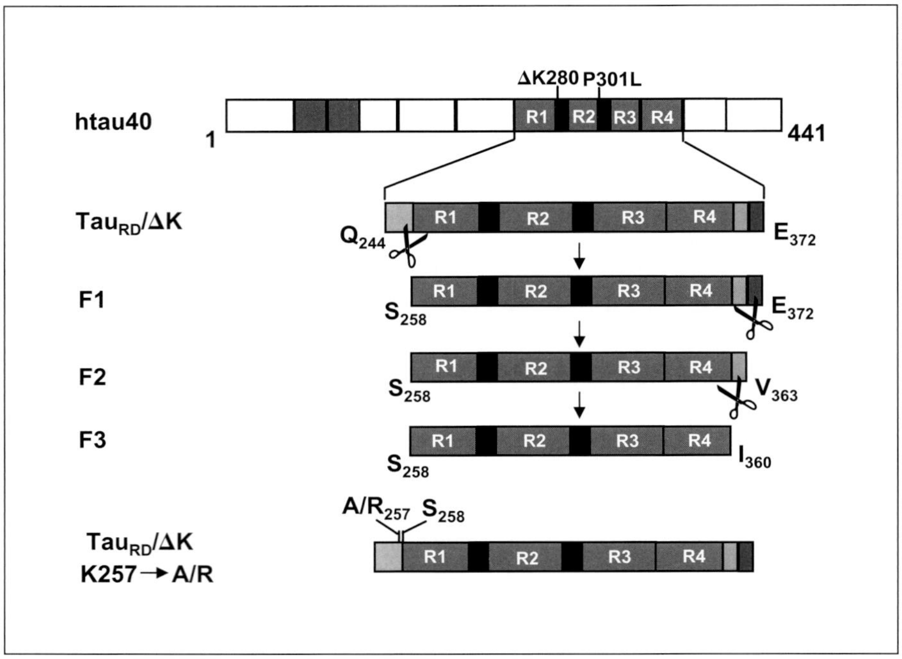

Fig. 1. Diagram of Tau, Tau fragments, and cleavage sites. Top: Tau isoform htau40 and positions of FTDP17 mutations ΔK280 and P301L. Bottom: repeat domain Tau_{RD}/ΔK (M-Q_{244}-E_{372}) and fragments F1, F2, F3. Scissors indicate cleavage sites behind K257 and near residue 360. The cleavage near the N-terminus is prevented if K257 is replaced by A or R; this also prevents the subsequent cleavages. The assembly-promoting hexapeptide motifs at the beginning of R2 and R3 are shown in black.

Color version available online

The ΔK280 mutation has been described for several cases of FTDP-17 [12–14]. The mutation is enigmatic because on the mRNA level the mutation lies within exon 10 and favors the exclusion of this exon by alternative splicing, due to the disruption of an existing exon splicing enhancer [15]. This results in Tau isoforms having only three repeats (R1, R3, R4) but lacking R2, encoded by exon 10 (in contrast to many other FTDP17 mutations which favor inclusion of exon 10 and therefore lead to four-repeat Tau isoforms). Thus, theoretically, one would not expect any protein carrying the ΔK280 mutation, and therefore the enhanced β-propensity should not become apparent on the protein level. In practice, the fraction of the more amyloidogenic mutant four-repeat Tau is reduced but still substantial enough to account for an increased level of aggregates.

Independently of the situation in the human brain, the high β-propensity of the ΔK280 mutant Tau makes it an interesting option for developing cell and mouse models of Tau aggregation. We developed mouse models expressing either full-length Tau, or only the repeat domain [16, 17]. The shorter construct offers the advantage of developing aggregates much more rapidly, due to the fact that the repeat domain represents the assembly unit of PHFs, whereas the N- and C-terminal flanking domains tend to retard aggregation. In the case of the short-lived cell models, full-length Tau-ΔK280 does not lead to aggregates, but the repeat domain Tau_{RD}-ΔK280 does. This opened an opportunity to investigate the mechanism of aggregation in more detail [9, 18]. As shown below, aggregation is preceded by proteolytic processing which generates fragments with an even higher amyloidogenicity. Furthermore, since aggregation is reversible when the expression of the protein is switched off, the cell model allows one to study the pathway of degradation. Here, we show that this occurs mainly by the autophagy-lysosomal pathway.

Results and Discussion

Figure 1 illustrates the relationship between full-length Tau (carrying the FTDP17 mutation ΔK280), the repeat domain with four repeats (Tau_{RD}/ΔK), and the fragments generated by successive cleavage by intracellular proteolysis. The first cleavage occurs before residue S258 generating fragment F1, the second after V363 generating F2, and the third after I360 generating F3. The proteins Tau_{RD}/ΔK and its first cleavage product F1 aggregate rather slowly, but fragments F2 and especially F3 are much more amyloidogenic and rapidly lead to aggregates which can be detected in the sarkosyl-insoluble pellet.

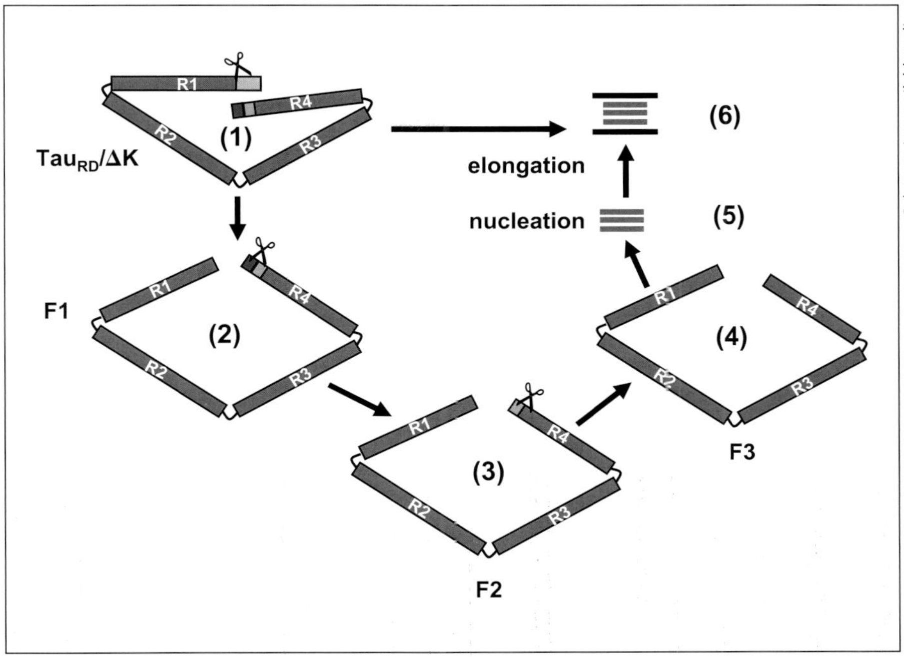

Fig. 2. Model of Tau$_{RD}$ conformation explaining the sequential cleavage. In the model, the N-terminal region protects the C-terminal part (state 1). Cleavage near the N-terminus (state 2) removes the protection and allows cleavages near the C-terminus (states 3, 4). The fragment F3 thus generated can aggregate by itself and nucleate PHFs (state 5) and then also coaggregates with Tau$_{RD}$/ΔK or full-length Tau if present (state 6).

Color version available online

The first cleavage (K257-S258) can be prevented by mutating the surrounding residues, suggesting a protease with the target specificity similar to thrombin (a serine protease); and indeed the cleavage can be prevented by the thrombin inhibitor PPACK. Surprisingly, the cleavage can also be prevented if one eliminates the β-propensity in the hexapeptide motifs (275-VQIINK-280 and 306-VQIVYK-311) by inserting prolines (e.g. I277P and I308P). This means that an extended, β-like conformation of the polypeptide chain in the hexapeptide motifs is necessary for the first cleavage, although the cleavage site is ~20 residues upstream of the hexapeptide motif. Even more surprising is the fact that the second and third cleavages (near the C-terminus, generating F2 and F3) occurs only after the first one. These observations suggest that the repeat domain must have a particular conformation, such that the N-terminal part protects the C-terminal part against proteolytic attack. These relationships are diagrammed in figure 2.

Once the fragment F3 is generated by processing near the N- and C-terminus, it begins to aggregate because of its high β-propensity. Consequently, F3 accumulates almost entirely in the sarkosyl-insoluble fraction. By contrast, the parent protein and fragment F1 are mostly found in the soluble fraction. F2 is short-lived since it is rapidly converted to F3, and is found in the insoluble pellet. The important feature of this process is that the nuclei of F3 aggregation can induce the intact parent protein to coaggregate, so that this begins to appear in the insoluble fraction as well. More generally, even full-length Tau molecules can participate in the coaggregation, in spite of their inherent high solubility which would otherwise prevent it from becoming aggregated. This is akin to the heterologous nucleation of rain drops in a humid atmosphere by dust particles.

One important question addressed in this study concerns the reversibility of aggregation. When the expression of the exogenous Tau is allowed to proceed (in the presence of doxycyclin), aggregates continue to accumulate until the cells die after 11 days. However, when the expression of foreign Tau is first induced for several days and then discontinued (by withdrawal of doxycyclin), the fraction of soluble foreign Tau gradually disappears within 6 days, as expected. Surprisingly, the fraction of aggregated Tau disappears as well over a similar time period. This means that the cell still possesses the ability to dispose of the aggregates, and suggests that the aggregates are more dynamic than expected.

We next searched for the mechanism by which the cell clears the aggregates. Several models can be envisaged. One is the regulated disassembly by a change in the state of the cell. This would be akin to the dissolution of other cellular polymers, e.g. physiological ones (disassembly of microtubules upon completion of mitosis) or pathologi-

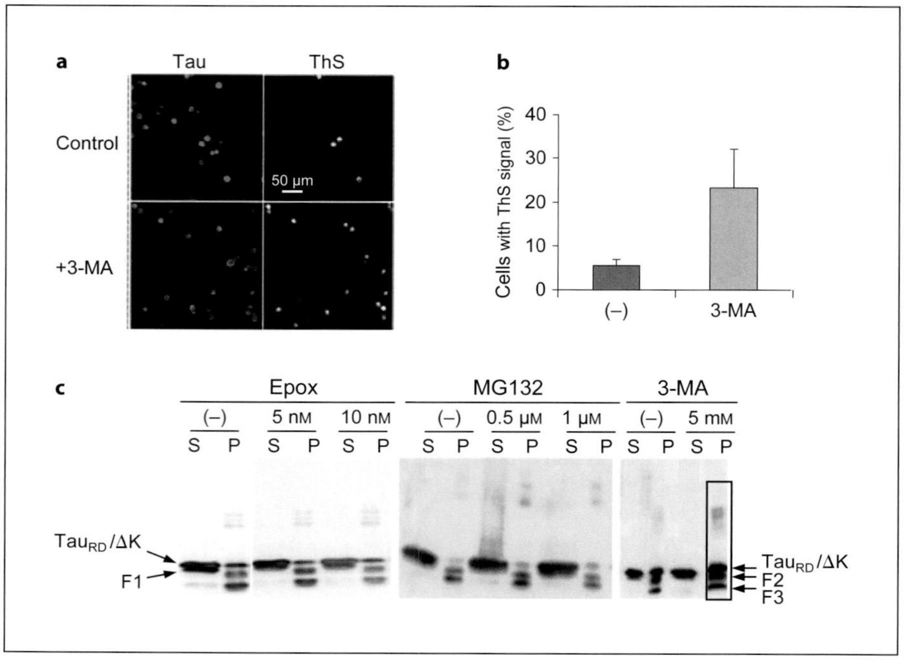

Fig. 3. Degradation of aggregates involves autophagy but not the proteasome. **a** Thioflavin S (ThS) staining of N2a cells showing the influence of the autophagy inhibitor with 3-methyladenine (3-MA) on the aggregation of $Tau_{RD}/\Delta K$. Left: Tau expression of cells is visualized by antibody. Right: thioflavin S staining of aggregates. **b** Quantification of thioflavin S-positive cells, which increase ~5-fold by 3-MA. **c** Blot analysis of effects of proteasomal inhibitors (epoxomicin or MG132) or macroautophagy inhibitors (3-MA) on the degradation of $Tau_{RD}/\Delta K$. N2a cells overexpressing $Tau_{RD}/\Delta K$ were treated with these inhibitors for 5 days. Lanes labeled P (pellet) denote sarkosyl-insoluble Tau species, S (supernatant) indicates soluble proteins. Note that 3-MA but not MG132 or epoxomicin inhibits the cleavage and aggregation of $Tau_{RD}/\Delta K$ (see increase in Tau, Tau fragments and high-molecular-weight species in the box on the right).

Color version available online

cal ones (disassembly of hemoglobin S fibers upon binding of oxygen). A second mechanism is the degradation by cytosolic proteases, such as proteasomes and associated proteases [19]. A third mechanism is the sequestration of the polymers by autophagic vesicles and subsequent degradation in the lysosomes. A fourth mechanism would be the exocytosis into the extracellular environment. All of these mechanisms may take place simultaneously. However, our studies with different inhibitors indicate that the largest contribution comes from macroautophagy, as illustrated in figure 3. It shows that the inhibition of macroautophagy by 3-MA leads to a strong accumulation of Tau aggregates, whereas the inhibition of proteasomes by MG-132 or epoxomicin has no major effect [20]. Note that this result holds in particular for Tau aggregates, whereas soluble Tau may be digested by proteasomes, as suggested by several authors [21, 22].

Finally, one should note that the reversibility of Tau aggregation in cells suggests that it should be possible to prevent them by aggregation inhibitor compounds. This is indeed the case, using compounds that were identified by an in vitro screen for such inhibitors [23, 24]. Treatment of the cells with inhibitors not only reduces aggregation, but also the toxicity of Tau which closely correlates with aggregation. Thus, future research will be aimed at testing and delivering aggregation inhibitors to cells and Tau-transgenic animals. Other approaches to lower aggregates seem possible as well, for example the inhibition of proteases that generate amyloidogenic fragments, or the activation of autophagy by rapamycin [25, 26]. Our recent results showed that cathepsin L, a lysosomal protease, contributes to the generation of aggregation-prone fragments F2 and F3 (fig. 1, 2), indicating that the lysosome plays a complex role in both the generation of aggregates and their removal [20].

Acknowledgements

We thank S. Hübschmann and I. Lindner for preparing Tau proteins. This work was supported by Max-Planck-Gesellschaft, Deutsche Forschungsgemeinschaft, Breuer-Foundation, Volkswagen Foundation, and EU/FP7 through the Memosad consortium.

References

1 Drubin DG, Feinstein SC, Shooter EM, Kirschner MW: Nerve growth factor-induced neurite outgrowth in PC12 cells involves the coordinate induction of microtubule assembly and assembly-promoting factors. J Cell Biol 1985;101:1799–1807.

2 Binder LI, Frankfurter A, Rebhun LI: The distribution of tau in the mammalian central nervous system. J Cell Biol 1985;101:1371–1378.

3 Lee G, Cowan N, Kirschner M: The primary structure and heterogeneity of tau protein from mouse brain. Science 1988;239:285–288.
4 Lee VM, Goedert M, Trojanowski JQ: Neurodegenerative tauopathies. Annu Rev Neurosci 2001;24:1121–1159.
5 Garcia ML, Cleveland DW: Going new places using an old MAP: tau, microtubules and human neurodegenerative disease. Curr Opin Cell Biol 2001;13:41–48.
6 Schneider A, Mandelkow E: Tau-based treatment strategies in neurodegenerative diseases. Neurotherapeutics 2008;5:443–457.
7 Lewis J, McGowan E, Rockwood J, Melrose H, Nacharaju P, Van Slegtenhorst M, Gwinn-Hardy K, Paul Murphy M, Baker M, Yu X, Duff K, Hardy J, Corral A, Lin WL, Yen SH, Dickson DW, Davies P, Hutton M: Neurofibrillary tangles, amyotrophy and progressive motor disturbance in mice expressing mutant (P301L) tau protein. Nat Genet 2000; 25:402–405.
8 Baum L, Seger R, Woodgett JR, Kawabata S, Maruyama K, Koyama M, Silver J, Saitoh T: Overexpressed tau protein in cultured cells is phosphorylated without formation of PHF: implication of phosphoprotein phosphatase involvement. Brain Res Mol Brain Res 1995; 34:1–17.
9 Khlistunova I, Biernat J, Wang Y, Pickhardt M, von Bergen M, Gazova Z, Mandelkow E, Mandelkow EM: Inducible expression of Tau repeat domain in cell models of tauopathy: aggregation is toxic to cells but can be reversed by inhibitor drugs. J Biol Chem 2006; 281:1205–1214.
10 Barghorn S, Zheng-Fischhofer Q, Ackmann M, Biernat J, von Bergen M, Mandelkow EM, Mandelkow E: Structure, microtubule interactions, and paired helical filament aggregation by tau mutants of frontotemporal dementias. Biochemistry 2000;39:11714–11721.
11 von Bergen M, Barghorn S, Li L, Marx A, Biernat J, Mandelkow EM, Mandelkow E: Mutations of tau protein in frontotemporal dementia promote aggregation of paired helical filaments by enhancing local beta-structure. J Biol Chem 2001;276:48165–48174.
12 Rizzu P, Van Swieten JC, Joosse M, Hasegawa M, Stevens M, Tibben A, Niermeijer MF, Hillebrand M, Ravid R, Oostra BA, Goedert M, van Duijn CM, Heutink P: High prevalence of mutations in the microtubule-associated protein tau in a population study of frontotemporal dementia in the Netherlands. Am J Hum Genet 1999;64:414–421.
13 van Swieten JC, Bronner IF, Azmani A, Severijnen LA, Kamphorst W, Ravid R, Rizzu P, Willemsen R, Heutink P: The DeltaK280 mutation in MAP tau favors exon 10 skipping in vivo. J Neuropathol Exp Neurol 2007; 66:17–25.
14 Momeni P, Pittman A, Lashley T, Vandrovcova J, Malzer E, Luk C, Hulette C, Lees A, Revesz T, Hardy J, de Silva R: Clinical and pathological features of an Alzheimer's disease patient with the MAPT DeltaK280 mutation. Neurobiol Aging 2009;30:388–393.
15 D'Souza I, Poorkaj P, Hong M, Nochlin D, Lee VM, Bird TD, Schellenberg GD: Missense and silent tau gene mutations cause frontotemporal dementia with parkinsonism-chromosome 17 type, by affecting multiple alternative RNA splicing regulatory elements. Proc Natl Acad Sci USA 1999;96: 5598–5603.
16 Eckermann K, Mocanu MM, Khlistunova I, Biernat J, Nissen A, Hofmann A, Schonig K, Bujard H, Haemisch A, Mandelkow E, Zhou L, Rune G, Mandelkow EM: The beta-propensity of Tau determines aggregation and synaptic loss in inducible mouse models of tauopathy. J Biol Chem 2007;282:31755–31765.
17 Mocanu MM, Nissen A, Eckermann K, Khlistunova I, Biernat J, Drexler D, Petrova O, Schonig K, Bujard H, Mandelkow E, Zhou L, Rune G, Mandelkow EM: The potential for beta-structure in the repeat domain of tau protein determines aggregation, synaptic decay, neuronal loss, and coassembly with endogenous Tau in inducible mouse models of tauopathy. J Neurosci 2008;28:737–748.
18 Wang YP, Biernat J, Pickhardt M, Mandelkow E, Mandelkow EM: Stepwise proteolysis liberates tau fragments that nucleate the Alzheimer-like aggregation of full-length tau in a neuronal cell model. Proc Natl Acad Sci USA 2007;104:10252–10257.
19 Karsten SL, Sang TK, Gehman LT, Chatterjee S, Liu J, Lawless GM, Sengupta S, Berry RW, Pomakian J, Oh HS, Schulz C, Hui KS, Wiedau-Pazos M, Vinters HV, Binder LI, Geschwind DH, Jackson GR: A genomic screen for modifiers of tauopathy identifies puromycin-sensitive aminopeptidase as an inhibitor of tau-induced neurodegeneration. Neuron 2006;51:549–560.
20 Wang Y, Martinez-Vincente M , Krüger U, Kaushik S, Wong E, Mandelkow EM, Cuervo AM, Mandelkow E: Tau fragmentation, aggregation and clearance: the dual role of lysosomal processing. Hum Mol Genet 2009; 18:4153–4170.
21 Petrucelli L, Dickson D, Kehoe K, Taylor J, Snyder H, Grover A, De Lucia M, McGowan E, Lewis J, Prihar G, Kim J, Dillmann WH, Browne SE, Hall A, Voellmy R, Tsuboi Y, Dawson TM, Wolozin B, Hardy J, Hutton M: CHIP and Hsp70 regulate tau ubiquitination, degradation and aggregation. Hum Mol Genet 2004;13:703–714.
22 Shimura H, Schwartz D, Gygi SP, Kosik KS: CHIP-Hsc70 complex ubiquitinates phosphorylated tau and enhances cell survival. J Biol Chem 2004;279:4869–4876.
23 Pickhardt M, Biernat J, Khlistunova I, Wang YP, Gazova Z, Mandelkow EM, Mandelkow E: N-phenylamine derivatives as aggregation inhibitors in cell models of tauopathy. Curr Alzheimer Res 2007;4:397–402.
24 Bulic B, Pickhardt M, Schmidt B, Mandelkow EM, Waldmann H, Mandelkow E: Development of tau aggregation inhibitors for Alzheimer's disease. Angew Chem Int Ed Engl 2009;48:1740–1752.
25 Berger Z, Ravikumar B, Menzies FM, Oroz LG, Underwood BR, Pangalos MN, Schmitt I, Wullner U, Evert BO, O'Kane CJ, Rubinsztein DC: Rapamycin alleviates toxicity of different aggregate-prone proteins. Hum Mol Genet 2006;15:433–442.
26 Cuervo AM: Autophagy and aging: keeping that old broom working. Trends Genet 2008; 24:604–612.

Disease Models

Neuro-degenerative Diseases

Neurodegenerative Dis 2010;7:108–111
DOI: 10.1159/000285517

Published online: February 18, 2010

Silencing/Overexpressing Selected Genes as a Model of Sporadic Parkinson's Disease

Tali Fishman-Jacob Moussa B.H. Youdim Silvia A. Mandel

Eve Topf Center for Neurodegenerative Diseases Research and Department of Molecular Pharmacology, Faculty of Medicine, Technion, Haifa, Israel

Key Words
Sporadic Parkinson's disease · Cell culture model · SKP1, Cullin, F-box complex · Cell cycle · Short hairpin RNA · Dopaminergic markers

Abstract
Background: High-throughput gene-based platform studies in human postmortem substantia nigra (SN) from sporadic Parkinson's disease (PD) cases have revealed significant dysregulation of genes involved in biological processes linked to previously established neurodegenerative mechanisms in both sporadic and hereditary PD. ***Objective:*** Our study aimed to develop a new genetic model of PD by modulating the expression of single genes that were found to be most significantly affected in SN of sporadic PD. ***Methods:*** SN-derived cell line (SN4741 cells) was infected with short hairpin RNA lentiviruses carrying different gene-specific sequences. ***Results:*** Silencing of the E3 ligase ubiquitin *SKP1A* resulted in a decline in the expression of dopaminergic phenotypic markers together with progression into an aberrant cell cycle and death. Furthermore, added knockout of the dopamine-metabolizing enzyme aldehyde dehydrogenase, found almost absent in sporadic PD SN pars compacta, exacerbated the vulnerability of *SKP1A*-silenced neurons to MPP^+ and neurotrophin deprivation. ***Conclusion:*** Future studies should focus on a careful consideration of crucial dopaminergic gene network interactions as emerged from human sporadic PD, which will serve as a basis for the development of a slowly progressive genetic animal model of sporadic PD, with the potential of evaluating drugs with 'disease-modifying activity'.

Molecular Pathogenic Mechanisms of Parkinson's Disease

Parkinson's disease (PD) may be the second most common neurodegenerative disease after Alzheimer's disease, featuring an incidence that increases with age and a higher prevalence in the male population. PD is a multifactorial disease, and several factors related to genes, age, sex, and environment may increase the risk to contract the disease. The pathological hallmark of PD is represented by degeneration of the nigrostriatal dopaminergic neurons associated with the presence of intracytoplasmatic inclusions of ubiquitin and α-synuclein denominated Lewy bodies. It is interesting to note that the motor symptoms characterizing the disease are manifested once degeneration of the dopaminergic nigrostriatal pathway has reached at least 70–80% [1]. Numerous recent studies

KARGER

Fax +41 61 306 12 34
E-Mail karger@karger.ch
www.karger.com

1660–2854/10/0073–0108$26.00/0

Accessible online at:
www.karger.com/ndd

Silvia Alicia Mandel
Department of Molecular Pharmacology, Faculty of Medicine
Technion, Efron St., PO Box 9697
IL–31096 Haifa (Israel)
Tel. +972 4829 5289, Fax +972 4851 3145, E-Mail mandel@tx.technion.ac.il

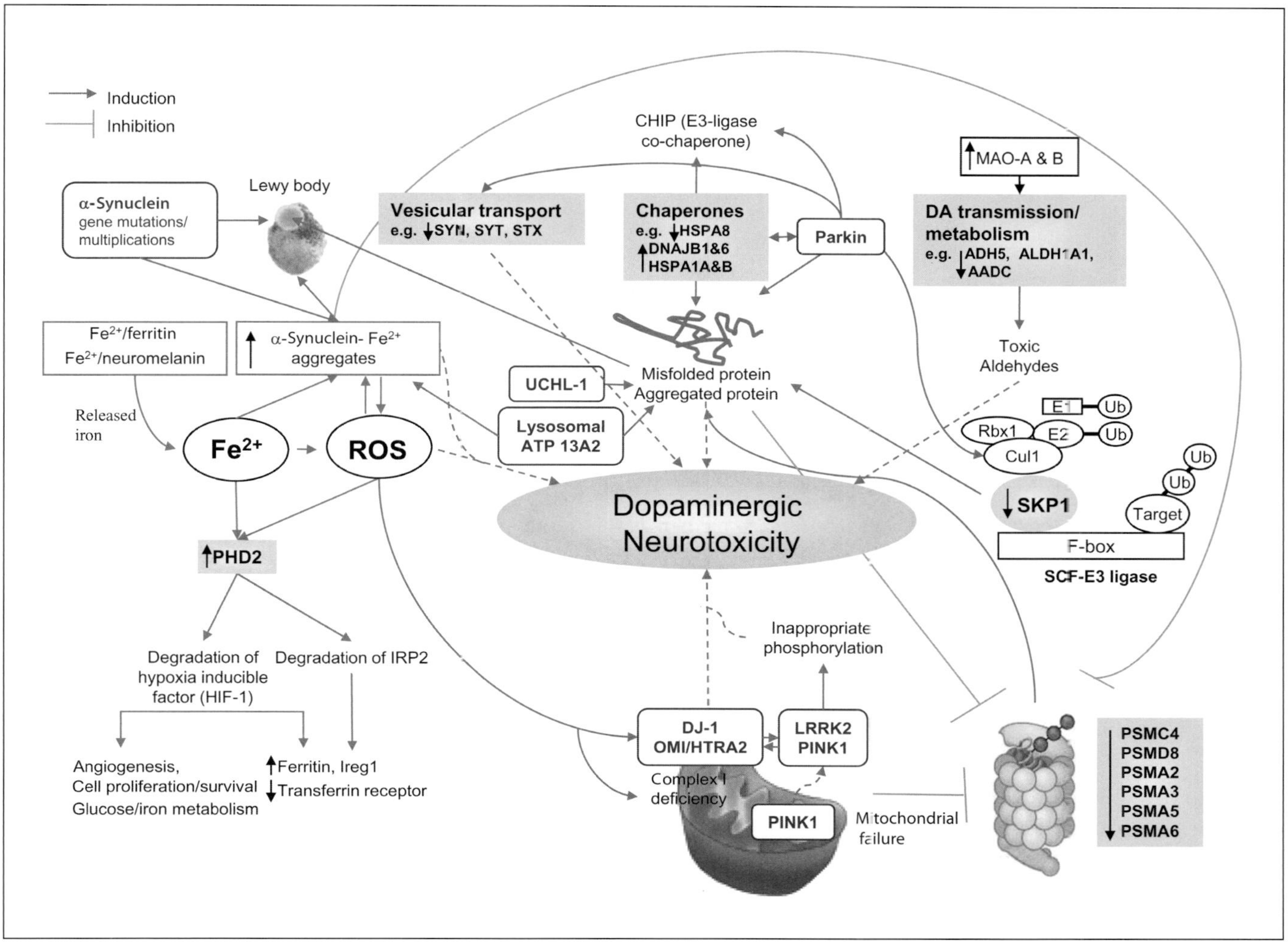

Color version available online

Fig. 1. Molecular cascades of dopaminergic neurotoxicity in human parkinsonian SN. Gene expression profiling studies in human postmortem PD SN share the identification of similar functional classes, including DA metabolism and transmission, vesicular transport, cytoskeleton and protein handling/degradation. The decrease in SKP1A (a ubiquitin E3 ligase component), chaperones and proteasome subunits can lead to a general impairment in the normal degradation of wide arrays of proteins, which may include activators of cell cycle, α-synuclein, parkin, iron regulatory protein 2 (IRP2), and hypoxia-inducible factor (HIF). Reductions in ALDH and alcohol dehydrogenase can cause accumulation of neurotoxic aldehydes and promote neuronal death. Neurodegeneration can also result from impaired iron transport across the blood-brain barrier, release of iron from ferritin or neuromelanin and induction of oxidative stress in the SNpc DA-containing neurons. Free (labile) iron can cause aggregation of α-synuclein and degradation of IRP2 via activation of prolyl-4-hydroxylase (encoded by EGLN1), which is a key iron and oxidative stress sensor. This in turn results in proteasomal degradation of HIF and IRP2, and a decrease in prosurvival genes. The various familial PD-associated genes (e.g. α-synuclein, parkin, *DJ-1*, *LRRK2*, *OMI/HTRA2*, *ATP 13A2*) have been intercalated at different molecular pathways to illustrate potential cross-talk sites common to sporadic and hereditary PD. ADH = Alcohol dehydrogenase; MAO = monoamine oxidase. Adapted from Halperin et al. [16].

have demonstrated the involvement of several other neurotransmitters, including acetylcholine, noradrenaline, glutamate and adenosine [2].

Recent approaches using smart advanced biotechnology have confirmed, extended and altered our current view on the molecular pathways underlying the etiology and pathology of PD. Microarray-assisted large-scale transcriptomic studies in human postmortem substantia nigra (SN) from sporadic PD have revealed significant dysregulation of genes involved in biological processes

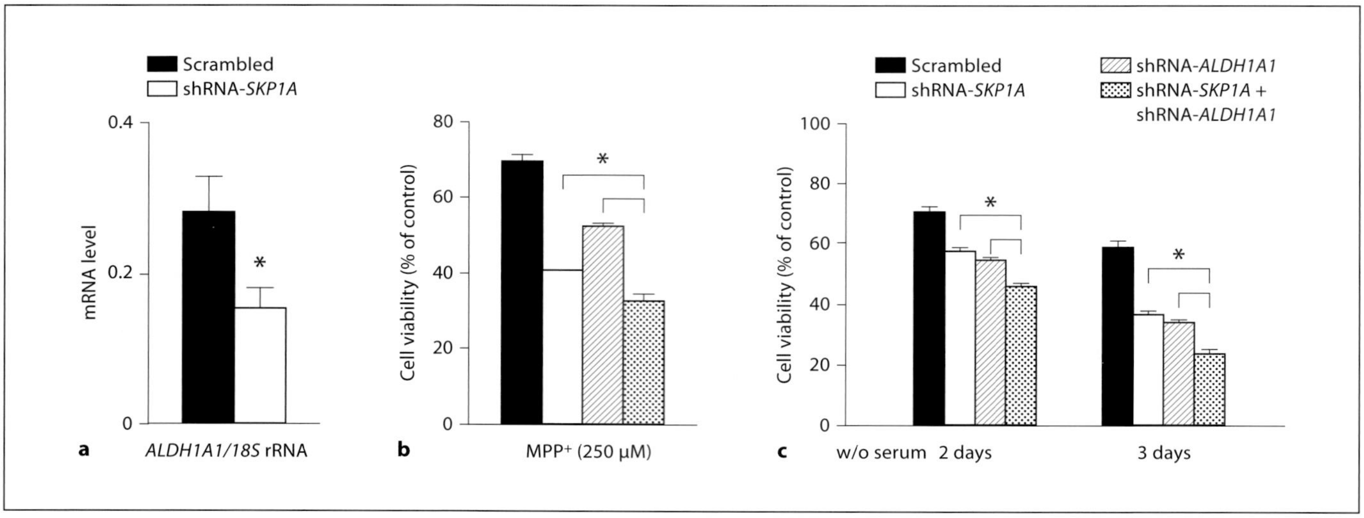

Fig. 2. Effect of RNA interference-mediated *SKP1A* and/or *ALDH1A1* inhibition on cell survival. **a** Following infection with *SKP1A* shRNA or scrambled vector, SN4741 cells were seeded in 2% fetal calf serum (FCS)-containing medium for 48 h, and the mRNA levels of *ALDH1A1* were quantified by Q-PCR. The relative expression was assessed by normalizing to 18S-rRNA. * $p < 0.01$ versus scrambled vector. *SKP1A+ALDH1A1* shRNAs double-infected SN4741 cells were seeded in 10% FCS-containing medium for 24 h, and then fresh medium with 0.5% FCS and MPP^+ was added for an additional 48 h (**b**), or seeded in 2% FCS-containing medium for 24 h, and subsequently deprived of serum support for a period of 2–3 days (**c**). * $p < 0.01$ versus each individual shRNA.

linked to protein aggregation and catabolism, mitochondrial dysfunction, oxidative stress, cell cycle, vesicle trafficking, synaptic transmission, dopamine (DA) metabolism and cell adhesion/cytoskeleton maintenance [3]. One of them, *SKP1A* (p19, S-phase kinase-associated protein 1A), has been found significantly decreased in the SN pars compacta (SNpc) of postmortem sporadic parkinsonian brains compared to age-matched controls at the gene and protein level [4, 5]. Skp1 is a component of the largest class of E3 ubiquitin ligases, functioning within modular multiprotein Skp1, Cullin-1, F-box (SCF) protein for substrate recognition, and Rbx1 [6, 7]. Together with *SKP1A*, a reduced expression of *HSPA8* gene was observed in the parkinsonian SNpc, also involved in protein ubiquitination and degradation. *HSPA8* encodes the 70-kDa heat-shock cognate protein named Hsc-70, a chaperone responsible for recognizing unfolded or aberrant proteins [4, 5] (see fig. 1 for a general overview of the major molecular changes in the SN of sporadic PD, highlighting candidate genes identified by the various research groups). Ubiquitination and proteasomal-mediated protein handling defects are thought to be common features in PD and other chronic neurodegenerative diseases such as Alzheimer's disease, amyotrophic lateral sclerosis and Huntington disease and in ageing [8, 9]. A role for the ubiquitin proteasome system in PD pathogenesis has received support from the finding that mutations in the E3 ubiquitin ligase parkin, cause early-onset, autosomal recessive PD, characterized by midbrain DA neuron loss [10].

The gene and protein expression levels of aldehyde dehydrogenase 1 family, member A1 *(ALDH1A1)*, was almost absent in SNpc of sporadic PD [4, 5]. In nonaffected individuals, this isoform is highly and specifically expressed in DA cells of the SN and ventral tegmental area [11], having a role in the neutralization of toxic aldehyde derivatives of DA (fig. 1). This is in line with the observation that striatal aldehyde dehydrogenase (ALDH) activity in 6-OHDA-treated rats [12] or in cats after electrical induced lesion [13] was significantly reduced. Aldehyde derivatives of DA metabolism are highly neurotoxic [14], and ALDH1 is the key enzyme for their metabolism to inert acidic metabolites [15].

A Genetic Model of Sporadic PD

A careful selection of genes identified as significantly affected in sporadic PD may offer a superior platform to future development of a reliable animal model of idiopathic PD. It has been proposed that subtle alterations in the kinetics of the different affected proteins in PD may have, during decades, a cumulative effect underlying the slowly progressive neurodegeneration of the DA-containing neuron. Resting on this assumption, we have recently knocked down *SKP1A* by means of short hairpin RNA (shRNA) lentiviruses in the mouse embryonic SN-derived dopaminergic cell line, SN4741. shRNA-mediated silencing of *SKP1A* increased the vulnerability of SN4741 cells to the DA neuron selective neurotoxin MPP^+, a dynamic producer of ROS, compared to nonsilenced (scrambled) cells [5], and decreased the gene expression of the dopaminergic marker *ALDH1A1* (fig. 2a). Furthermore, when *SKP1A*-deficient cells, but not shRNA-scrambled infected cells, were shifted to restrictive temperature differentiation conditions, a progressive lethality of more than 95% of cells was observed accompanied by severe cell cycle derangements [17]. This process was accompanied by the appearance of cytosolic round inclusion structures which stained positively for α-synuclein, TH, ubiquitin, proteasomal ATPase subunit PSMC4 and Hsc-70. Some cells exhibited single perinuclear gamma-tubulin-positive aggregates, reminiscent of LB-like inclusions termed aggresomes. To further investigate a potential intersection between *ALDH1A1* and *SKP1A*, the two genes were concurrently silenced by RNA interference. The double gene deficiency further exacerbated the susceptibility of the cells to neurotrophin deprivation and MPP^+ damage (fig. 2b, c). Thus, subtle alterations in one or more parameters of cell vitality/function as a result of multigene manipulation may elaborate an escalating lethal phenotype, culminating in DA neuron degeneration.

Conclusion

The results of the present study show that Skp1 deficiency leads to a lethal phenotype in arrested/postmitotic SN-derived cells, suggesting that Skp1 may play a crucial role at the interface between the cell cycle, differentiation and death. This observation links, for the first time, Skp1 to DA neuronal function and survival, suggesting an essential role in sporadic PD. These results have laid the basis for the development of a model of sporadic PD based on a gradual silencing and overexpression of selected genes with the potential of evaluating drugs with 'disease-modifying activity'.

References

1 Dauer W, Przedborski S: Parkinson's disease: mechanisms and models. Neuron 2003; 39:889–909.
2 Schapira AH, Bezard E, Brotchie J, Calon F, Collingridge GL, Ferger B, et al: Novel pharmacological targets for the treatment of Parkinson's disease. Nat Rev Drug Discov 2006; 5:845–854.
3 Mandel S, Amit T, Kalfon L, Youdim MB: Applying transcriptomic and proteomic knowledge to Parkinson's disease drug discovery. Exp Opin Drug Disc 2007;2:1225–1240.
4 Grunblatt E, Mandel S, Jacob-Hirsch J, Zeligson S, Amariglo N, Rechavi G, et al: Gene expression profiling of parkinsonian substantia nigra pars compacta; alterations in ubiquitin-proteasome, heat shock protein, iron and oxidative stress-regulated proteins, cell adhesion/cellular matrix and vesicle trafficking genes. J Neural Transm 2004;111: 1543–1573.
5 Mandel SA, Fishman T, Youdim MB: Gene and protein signatures in sporadic Parkinson's disease and a novel genetic model of PD. Parkinsonism Relat Disord 2007;13(suppl 3):242–247.
6 Feldman RM, Correll CC, Kaplan KB, Deshaies RJ: A complex of Cdc4p, Skp1p, and Cdc53p/cullin catalyzes ubiquitination of the phosphorylated CDK inhibitor Sic1p. Cell 1997;91:221–230.
7 Zheng N, Schulman BA, Song L, Miller JJ, Jeffrey PD, Wang P, et al: Structure of the Cul1-Rbx1-Skp1-f Boxskp2 Scf ubiquitin ligase complex. Nature 2002;416:703–709.
8 Ciechanover A, Brundin P: The ubiquitin proteasome system in neurodegenerative diseases: sometimes the chicken, sometimes the egg. Neuron 2003;40:427–446.
9 Dawson TM, Dawson VL: Molecular pathways of neurodegeneration in Parkinson's disease. Science 2003;302:819–822.
10 Kitada T, Asakawa S, Hattori N, Matsumine H, Yamamura Y, Minoshima S, et al: Mutations in the parkin gene cause autosomal recessive juvenile parkinsonism. Nature 1998; 392:605–608.
11 Galter D, Buervenich S, Carmine A, Anvret M, Olson L: Aldh1 mRNA: presence in human dopamine neurons and decreases in substantia nigra in Parkinson's disease and in the ventral tegmental area in schizophrenia. Neurobiol Dis 2003;14:637–647.
12 Agid Y, Javoy F, Youdim MB: Monoamine oxidase and aldehyde dehydrogenase activity in the striatum of rats after 6-hydroxydopamine lesion of the nigrostriatal pathway. Br J Pharmacol 1973;48:175–178.
13 Duncan RJ, Sourkes TL, Boucher R, Poirier LJ, Roberge A: Aldehyde dehydrogenase and monoamine oxidase in the striatum of cats with nigrostriatal lesions. J Neurochem 1972;19:2007–2010
14 Hjelle JJ, Petersen DR: Hepatic aldehyde dehydrogenases and lipid peroxidation. Pharmacol Biochem Behav 1983;18(suppl 1):155–160.
15 Mardh G, Vallee BL: Human class I alcohol dehydrogenases catalyze the interconversion of alcohols and aldehydes in the metabolism of dopamine. Biochemistry 1986;25:7279–7282.
16 Halperin I, Morelli M, Korczyn AD, Youdim MB, Mandel SA: Biomarkers for evaluation of clinical efficacy of multipotential neuroprotective drugs for Alzheimer's and Parkinson's diseases. Neurotherapeutics 2009;6:128–140.
17 Fishman-Jacob T, Reznichenko L, Youdim MBH, Mandel SA: A sporadic Parkinson disease model via silencing the ubiquitin-proteasome/E3-ligase component, SKP1A. J Biol Chem 2009;284:32835–32845.

Neuro-degenerative Diseases

Neurodegenerative Dis 2010;7:112–115
DOI: 10.1159/000285518

Published online: February 18, 2010

Prevalence and Impact of Cerebrovascular Lesions in Alzheimer and Lewy Body Diseases

Kurt A. Jellinger

Institute of Clinical Neurobiology, Vienna, Austria

Key Words

Alzheimer disease · Cerebrovascular lesions · Lewy body disease · Parkinson disease · Dementia with Lewy bodies

Abstract

Background: Data on the prevalence of cerebrovascular lesions (CVLs) and their impact on cognitive decline in Alzheimer disease (AD) and Lewy body disease are conflicting. ***Objective:*** Retrospective examination of the prevalence of CVL in a consecutive autopsy series. ***Material and Methods:*** 1,339 cases of autopsy-proven AD, Parkinson disease (PD), dementia with Lewy bodies (± AD), and 486 age-matched controls were examined according to standardized neuropathologic methods including immunohistochemistry. Diagnoses followed current consensus criteria, classification of CVLs and of cerebral amyloid angiopathy (CAA) in 5 grades [Acta Neurol Scand 2006;114:38–46; Acta Neuropathol 2005; 110:345–359]. ***Results:*** Lewy body variant of AD and AD showed significantly more frequent CVLs (91.9 and 67.8%) than the other groups (29.4 to 45.7%), with the highest frequency of severe CVLs (old, recent infarcts and hemorrhages) in AD (23.6%), but 2.0–8.3% in the other groups. Severe CAA was most frequent in AD and the Lewy body variant of AD (97.9 and 85%), less in PD (36%) and controls (30%). CAA was more frequent/severe in demented than in nondemented cases. CVLs in cortico-subcortical and hippocampal areas were most frequent in AD; subcortical CVLs (lacunes) in both AD and PD were more frequent than in controls. The incidence and severity of CVLs significantly correlated with neuritic Braak stages. Cognitive impairment was largely independent of coexisting CVLs, but related to the severity/location of AD and/or Lewy pathology. ***Conclusions:*** The present data confirm the importance of CVLs in AD and in dementia with Lewy bodies with severe AD, and the little impact of CVLs alone, but show a close association of CAA with clinical dementia associated with AD pathology.

Introduction

Cerebrovascular lesions (CVLs) frequently occur in aged brains, coexist in both Alzheimer disease (AD) and Parkinson disease (PD), and are less common in dementia with Lewy bodies (DLB [1–3]), but the results of epidemiological and clinicopathological studies on the impact on these disorders are controversial. Neurovascular dysfunction has a major role in the pathogenesis of AD [4] and CVLs show synergistic effects on the development of parkinsonism [5]. Seen in 40–80% of aged, AD and PD brains, they may be important for the development of cognitive decline [1, 2, 6–9], whereas in patients with CVLs, the densities of plaques and tangles were

KARGER

Fax +41 61 306 12 34
E-Mail karger@karger.ch
www.karger.com

1660–2854/10/0073–0112$26.00/0

Accessible online at:
www.karger.com/ndd

Kurt A. Jellinger, MD
Institute of Clinical Neurobiology
Kenyongasse 18
AT–1070 Vienna (Austria)
Tel./Fax +43 1 526 6534, E-Mail kurt.jellinger@univie.ac.at

lower than in 'pure' AD for every given level of cognitive deficit [10]. These and other data suggest that CVLs contribute to cognitive impairment by an additive effect to AD pathology. Cerebral amyloid angiopathy (CAA), the severity and distribution of which are strongly influenced by AD pathology [11, 12], is also related to cognitive impairment in both AD, PD and the Lewy body variant of AD (LBV/AD) [1, 13]. This study retrospectively compares the prevalence of CVLs in a large autopsy series.

Material and Methods

The prevalence of CVLs was assessed semiquantitatively in 621 autopsy-proven cases of AD (191 male, 430 female, aged 60–101, mean 83.2 ± 7.6 years), 612 PD cases (267 male, 345 female; demented mean MMSE 15.0 ± 2.2, and nondemented mean MMSE 24.7 ± 3.2; aged 52–96, mean 75.9 ± 8.2 years); 106 DLB cases (mean age 78.6 ± 6.3 years; mean MMSE 13.5 ± 3.1), of whom 58 were of the diffuse DLB type (DDLB; mean AD Braak stage 2.9, mean age 77.9 ± 7.4 years; mean MMSE 17 ± 4.0), and 48 were of the DLB+AD or LBV/AD type (mean Braak stage 5.0; mean age 79.3 ± 6.8 years; mean MMSE 1.3 ± 0.1), and 485 controls (219 male, 267 female; age 60–101, mean 79.0 ± 7.6 years; mean Braak stage 2.2; MMSE >27). Neuropathologic assessment was performed according to standard protocols. Paraffin-embedded blocks from multiple brain regions (frontal, temporal, occipital cortex, hippocampus, basal ganglia, pons, medulla oblongata) were examined using routine stains, including immunohistochemistry for tau, Aβ, GFAP and α-synuclein. CVLs were classified semiquantitatively according to grades shown in table 1; CAAs were graded according to Olichney et al. [14] and Attems [15]. Statistical methods correlating the different lesions were Spearman's rank correlation coefficient and Mann-Whitney U test.

Results

The highest frequency of CVLs was found in LBV/AD and in AD (91.8 and 67.8%), which was significantly greater than in the other groups, with the lowest incidence in controls (29.4%), while PD and DDLB showed similar negative results (table 2). Minor vascular pathology was most frequent in LBV/AD and DDLB (47.9 and 32.9%). Moderate CVLs were significantly more frequent in LBV/AD and AD (42 and 31.7%), but much less in DDLB and controls than in PD. Severe CVLs (old/recent infarcts and hemorrhages) were most frequent in AD (23.6%), similar in PD, DDLB and controls (8.8–5.4%) and least frequent in DDLB (2%). In both AD and PD, subcortical vascular lesions were most frequent as were cortico-subcortical infarcts and hippocampal sclerosis in

Table 1. Classification of cerebrovascular pathology

0	No concomitant CVLs
1+	Minimal CVLs: 1–2 small lacunes, mild-moderate CAA, with/without mild CVLs, mild leukoencephalopathy
2+	Moderate CVLs: >2 lacunes, severe subcortical lacunar state, severe CAA with moderate CVLs, diffuse WMLs
3+	Severe CVLs: (a) Old infarcts, multiple old microinfarcts or hemorrhages, hippocampal sclerosis; (b) acute ischemic infarcts, hemorrhages (<1–2 days old)

WMLs = White matter lesions.

Table 2. Frequency (%) and severity of cerebrovascular pathology in various disorders

	No CVP	CVP severity				CVP total
		1+	2+	3a+	3b+	
Controls	70.6*	14.4	9.7	3.8	1.6	29.4
PD	57.8*	17.5	16.4	6.2	2.1	42.2
DDLB	54.7*	32.9	5.2	5.2	2.0	45.3
LBV/AD	8.1	47.9	42.0	2.0	0	91.9
AD	32.2*	12.5	31.7	17.2	6.4	67.8

Underlined values: p < 0.01 vs. other values in same column; * p < 0.01 vs. LBV/AD. CVP = Cerebrovascular pathology.

Table 3. Frequency (%) of CVLs (infarcts, hemorrhages) in various brain regions

	Controls (n = 486)	DLB (n = 103)	PD (n = 612)	AD (n = 621)
Cortical	0.8	1.0	0.1	3.0
Subcortical + lacunes	8.7	5.8	21.9*	27.9*
Corticosubcortical	1.9	1.9	4.1	10.3**
Hippocampus	0.2	0	0.1	2.7**
Brainstem	0.8	0	0.5	0.8
Cerebellum	0.2	0	0.5	1.0

* p < 0.01 vs. controls and DLB; ** p < 0.01 vs. controls and DLB.

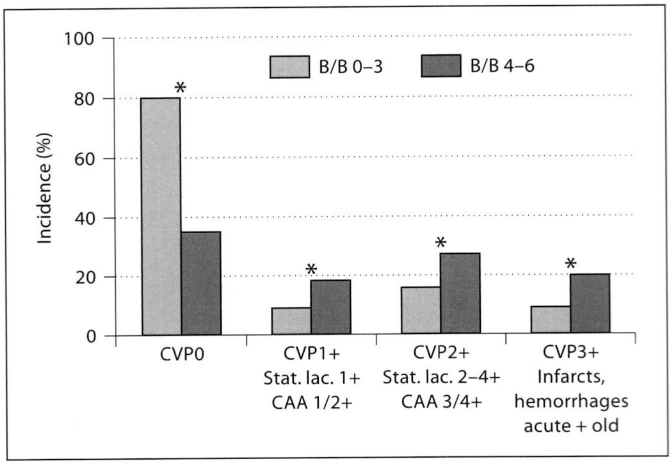

Fig. 1. Relation between Braak stages and CVLs in aged brain (AD: n = 621, PD: n = 612, controls: n = 468, total: n = 1,339; mean age: 79.3 years). DLB cases (n = 103) were not included. * $p < 0.01$. CVP = Cerebrovascular pathology.

AD (table 3). Brain weight in AD and controls was not significantly different (data not shown), but the incidence and severity of CVLs in aged brain, similar to a previous smaller study [3], increased with higher neuritic Braak stages (fig. 1).

The prevalence and severity of CAA increased (in the ascending order) in aged controls (total 30%, 20% severe), PD (total 35%, 6% severe), DDLB (total 41%, 5% severe), LBV/AD (total 85%, 35% severe) and AD (total 97.7%, 75% severe). In 75% of AD patients, hemorrhages were associated with severe and in 10% with mild/moderate CAA; only 20% of infarcts were associated with severe CAA.

In the Lewy body disease group, lack of CVLs was more frequent in nondemented patients with PD (PDND; 70 vs. 41%), without differences between PD dementia (PDD) and DLB. PDD patients, however, showed more frequent severe CVLs than PDND and DLB patients. PDD patients showed significantly higher AD Braak stages, cortical Aβ plaque load, and more frequent and severe CAA [1].

Discussion

The present study confirms significantly higher prevalence of cerebrovascular pathology in AD and LBV/AD than in PD, DDLB and aged controls, severe acute and old infarcts and hemorrhages being most frequent in AD (often due to severe CAA), but very rare in LBV/AD. The frequency and degree of coexistent CVLs were significantly related to Braak stages, and CAA also increased with neuritic AD pathology, being most frequent in progressed stages of AD and LBV/AD (DLB+AD; 97.7 and 85%). A recent study showed significantly more severe cortical Aβ plaque load and CAA in DLB+AD and PDD than in PD without dementia [1].

These data not only suggest a strong association of CAA with neuritic AD pathology but do not support CAA as an independent risk factor for cognitive decline [10, 16], except in a small subgroup of dementia patients lacking neuritic AD pathology. Cognitive impairment in DLB, PD and, in particular, AD appears to be largely independent of coexisting cerebrovascular pathology, except for severe multifocal lesions, but is overwhelmed by the severity and extent of neuritic AD and/or Lewy pathology. The thresholds of Alzheimer and vascular lesions in dementia highly depend on the lesion type and location, and the severity of AD-related pathology [17].

Despite increasing evidence indicating synergistic/additive effects of both vascular and AD pathologies and a similar frequency and severity of CVLs in PD and DLB without severe AD pathology, the molecular and pathophysiological background of CVLs in the progression of neurodegeneration and development of cognitive decline in these disorders awaits further elucidation.

References

1 Jellinger KA, Attems J: Prevalence and impact of vascular and Alzheimer pathologies in Lewy body disease. Acta Neuropathol 2008;115:427–436.
2 Jellinger KA, Attems J: Prevalence and impact of cerebrovascular pathology in Alzheimer's disease and parkinsonism. Acta Neurol Scand 2006;114:38–46.
3 Jellinger KA, Mitter-Ferstl E: The impact of cerebrovascular lesions in Alzheimer disease – a comparative autopsy study. J Neurol 2003;250:1050–1055.
4 Zlokovic BV, Deane R, Sallstrom J, Chow N, Miano JM: Neurovascular pathways and Alzheimer amyloid beta-peptide. Brain Pathol 2005;15:78–83.
5 Thanvi B, Lo N, Robinson T: Vascular parkinsonism – an important cause of parkinsonism in older people. Age Ageing 2005;34:114–119.

6 Giannakopoulos P, Gold G, Kovari E, von Gunten A, Imhof A, Bouras C, Hof PR: Assessing the cognitive impact of Alzheimer disease pathology and vascular burden in the aging brain: the Geneva experience. Acta Neuropathol 2007;113:1–12.
7 Schneider JA, Boyle PA, Arvanitakis Z, Bienias JL, Bennett DA: Subcortical infarcts, Alzheimer's disease pathology, and memory function in older persons. Ann Neurol 2007; 62:59–66.
8 Petrovitch H, Ross GW, Steinhorn SC, Abbott RD, Markesberry W, Davis DG, Nelson J, Hardman J, Masaki KH, Vogt MR, Launer LJ, White LR: AD lesions and infarcts in demented and non-demented Japanese-American men. Ann Neurol 2005;57:98–103.
9 Troncoso JC, Zonderman AB, Resnick SM, Crain B, Pletnikova O, O'Brien RJ: Effect of infarcts on dementia in the Baltimore longitudinal study of aging. Ann Neurol 2008;64: 168–176.
10 Zekry D, Duyckaerts C, Belmin J, Geoffre C, Herrmann F, Moulias R, Hauw JJ: The vascular lesions in vascular and mixed dementia: the weight of functional neuroanatomy. Neurobiol Aging 2003;24:213–219.
11 Attems J, Jellinger KA, Lintner F: Alzheimer's disease pathology influences severity and topographical distribution of cerebral amyloid angiopathy. Acta Neuropathol (Berl) 2005;110:222–231.
12 Thal DR, Griffin WS, de Vos RA, Ghebremedhin E: Cerebral amyloid angiopathy and its relationship to Alzheimer's disease. Acta Neuropathol 2008;115:599–609.
13 Jellinger KA, Attems J: Cerebral amyloid angiopathy in Lewy body disease. J Neural Transm 2008;115:473–482.
14 Olichney JM, Hansen LA, Galasko D, Saitoh T, Hofstetter CR, Katzman R, Thal LJ: The apolipoprotein E epsilon 4 allele is associated with increased neuritic plaques and cerebral amyloid angiopathy in Alzheimer's disease and Lewy body variant. Neurology 1996;47: 190–196.
15 Attems J: Sporadic cerebral amyloid angiopathy: pathology, clinical implications, and possible pathomechanisms. Acta Neuropathol 2005;110:345–359.
16 Tian J, Shi J, Mann DM: Cerebral amyloid angiopathy and dementia. Panminerva Med 2004;46:253–264.
17 Gold G, Giannakopoulos P, Herrmann FR, Bouras C, Kovari E: Identification of Alzheimer and vascular lesion thresholds for mixed dementia. Brain 2007;130:2830–2836.

Relationship Between Cerebrovascular Lesions and Primary Neurodegenerative Diseases

Neuro-degenerative Diseases

Neurodegenerative Dis 2010;7:116–121
DOI: 10.1159/000285520

Published online: February 18, 2010

The Vascular Hypothesis of Alzheimer's Disease: Bench to Bedside and Beyond

Jack C. de la Torre

Banner Sun Health Research Institute, Sun City, Ariz., USA

Key Words
Echocardiography · Carotid artery ultrasound · Vascular hypothesis of Alzheimer's disease · Cerebral hypoperfusion · Cardiovascular disease · Intima media thickness · Carotid artery stenosis

Abstract
The vascular hypothesis of Alzheimer's disease (AD) which we first proposed in 1993, has become a useful concept in identifying vascular risk factors for AD or vascular dementia that can be modified through appropriate treatment to prevent, reduce or delay the onset of cognitive impairment and dementia onset. Among the more than two dozen vascular risk factors already identified for AD, are cardiovascular disease and carotid artery atherosclerosis, which may exert their pathology by chronically lowering cerebral hypoperfusion during aging. We propose and plan to initiate a clinical study to screen middle-aged, cognitively intact individuals, with carotid artery ultrasound and echocardiography to identify potentially progressive pathology in the heart and carotid artery that is considered modifiable with optimal medical treatment. This clinical strategy, if found effective in preventing pathologic conditions suspected of contributing to severe cognitive impairment, could significantly reduce AD prevalence if applied on a wide scale and help promote healthier mental and physical aging while providing a compelling economic benefit to society.

Introduction

The search for a cure for sporadic Alzheimer's disease (AD) has been elusive in the past 100 years due to a major difficulty. The loss of cognitive functions in AD patients is irrevocable because the neurons that formerly controlled these functions are likely dead and dead neurons can not be brought back to life. Inexplicably, some pharmaceutical houses have challenged this 'biological rule' by giving AD patients drugs claimed to rescue dead neurons by reducing Aβ load or clearance from the brain. This attempt to pharmacologically reverse AD symptoms or somehow affect disease outlook has ended in repeated failure during clinical trials of drugs such as AlzheMed (tramiprosate), Flurizan (tarenflurbil), AN-1792, Elan 301 and 302 (bapineuzimab). It is therefore baffling to see the same concept tested clinically over and over again while somehow expecting a different result to occur. Observers of this phenomenon may try to guess how, after more than 12,000 published papers on the role of Aβ on AD in the last 20 years, the amyloid cascade hypothesis continues to run on empty. A clue to this puzzling tactic may be found in Einstein's cynical maxim 'if the facts don't fit the theory, change the facts'.

Since neurogenesis, stem cell or other research breakthrough to replace dead neurons is still a distant prospect as a relevant solution, development of techniques that can be presently applied to reduce AD prevalence may be a more pragmatic clinical approach.

KARGER

Fax +41 61 306 12 34
E-Mail karger@karger.ch
www.karger.com

1660–2854/10/0073–0116$26.00/0

Accessible online at:
www.karger.com/ndd

J.C. de la Torre, MD, PhD
Center for Alzheimer's Research
Banner Sun Health Research Institute
Sun City, AZ 85351 (USA)
Tel. +1 760 703 0585, E-Mail jcdelatorre@comcast.net

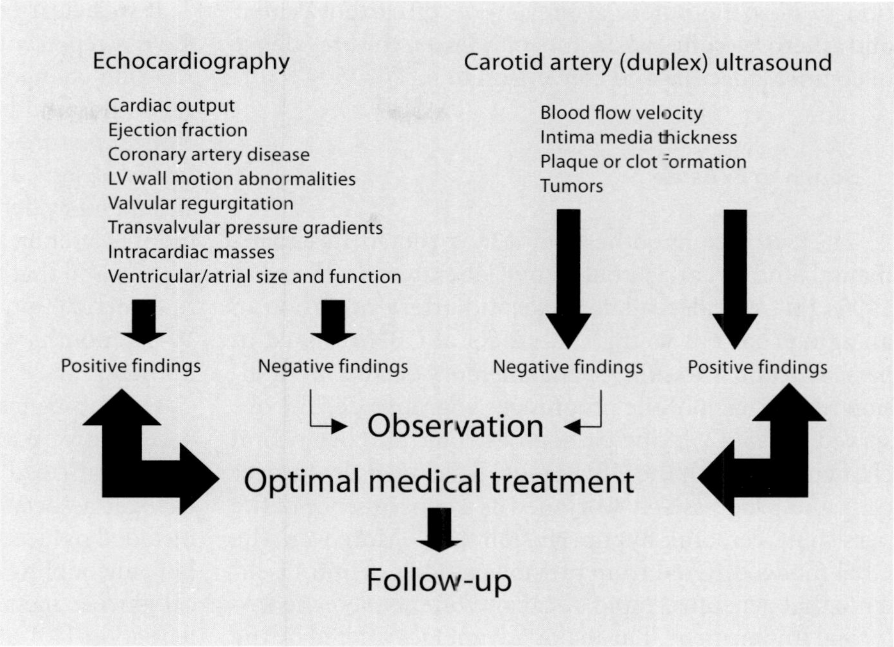

Fig. 1. Clinical flowchart for screening patients with echocardiography and carotid artery (duplex) ultrasound. Note the number of cardiovascular and carotid artery deficits that can be identified with both techniques and the possibility of using OMT and follow-up after treatment in the event positive pathologic findings are recorded. When negative pathologic findings are recorded, the patient can be monitored periodically (observation). LV = Left ventricular.

Consequently, *prevention*, rather than a *cure* of AD, appears as a more realistic stratagem to offset the catastrophic impact of this dementia whose incidence by 2050 is expected to approach nearly a million people per year in the US alone, with a total estimated prevalence of 11–16 million people affected [1].

The vascular hypothesis of AD, first proposed by us in 1993 [2], has become a mother lode of interdisciplinary research involving mainly the brain, the heart and the circulation [3–13]. The collective evidence supporting the vascular hypothesis offers the possibility of targeting vascular risk factors for AD and vascular dementia (VaD) by preventing, delaying or reversing further progression and inherent cognitive deterioration that often precede AD and VaD [14]. Following our proposal in 1993, we observed in 1994 that conditions such as advanced aging, a former head injury, apoE4 genotype, etc, were *risk factors* for AD by virtue of their lowering blood flow to the brain [15]. Since then, several dozen heterogeneous AD vascular risk factors have been reported [6, 8], including atherosclerosis and cardiovascular disease [16–22], which is the focus of this review.

A lowered prevalence of cognitive impairment by prevention or delay of atherosclerosis and cardiovascular disease in cognitively intact, middle-aged individuals may now be a rational clinical goal much like early detection and prevention of cancer using colonoscopy and mammography. We propose that this strategy may be feasible by screening with carotid artery ultrasound and echocardiography (CAUSE) [23, 24].

These screening tools are useful because they are noninvasive, cost-effective, easily applied within a 90-min session, relatively accurate procedures and pose no inherent harmful effects. More specifically, these tools can help identify patients most likely to develop progressive cognitive decline during aging as a result of mild but persistent chronic brain hypoperfusion (CBH), a reactive process that can develop decades after long-term cardiovascular and carotid artery pathology from suboptimal delivery of blood flow to the brain. Following screening with CAUSE and after careful analysis of each case, optimal medical treatment (OMT) may be recommended in patients who show subclinical evidence of carotid or cardiovascular pathology (fig. 1). OMT is defined as any medically sound therapy considered clinically indicated to prevent, delay, or reverse a condition or disease that if left alone, will likely result in worsening damage and complications. For example, antihypertensive treatment to prevent or delay premature death or organ damage is the preferred medical treatment for persistent hypertension.

In this brief review, the bench-to-bedside research that led to the vascular hypothesis of AD and what lessons can be learned from such research will be discussed in relation to how the potential prevention of cardiovascular and atherosclerotic risk factors may lessen the prevalence of cognitive decline and conversion to AD or VaD.

Bench to Bedside

The vascular hypothesis of AD is rooted in experimental studies carried out in our laboratory in the early 1990s that revealed bilateral carotid artery occlusion in an aging (but not young) rat model of CBH resulted in *persistent* and *worsening* spatial memory decline, a condition reminiscent of the progressive cognitive decline observed in AD [25]. The pathophysiologic and behavioral changes seen with the CBH model developed slowly over time and progressively worsened as a consequence of the persistent cerebral hypoperfusion [26]. Moreover, the CBH model differed from previous models of brain ischemia that generated rapid, focal and often severe, neurological impairment. The major advantages offered by the CBH model were the resulting progressive unfolding of the spatial memory decline and the expanding cascade of abnormal biochemical and subcellular events that preceded the memory loss and led eventually to cortical atrophy and death [27]. Thus, the slowly emerging pathology could be chronologically examined over many months allowing a clinical picture to develop that revealed the onset of anatomic, physiologic and memory abnormalities affecting the brain cells at the cellular and molecular level [28].

The cellular-molecular events initially targeted the ischemic-sensitive hippocampal CA1 brain cells and the posterior parietal cortex [14, 25–27], mimicking the neuropathologic process seen in early AD [29–31]. Aging rats subjected to CBH showed an immediate 34% hippocampal blood flow reduction [25] and the following sequential events: (a) impaired neuronal energy metabolism [32, 33], (b) astrocytosis [26], (c) oxidative stress [14, 33], (d) reduced protein synthesis and increased protein abnormalities [34], (e) spatial memory loss [25–27], (f) endothelial cell damage affecting vascular nitric oxide [35], (g) Aβ1–42 upregulation [35], (h) overexpression of G protein-coupled receptor kinase 2, an indicator of oxidative stress and cardiac ischemia and early marker of AD [36], and (i) brain atrophy and death [32]. Most surprisingly, the early hypometabolic changes after CBH occurred in the *absence* of *senile plaque* formation and *neurofibrillary tangles*, the hallmark pathologic deposits of AD. There was also no evidence of gray-white matter ischemic stroke damage [26].

It was clear from these findings that the CBH model did not represent VaD-like changes but rather resembled AD-like changes that ultimately involved atrophic, degenerative and progressive pathology that simulated the clinical picture characterizing AD [25–36].

We observed that the early cerebral hypometabolism and memory deficits seen soon after CBH were followed months later by the slow emergence of CA1 neurodegeneration and that the 'sole' trigger that generated the eventual corticohippocampal atrophy which developed after 10–12 months was CBH [32, 37], equivalent to about 18 human years.

Our lab-bench findings of severe cognitive and neurodegenerative pathology in aging rats subjected to CBH were confirmed by others [38, 39]. Some of the main changes associated with CBH in rats reported by others included reduced acetylcholine levels in the hippocampus [40], uncoupling of regional cerebral blood flow and cortical glucose metabolism [41, 42], impaired long-term potentiation [43] and downregulation of protein synthesis reflected by depressed mRNA microtubule associated protein-2, a marker of neurodegeneration [44]. These and our own data indicated that experimental CBH in aging rats led to symptoms and signs reminiscent of the pathologic process seen prior to and during the development of AD.

If no neuropathological 'hallmarks' of AD or VaD were present after CBH in the aging rats, what did their progressive cognitive and degenerative pathology reflect? Could it be that plaque or tangle deposits do not play a central role in the pathophysiology of AD (like rats) and CBH generated from vascular risk factors is the main trigger (like rats) of the neurodegenerative cascade during advanced aging? In support of the first part of this notion, a number of studies have indicated that substantial Aβ burden can be found in cognitively intact older people even though the plaque and tangle distribution, density and topographical progression of these 'hallmark' deposits is the same as that seen in symptomatic AD patients [45–48]. Significant Aβ brain deposition does not appear to be associated with worse cognitive function [49]. In addition, virtual clearing of plaques from human brain with Aβ42 immunization does not prevent progressive neurodegeneration or the advancing severity of AD [50].

Beyond the Bedside

The concept that AD may be a vascular disorder with neurodegenerative consequences [2, 51] has offered a verifiable explanation into the nature of this disorder and opened the authentic possibility of preventing AD by targeting its reported vascular risk factors, such as cardiovascular disease and atherosclerosis [16, 22]. We have previously discussed the application and benefits of CAUSE in the prevention-by-detection of severe cognitive impairment from cardiac-carotid pathology [23, 24], and for brevity's sake will only refer to this technology in a clinical flowchart (fig. 1).

The ability to accurately measure cardiac function and carotid artery pathology using CAUSE in asymptomatic or symptomatic individuals is important in clinical practice because it may detect functional and structural abnormalities at an early stage that may progress irreversibly in severity if left untreated. CAUSE, like colonoscopies that are used to prevent cancer, would be less costly than a colonoscopy and would offer the possibility of treating a preventable disorder at a stage when intervention may be most effective. There is presently no clinical screening test that can identify potential candidates at risk of cognitive dysfunction and dementia in a population who have no apparent symptoms of the diseases being screened. CAUSE may offer this possibility. Once individuals with carotid artery-cardiac pathology are identified, additional diagnostic tests can be performed to try and confirm the ultrasound findings with greater certainty.

Figure 1 shows a clinical plan to screen cognitively intact middle-aged individuals for subclinical cardiovascular disease and carotid artery atherosclerosis that can slow or prevent CBH, a presumed promoter of cognitive decline. The plan calls for early OMT when indicated, to try and prevent further progression of specific cardiovascular and carotid artery deficits identified using CAUSE (fig. 1). If OMT is not indicated, the practitioner may recommend lifestyle changes to the patient which can foster a healthier mental and physical outlook [52].

It is reasonable to assume that OMT which can prevent or delay the rate of disease progression, would also improve the identified pathological deficit, whether it is regression or stabilization of carotid artery plaque formation, intima media thickness or a cardiovascular abnormality detected by echocardiography.

Although a number of studies have linked cardiovascular disease and atherosclerosis with cognitive decline [3, 4, 6, 7, 10, 11, 46], and with AD or VaD [6, 8, 12, 16, 18, 20, 50, 53, 54], it remains speculative at present to assume that screening and treating these conditions before they become symptomatic will have a significant impact on the number of new dementia cases recorded annually. The clinical plan to screen individuals with CAUSE and when indicated, start early OMT or patient monitoring to prevent or delay further progression of specific cardiovascular-carotid artery pathology, could, if validated, significantly help reduce the prevalence of AD and VaD in the years to come. For these reasons, a feasibility study such as we have proposed [23, 24], needs to be done to test the merit and practicality of CAUSE screening in cognitively intact individuals. On the other hand, if nothing is done, or if clinical trials can only repeat past clinical failures, progress in dementia research will continue at a glacial pace. It is important to remember that a 5-year delay in the onset of AD could reduce the prevalence of AD by 50% [55] and the relative annual costs presently estimated at 100 billion dollars in the US alone [1]. We are therefore planning to test the merit of CAUSE in a preliminary clinical study of cognitively healthy, middle-aged population and offer this discussion for investigators to consider this clinical strategy.

Acknowledgment

This research was supported by an Investigator-Initiated Research Grant from the Alzheimer's Association.

References

1 Alzheimer's Association: 2009 Alzheimer's disease facts and figures. Alzheimers Dement 2009;5:234–270.
2 de la Torre JC, Mussivand T: Can disturbed brain microcirculation cause Alzheimer's disease? Neurol Res 1993;15:146–153.
3 Caselli RJ, Chen K, Lee W, Alexander GE, Reiman EM: Correlating cerebral hypometabolism with future memory decline in subsequent converters to amnestic pre-mild cognitive impairment. Arch Neurol 2008;65:1231–1236.
4 Roher AE, Esh C, Kokjohn TA, Kalbak W, Luhers DC, Seward JD, Sue LI, Beach TG: Circle of Willis atherosclerosis is a risk factor for sporadic Alzheimer's disease. Arterioscler Thromb Vasc Biol 2003;23:2055–2062.
5 Milionis HJ, Florentin M, Giannopoulos S: Metabolic syndrome and Alzheimer's disease: a link to a vascular hypothesis? CNS Spectr 2008;13:606–613.

6 Helzner E, Luchsinger J, Scarmeas N, Cosentino S, Brickman A, Glymour M, Stern Y: Contribution of vascular risk factors to the progression in Alzheimer disease. Arch Neurol 2009;66:343–348.
7 Aguero-Torres H, Kivipelto M, von Strauss E: Rethinking the dementia diagnoses in a population-based study: what is Alzheimer's disease and what is vascular dementia? A study from the Kungsholmen project. Dement Geriatr Cogn Disord 2006;22:244–249.
8 Breteler MM: Vascular risk factors for Alzheimer's disease: an epidemiological study. Neurobiol Aging 2000;21:153–160.
9 Dede DS, Yavuz B, Yavuz BB, Cankurtaran M, Halil M, Ulger Z, Cankurtaran ES, Aytemir K, Kabakci G, Ariogul S: Assessment of endothelial function in Alzheimer's disease: is Alzheimer's disease a vascular disease? J Am Geriatr Soc 2007;55:1613–1617.
10 Beach TG, Wilson JR, Sue LI, Newell A, Poston M, Cisneros R, Pandya Y, Esh C, Connor DJ, Sabbagh M, Walker DG, Roher AE: Circle of Willis atherosclerosis: association with Alzheimer's disease, neuritic plaques and neurofibrillary tangles. Acta Neuropathol 2007;113:13–21.
11 Ruitenberg A, den Heiker T, Bakker SL: Cerebral hypoperfusion and clinical onset of dementia: the Rotterdam study. Ann Neurol 2005;57:789–794.
12 Lindsay J, Laurin D, Verreault R, et al: Risk factors for Alzheimer's disease: a prospective analysis from the Canadian Study of Health and Aging. Am J Epidemiol 2002;156:445–453.
13 de la Torre JC: How do heart disease and stroke become risk factors for Alzheimer's disease? Neurol Res 2006;28:637–644.
14 de la Torre JC, Cada A, Nelson N, Davis G, Sutherland RJ, Gonzalez-Lima F: Reduced cytochrome oxidase and memory dysfunction after chronic brain ischemia in aged rats. Neurosci Lett 1997;223:165–168.
15 de la Torre JC: Impaired brain microcirculation may trigger Alzheimer's disease. Neurosci Behav Rev 1994;18:397–401.
16 Hofman A, Breteler MM, Bots ML, Slooter AJ, van Harskamp F: Atherosclerosis, apolipoprotein E and prevalence of dementia and Alzheimer's disease in the Rotterdam Study. Lancet 1997;349:151–154.
17 Casserly I, Topol E: Convergence of atherosclerosis and Alzheimer's disease: inflammation, cholesterol, and misfolded proteins. Lancet 2004;363:1139–1146.
18 van Oijen M, de Jong FJ, Witteman JC, Hofman A, Koudstaal PJ, Breteler MM: Atherosclerosis and risk for dementia. Ann Neurol 2007;61:403–410.
19 de la Torre JC: Is Alzheimer's a neurodegenerative or a vascular disorder? Data, dogma and dialectics. Lancet Neurol 2004;3:184–190.
20 Whitmer RA, Sidney S, Selby J, Johnston SC, Yaffe K: Midlife cardiovascular risk factors and risk of dementia in late life. Neurology 2005;64:277–281.
21 Kilander L, Andren B, Nyman H, Lind L, Boberg M, Lithell H: Atrial fibrillation is an independent determinant of low cognitive function: a cross-sectional study in elderly men. Stroke 1998;29:1816–1820.
22 Zuccalà G, Cattel C, Manes-Gravina E, Di Niro MG, Cocchi A, Bernabei R: Left ventricular dysfunction: a clue to cognitive impairment in older patients with heart failure. J Neurol Neurosurg Psychiatry 1997;3:509–512.
23 de la Torre JC: Alzheimer's disease prevalence can be lowered with non-invasive testing. J Alzheimers Dis 2008;14:353–359.
24 de la Torre JC: Carotid artery ultrasound and echocardiography (CAUSE) testing to lower the prevalence of Alzheimer's disease. J Stroke Cerebrovasc Dis 2009;18:319–328.
25 de la Torre JC, Fortin T, Park G, Butler K, Kozlowski P, Pappas B, de Socarraz H, Saunders J, Richard M: Chronic cerebrovascular insufficiency induces dementia-like deficits in aged rats. Brain Res 1992;582:186–195.
26 de la Torre JC, Fortin T, Park Saunders J, Kozlowski P, Butler K, de Socarraz H, Pappas B, Richard M: Aged but not young rats develop metabolic, memory deficits after chronic brain ischemia. Neurol Res 1992; 14(suppl):177–180.
27 de la Torre JC, Fortin T, Park G, Pappas B, Saunders J, Richard M: Brain blood-flow restoration 'rescues' chronically damaged rat CA1 neurons. Brain Res 1993;623:6–15.
28 de la Torre JC, Pappas BA, Fortin T, Keyes M, Davidson C: Progressive neurodegeneration in rat brain after chronic 3-VO or 2-VO; in Fiskum G (ed): Neurodegenerative Diseases. New York, Plenum Press, pp 77–84, 1996.
29 Matsuda H: The role of neuroimaging in mild cognitive impairment. Neuropathology 2007;27:570–577.
30 Rodriguez G, Vitali P, Calvini P, Bordoni C, Girtler N, Taddei G, Mariani G, Nobili F: Hippocampal perfusion in mild cognitive impairment. Psychiatry Res 2000;100:65–74.
31 Mosconi L, Mistur R, Switalski R, Tsui WH, Glodzik L, Li Y, Pirraglia E, De Santi S, Reisberg B, Wisniewski T, de Leon MJ: FDG-PET changes in brain glucose metabolism from normal cognition to pathologically verified Alzheimer's disease. Eur J Nucl Med Mol Imaging 2009;36:811–822.
32 de la Torre JC, Fortin T, Saunders J: Correlates between NMR spectroscopy, diffusion weighted imaging and CA1 morphometry following chronic brain ischemia. J Neurosci Res 1995;41:238–245.
33 Cada A, de la Torre JC, Gonzalez-Lima F: Chronic cerebrovascular ischemia in aged rats: effects of brain metabolic capacity and behavior. Neurobiol Aging 2000;21:225–234.
34 Abdollahian NP, Cada A, Gonzalez-Lima F, de la Torre JC: Cytochrome oxidase: a predictive marker of neurodegeneration; in Gonzalez-Lima F (ed): Cytochrome Oxidase in Neuronal Metabolism and Alzheimer's Disease. New York, Plenum Press, 1998, pp 233–261.
35 de la Torre JC, Aliev G: Inhibition of vascular nitric oxide after rat chronic brain hypoperfusion: spatial memory and immunocytochemical changes. J Cerebral Blood Flow Metab 2005;25:663–672.
36 Obrenovich ME, Smith MA, Siedlak SL, Chen SG, de la Torre JC, Perry G: Overexpression of GRK2 in Alzheimer disease and in a chronic hypoperfusion rat model is an early marker of brain mitochondrial lesions. Neurotox Res 2000;10:43–56.
37 De Jong GI, Farkas E, Stienstra CM, Plass JR, Keijser JN, de la Torre JC, Luiten PG: Cerebral hypoperfusion yields capillary damage in the hippocampal CA1 area that correlates with spatial memory impairment. Neuroscience 1999;91:203–210.
38 Sopala M, Danysz W: Chronic cerebral hypoperfusion in the rat enhances age-related deficits in spatial memory. J Neural Transm 2001;108:1445–1456.
39 Farkas E, Luiten PG: Cerebral microvascular pathology in aging and Alzheimer's disease. Prog Neurobiol 2001;64:575–611.
40 Ni JW, Matsumoto K, Li HB, Murakami Y, Watanabe H: Neuronal damage and decrease of central acetylcholine level following permanent occlusion of bilateral common carotid arteries in rat. Brain Res 1995;673:290–296.
41 Otori T, Katsumata T, Muramatsu H, Kashiwagi F, Katayama Y, Terashi A: Long-term measurements of cerebral blood flow and metabolism in a rat chronic hypoperfusion model. Clin Exp Pharmacol Physiol 2003;30: 266–272.
42 Tsuchiya M, Sako K, Yura S, Yonemasu Y: Local cerebral glucose utilisation following acute and chronic bilateral carotid artery ligation in Wistar rats: relation to changes in local cerebral blood flow. Exp Brain Res 1993;95:1–7.
43 Sekhon LH, Spence I, Morgan MK, Weber NC: Chronic cerebral hypoperfusion inhibits its calcium-induced long-term potentiation in rats. Stroke 1997;28:1043–1048.
44 Liu HX, Zhang JJ, Zheng P, Zhang Y: Altered expression of MAP-2, GAP-43, and synaptophysin in the hippocampus of rats with chronic cerebral hypoperfusion correlates with cognitive impairment. Brain Res Mol Brain Res 2005;139:169–177.
45 Schmitt FA, Davis DG, Wekstein DR, Smith CD, Ashford JW, Markesbery WR: 'Preclinical' AD revisited: neuropathology of cognitively normal older adults. Neurology 2000; 55:370–376.

46 Knopman DS, Parisi JE, Salviati A, Floriach-Robert M, Boeve BF, Ivnik RJ, Smith GE, Dickson DW, Johnson KA, Petersen LE, McDonald WC, Braak H, Petersen RC: Neuropathology of cognitively normal elderly. J Neuropathol Exp Neurol 2003;62:1087–1095.
47 Giannakopoulos P, Herrmann FR, Bussire T, et al: Tangle and neuron numbers, but not amyloid load, predict cognitive status in Alzheimer's disease. Neurology 2003;60:1495–1500.
48 Davis DG, Schmitt FA, Wekstein DR, Markesbery WR: Alzheimer neuropathologic alterations in aged cognitively normal subjects. J Neuropathol Exp Neurol 1999;58:376–388.
49 Aizenstein HJ, Nebes RD, Saxton JA, Price JC, Mathis CA, Tsopelas ND, Ziolko SK, James JA, Snitz BE, Houck PR, Bi W, Cohen AD, Lopresti BJ, DeKosky ST, Halligan EM, Klunk WE: Frequent amyloid deposition without significant cognitive impairment among the elderly. Arch Neurol 2008;65:1509–1517.
50 Holmes C, Boche D, Wilkinson D, Yadegarfar G, Hopkins V, Bayer A, Jones RW, Bullock R, Love S, Neal JW, Zotova E, Nicoll JA: Long-term effects of Abeta42 immunisation in Alzheimer's disease: follow-up of a randomised, placebo-controlled phase I trial. Lancet 2008;372:216–223.
51 de la Torre JC: Critically attained threshold of cerebral hypoperfusion (CATCH): can it cause Alzheimer's disease? Ann NY Acad Sci 2000;903:424–436.
52 Solfrizzi V, Capurso C, D'Introno A, Colacicco AM, Santamato A, Ranieri M, Fiore P, Capurso A, Panza F: Lifestyle-related factors in predementia and dementia syndromes. Expert Rev Neurother 2008;8:133–158.
53 Singh-Manoux A, Sabia S, Lajnef M, Ferrie JE, Nabi H, Britton AR, Marmot MG, Shipley MJ: History of coronary heart disease and cognitive performance in midlife: the Whitehall II study. Eur Heart J 2008, Epub ahead of print.
54 Zhiyou C, Yong Y, Shanquan S, Jun Z, Liangguo H, Ling Y, Jieying L: Upregulation of BACE1 and beta-amyloid protein mediated by chronic cerebral hypoperfusion contributes to cognitive impairment and pathogenesis of Alzheimer's disease. Neurochem Res 2009;34:1226–1235.
55 Brookmeyer R, Gray S, Kawas C: Projections of Alzheimer's disease in the United States and the public health impact of delaying disease onset. Am J Public Health 1998;88:1337–1342.

Neurodegenerative Diseases

Neurodegenerative Dis 2010;7:122–126
DOI: 10.1159/000285521

Published online: February 18, 2010

Vascular Dementia and Alzheimer's Disease – Are We in a Dead-End Road?

Margherita Cavalieri[a, e] Christian Enzinger[b, c] Katja Petrovic[a] Aga Pluta-Fuerst[b] Nina Homayoon[a] Helena Schmidt[d] Franz Fazekas[b] Reinhold Schmidt[a]

[a]Division of Special Neurology, Department of Neurology, [b]Division of General Neurology, Department of Neurology, [c]Division of Neuroradiology, Department of Radiology, and [d]Institute of Molecular Biology and Biochemistry, Medical University of Graz, Graz, Austria; [e]Section of Internal Medicine, Gerontology and Geriatrics, Department of Clinical and Experimental Medicine, University of Ferrara, Ferrara, Italy

Key Words

Vascular dementia · Brain imaging · Diagnostic criteria · Surrogate marker

Abstract

Background: Diagnostic criteria separating vascular dementia from other dementias, particularly Alzheimer's disease (AD) neglect the real world in which most AD cases present with at least some vascular brain lesions. Most importantly, vascular lesions, even if subtle, exert significant effects on the patients' cognitive functioning if they coexist with AD pathology. ***Objectives:*** To emphasize the need for an integrative dementia concept in which the vascular component represents an important end point in trial planning and a possibility for disease modification along the whole spectrum of combined vascular and primary degenerative pathology. ***Methods:*** Review of the literature on possible surrogate markers to study the contribution of vascular brain damage in dementia. ***Results:*** The longitudinal change in volume of white matter lesions is the best elaborated putative surrogate marker for the study of the vascular component in dementia. Validation of the role of lacunes and microbleeds as surrogate end points is poor. Loss of brain volume is an important adjunct outcome measure even though the vascular origin of atrophy remains uncertain. ***Conclusions:*** A focus on pure vascular dementia distracts from the importance of vascular factors in dementia. Consideration of the vascular component in future clinical trials will improve our pathophysiological understanding and provide options for treatment.

Introduction

While a clear-cut distinction between vascular dementia (VaD) and Alzheimer's disease (AD) has been adopted by agencies approving medication for dementia treatment, it largely ignores data suggesting not only a considerable overlap but also a mutual interference between vascular and neurodegenerative processes in the context of dementia [1, 2]. This has been realized since the 1990s, and historically several steps have been undertaken to acknowledge the interference between vascular and primary degenerative processes in the development of dementia. The introduction of the term 'vascular cognitive impairment' (VCI) represented an important advancement as it abandoned the 'alzheimerized' concept of VaD and shifted from an arbitrary AD dementia threshold to a cognitive continuum [3]. Recognition of different subtypes of VCI, e.g. cortical VCI and subcorti-

KARGER

Fax +41 61 306 12 34
E-Mail karger@karger.ch
www.karger.com

1660–2854/10/0073–0122$26.00/0

Accessible online at:
www.karger.com/ndd

Prof. Reinhold Schmidt
Division of Special Neurology, Department of Neurology, Medical University of Graz
Auenbruggerplatz 22, AT–8036 Graz (Austria)
Tel. +43 316 385 83397, Fax +43 316 385 14178
E-Mail reinhold.schmidt@medunigraz.at

cal VCI, represented another crucial development which has been adopted in diagnostic criteria for VaD but still remained unappreciated in most randomized trials [4]. Subsequently, subcortical ischemic vascular disease (SIVD) was recognized as the prototype of VCI and clinical criteria for SIVD were developed [5]. Research criteria considering white matter hyperintensities and lacunar infarcts both as diagnostic markers and as disease surrogates of SIVD have also been proposed [6].

In line with the above-mentioned historical developments, this review advocates for a better appreciation of an integrative conceptual approach which more likely reflects the real world situation, and highlights that the separation between vascular disease and primary degenerative disease might even obviate further progress in the development of VaD treatment. The review proposes new approaches to circumvent these problems.

Diagnostic Criteria of VaD

While the DSM-IV [7] and ICD-10 [8] criteria for VaD completely spare out evidence from imaging, and also do not define the causal relationship between focal signs and symptoms and dementia, the NINDS-AIREN criteria [9] overcome these limitations. Thus, they include information derived from computed tomography or magnetic resonance imaging (MRI) on underlying ischemic brain damage, and also require a temporal relationship between focal neurologic signs and symptoms and dementia. Within these criteria, the detection of vascular lesions of specific topography and severity on brain computed tomography/MRI represents the mainstay – absence of vascular lesions rules out probable VaD.

Striving for identification of ischemic lesions causally linked to VaD undoubtedly constituted a major progress over previous criteria, yet the NINDS-AIREN criteria obviously aim at delineating a pure VaD group. They tend to include traditional poststroke patients and episodic memory/medial temporal lobe impairment patients and miss the dysexecutive SIVD phenotype. This might be one explanation for negative results in randomized controlled trials on patients with NINDS-AIREN criteria-diagnosed VaD. Another drawback is the required temporal relationship between focal neurological signs and dementia resulting in a tendency to exclude patients with nonacute vascular lesions that give rise to progressive cognitive impairment. Implementing the radiologic part of these criteria in the diagnostic workup also poses a challenge to readers.

This view is supported by an interobserver study indicating that considerable interreader variability exists and that operationalization helps the experienced reader but has no effect on inexperienced MRI readers, which applies to most clinicians working in daily routine [10]. There is clearly a need for educational programs on MRI reading when implementing NINDS-AIREN criteria for a diagnosis of VaD.

The Case for Integrative Concepts

Besides obvious difficulties with the interpretation of detailed VaD criteria, it is probably the dichotomic concept of all existing criteria that is responsible for the relative paucity of research towards development of treatment in this field.

There is broad evidence for a common coexistence of a vascular component in primary degenerative dementia with interactive effects on dementia expression, a fact that has been neglected by all proposed VaD criteria, so far.

A post-mortem study on 102 college-educated women aged 76–100 years demonstrated that among participants meeting neuropathological criteria for AD, those with brain infarcts had poorer cognitive function and a higher prevalence of dementia than those without infarcts [11]. Further, the development of dementia in the absence of cerebral infarction requires a tangle burden eight times greater. In a prospective autopsy series of 87 patients with clinically diagnosed dementia, only 13% of patients clinically diagnosed as having VaD in fact had pure VaD at autopsy [12], and AD pathology is seen in more than 40% of patients meeting VaD criteria [13]. In the MRC-Cognitive Function and Aging Study, only 21% of AD cases had pure AD pathology [14].

This leaves us with a scenario of diagnostic criteria neglecting the real world in which a mixed pathology is common, and in which the interaction between vascular and neurodegenerative pathology is obviously important [11–14]. It is clear, however, that one of the two pathologies predominates in many cases and that the study of pure forms of the disorders, e.g. AD without vascular lesions, remains an important task both from a pathophysiological point of view and in trials. Nevertheless the development of diagnostic criteria moving from dichotomy to integrative etiology appears mandatory.

Subsequently, trial designs in VaD need to appreciate that it is virtually impossible to exclude a mixed pathology, and to assess the efficacy of treatment on both the

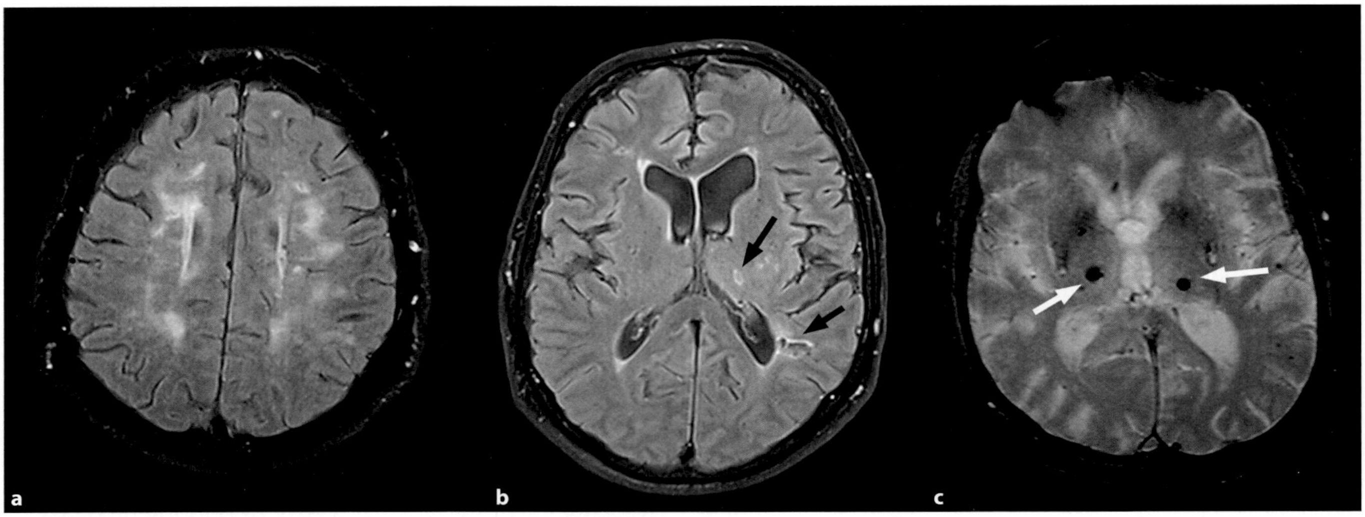

Fig. 1. Putative vascular imaging end points. **a** Confluent white matter lesions. **b** Lacunes in white matter and thalamus (black arrows). **c** Microbleeds (white arrows).

vascular and the degenerative component of dementia. The key question is whether and how we can tell that the vascular component contributes to the cognitive-behavioral phenotype of a given patient.

Longitudinal brain imaging will play a crucial role in better understanding the complex interplay of factors. Putative imaging surrogates such as small vessel disease-related brain abnormalities including white matter lesions, lacunes and microbleeds (fig. 1) must fulfill three important prerequisites [15]: there should be reasonable confidence that the observed tissue changes are 'vascular'; the rate of progression must be fast enough to observe therapeutic effects within a reasonable period of time, and the surrogate and clinical end point need to be correlated.

Possible Imaging End Points in VaD Trials

Progression of confluent white matter lesions is currently the best elaborated putative surrogate marker at least in trials focusing on subcortical VaD [16].

The literature on progression of white matter lesions and their association with cognitive decline has been reviewed recently by our group [16]. All subjects with confluent white matter lesions show progression beyond measurement error over a 6-year period, and based on the fast progression rate of confluent lesions it was estimated that only 195 patients would be required per treatment arm to demonstrate a 20% reduction in the rate of disease progression in a 3-year randomized trial. It is important to note that white matter lesion progression was consistently associated with cognitive decline and would thus fulfill the most crucial criterion of surrogate end points. Increase in white matter lesion volume correlates inversely with cognitive tests exploring general cognition, memory, conceptualization and visuopractical skills [16]. According to the LADIS experience, white matter lesions are not only related to cognition but also strongly predict the global functional decline of patients [17]. This is highly relevant for the use of white matter abnormalities as a surrogate marker because it was long debated whether these changes matter to the patient in terms of everyday functioning [18]. Lately, interventional studies started to incorporate white matter lesion volume as an outcome measure in their protocols. The MRI substudy of Perindopril Protection against Recurrent Stroke Study (PROGRESS) was the first investigation to report that an active blood pressure-lowering regimen can stop or delay lesion progression in patients with cerebrovascular disease [19]. The validation status of all other focal 'vascular' brain changes is much lower, longitudinal data are barely available for lacunes and absent for microbleeds.

Longitudinal brain volume change is another interesting candidate. In CADASIL, brain atrophy represents an important aspect of the disease process per se [20]. Substantial progression of brain volume loss also occurs in elderly individuals, but to a smaller extent, and relates to progression of white matter lesions and cognition. In the Austrian Stroke Prevention Study, there existed a complex interaction between brain parenchymal loss and progression of white matter damage [21]. Loss of brain volume should thus be included as an adjunct outcome measure besides white matter lesion load in future interventional trials irrespective of the fact that a vascular origin of atrophy remains uncertain. Regional atrophy measurements and assessment of cortical thickness in specific brain regions may help to better define the pattern of brain atrophy caused by vascular disease.

Executive Functioning – Another Tool to Study the Contribution of the Vascular Component

Impaired executive function, including shifting (the ability to shift between tasks and mental sets), updating (the ability to monitor information) and inhibition (the ability to inhibit dominant response) [22], is often described as the primary cognitive syndrome in VaD. Although this pattern may not apply to all patients with VaD, i.e., to multi-infarct dementia in which the type of cognitive impairment depends on the location of the lesions, a dysexecutive syndrome is the most prominent type of cognitive impairment in subcortical VaD. Lacunar infarcts and white matter abnormalities often occur in connecting pathways of frontal-subcortical circuits which mediate executive functioning, and lesions at any point may influence the integrity of the entire circuit with subsequent cognitive dysfunction [23].

Thus, testing performance in set shifting, verbal fluency, processing speed and working memory might represent an important instrument to tackle the impact of modifications of vascular factors on the clinical picture in dementia studies. Recently, recommendations for protocols for the investigation of patients with VCI have been proposed in a workshop of the NINDS and the Canadian Stroke Network [24]. It was suggested that the recommendations should cover a wide range of cognitive functions and be especially attuned to the assessment of executive abilities. However, these protocols vary in the time needed for their application and have to be validated before they can be used in clinical trials.

Implications beyond VaD

The strong interactive effect of vascular lesions on cognitive dysfunction in patients with AD strongly suggests that modification of the common vascular component even in patients with prevailing AD pathology allows for modification of the clinical course of dementia. In a scenario in which medication for treatment of AD provides modest symptomatic benefits at most, the control of vascular factors including treatment of risk factors and secondary stroke prevention represent important, although often neglected, strategies for preventing or slowing the progression of dementing illnesses.

References

1 Langa KM, Foster NL, Larson EB: Mixed dementia: emerging concepts and therapeutic implications. JAMA 2004;292:2901–2908.

2 Roman GC, Royall DR: A diagnostic dilemma: is 'Alzheimer's dementia' Alzheimer's disease, vascular dementia, or both? Lancet Neurol 2004;3:141.

3 O'Brien JT, Erkinjuntti T, Reisberg B, Roman G, Sawada T, Pantoni L, Bowler JV, Ballard C, DeCarli C, Gorelick PB, Rockwood K, Burns A, Gauthier S, DeKosky ST: Vascular cognitive impairment. Lancet Neurol 2003; 2:89–98.

4 Erkinjuntti T, Inzitari D, Pantoni L, Wallin A, Scheltens P, Rockwood K, Desmond DW: Limitations of clinical criteria for the diagnosis of vascular dementia in clinical trials. Is a focus on subcortical vascular dementia a solution? Ann NY Acad Sci 2000;903:262–272.

5 Erkinjuntti T, Inzitari D, Pantoni L, Wallin A, Scheltens P, Rockwood K, Roman G, Chui H, Desmond D: Research criteria for subcortical vascular dementia in clinical trials. J Neural Transm Suppl 2000;59:23–30.

6 Erkinjuntti T: Subcortical ischemic vascular disease and dementia. Int Psychogeriatr 2003;15(suppl 1):23–26.

7 American Psychiatric Association: DSM-IV. Diagnostic and Statistical Manual of Mental Disorders, ed 4th. Washington, American Psychiatric Association, 1994.

8 World Health Organization: The ICD-10 Classification of Mental and Behavioural Disorders. Diagnostic Criteria for Research. Geneva, World Health Organization, 1993.

9 Roman G, Tatemichi T, Erkinjuntti T, Cummings J, Masdeu J, Garcia J, Amaducci L, Orgogozo J, Brun A, Hofman A, Moody D, O'Brien M, Yamaguchi T, Grafman J, Drayer B, Bennet D, Fisher M, Ogata J, Kokmen E, Bermejo F, Wolf P, Gorelick P, Bick K, Pajeau A, Bell M, DeCarli C, Culebras A, Korczyn A, Bogousslavsky J, Hartman A, Scheinberg P: Vascular dementia: diagnostic criteria for research studies. Report of the NINDS-AIREN International Workshop. Neurology 1993;43:250–260.

10 Van Straaten E, Scheltens P, Knol D, van Buchem M, van Dijk E, Hofman P, Karas G, Kjartansson O, de Leeuw F, Prins N, Schmidt R, Visser M, Weinstein H, Barkhof F: Operational definitions for the NINDS-AIREN criteria for vascular dementia: an interobserver study. Stroke 2003;34:1907–1912.

11 Snowdon DA, Greiner LH, Mortimer JA, Riley KP, Greiner PA, Markesbery WR: Brain infarction and the clinical expression of Alzheimer disease. The Nun Study. JAMA 1997;277:813–817.

12 Nolan KA, Lino MM, Seligmann AW, Blass JP: Absence of vascular dementia in an autopsy series from a dementia clinic. J Am Geriatr Soc 1998;46:597–604.

13 Kalaria RN: Small vessel disease and Alzheimer's dementia: pathological considerations. Cerebrovasc Dis 2002;13(suppl 2):48–52.

14 Pathological correlates of late-onset dementia in a multicentre, community-based population in England and Wales. Neuropathology Group of the Medical Research Council Cognitive Function and Ageing Study (MRC CFAS). Lancet 2001;357:169–175.

15 Schmidt R, Scheltens P, Erkinjuntti T, Pantoni L, Markus H, Wallin A, Barkhof F, Fazekas F, for the European Task Force on Age-Related White Matter Changes: White matter lesion progression: a surrogate endpoint for trials in cerebral small vessel disease. Neurology 2004;63:139–144.

16 Schmidt R, Petrovic K, Ropele S, Enzinger C, Fazekas F: Progression of leukoaraiosis and cognition. Stroke 2007;38:2619–2625.

17 Inzitari D, Simoni M, Pracucci G, Poggesi A, Basile AM, Chabriat H, Erkinjuntti T, Fazekas F, Ferro JM, Hennerici M, Langhorne P, O'Brien J, Barkhof F, Visser MC, Wahlund LO, Waldemar G, Wallin A, Pantoni L: Risk of rapid global functional decline in elderly patients with severe cerebral age-related white matter changes: The LADIS study. Arch Intern Med 2007;167:81–88.

18 Schmidt R, Breteler M, Inzitari D, Fratiglioni L, Hofman A, Launer L, for the Neurologic Diseases in the Elderly Research Group: Prognosis with stroke in Europe: a collaborative study of population-based cohorts. Neurology 2000;54(suppl 5):S34–S37.

19 Dufouil C, Chalmers J, Coskun O, Besancon V, Bousser M, Guillon P, MacMahon S, Mazoyer B, Neal B, Woodward M, Tzourio-Mazoyer N, Tzourio C, PROGRESS MRI Substudy Investigators: Effects of blood pressure lowering on cerebral white matter hyperintensities in patients with stroke: the PROGRESS (Perindopril Protection against Recurrent Stroke Study) magnetic resonance imaging substudy. Circulation 2005;112: 1644–1650.

20 Peters N, Holtmannspotter M, Opherk C, Gschwendtner A, Herzog J, Samann P, Dichgans M: Brain volume changes in CADASIL: a serial MRI study in pure subcortical ischemic vascular disease. Neurology 2006;66: 1517–1522.

21 Schmidt R, Ropele S, Enzinger C, Petrovic K, Smith S, Schmidt H, Matthews PM, Fazekas F: White matter lesion progression, brain atrophy, and cognitive decline: The Austrian Stroke Prevention Study. Ann Neurol 2005; 58:610–616.

22 Miyake A, Friedman NP, Emerson MJ, Witzki AH, Howerter A, Wager TD: The unity and diversity of executive functions and their contributions to complex 'Frontal lobe' Tasks: a latent variable analysis. Cogn Psychol 2000;41:49–100.

23 Cummings JL: Frontal-subcortical circuits and human behavior. Arch Neurol 1993;50: 873–880.

24 Hachinski V, Iadecola C, Petersen RC, Breteler MM, Nyenhuis DL, Black SE, Powers WJ, DeCarli C, Merino JG, Kalaria RN, Vinters HV, Holtzman DM, Rosenberg GA, Wallin A, Dichgans M, Marler JR, Leblanc GG: National Institute of Neurological Disorders and Stroke-Canadian Stroke Network vascular cognitive impairment harmonization standards. Stroke 2006;37:2220–2241.

Neuro-degenerative Diseases

Neurodegenerative Dis 2010;7:127–130
DOI: 10.1159/000285522

Published online: February 18, 2010

Vascular Contribution to Dementia in Parkinson's Disease

Amos D. Korczyn

Sackler School of Medicine, Tel Aviv University, Ramat Aviv, Israel

Key Words
Parkinson's disease · Dementia · Vascular lesions

Abstract
Parkinson's disease is one of the most common neurodegenerative diseases. Although its motor symptoms are presently relatively well controlled, other manifestations are less well understood and poorly treated. Among these, the cognitive changes have a prominent role. Dementia is usually ascribed to changes in the nucleus basalis of Meynert and the cerebral cortex. This article discusses the possible contribution of vascular factors to the cognitive impairment in Parkinson's disease and its implication for the management.

Parkinson's disease (PD) is a common neurodegenerative disease. While its etiology has been debated for several decades, no clear consensus has emerged, and it is likely that the death of nigral dopaminergic neurons can be the result of several converging pathogenic mechanisms. Lewy bodies (LB) have been known for many years to play a central role in PD. Initially, they were looked at as markers of the disease process, but later a fierce debate erupted as to whether they are themselves pathogenic or reflect a protective process. It is only after the recognition that LB contain ubiquitin, a protein involved in transporting other proteins for reprocessing, that more light began to be shed on their role. This has been even more clearly defined after the identification of α-synuclein. This protein is also deposited in LB and its central role in PD pathogenesis is witnessed by the existence of mutations, duplications or triplications of the α-synuclein gene in some familial PD cases [1].

The importance of α-synuclein as a marker of neuronal degeneration in PD is credited to Del Tredici et al. [2] who demonstrated that beyond LB, α-synuclein deposits can be demonstrated in neurons, axons and dendrites ('Lewy neurites') in several brain areas, only some of which are dopaminergic. Moreover, Del Tredici et al. [2] further showed that the deposition of α-synuclein does not occur at random but rather follows an orderly manner, starting in the olfactory bulb and dorsal motor nucleus of the vagus, later extending rostrally in the brain stem, then the midbrain, until eventually reaching the cortex. These anatomical changes were demonstrated conveniently at the same time when nonmotor symptoms of PD attracted wider attention [3].

Dementia is common in advanced stages of PD and in fact it is likely that most if not all PD patients will eventually develop dementia if they survive long enough [4]. The existence of cognitive impairment has a strong impact on the quality of life of PD patients and their spouses and carers [5]. Nevertheless, its pathogenesis is still unclear.

In advanced stages of the disease, PD patients have cortical changes, including LB deposition in neurons. It

KARGER
Fax +41 61 306 12 34
E-Mail karger@karger.ch
www.karger.com

1660–2854/10/0073–0127$26.00/0

Accessible online at:
www.karger.com/ndd

Prof. Amos D. Korczyn
Sackler School of Medicine
Tel Aviv University
IL–69978 Ramat Aviv (Israel)
Tel. +972 3 697 4229, Fax +972 3 640 9113, E-Mail amoskor@post.tau.ac.il

Table 1. Pathologic contributors to cognitive changes in the Parkinson complex

Cholinergic loss due to nucleus basalis of Meynert lesions
Noradrenergic loss due to locus ceruleus lesions
Serotoninergic loss due to raphe lesions
Dopaminergic loss due to nigral lesions
Cortical dysfunction due to Lewy body deposition
Cortical dysfunction due to coexistent Alzheimer pathology
Cortical dysfunction due to coexistent vascular lesions
Cortical dysfunction due to coexistent nonspecific changes of aging

is unclear how exactly LB relate to the cognitive decline. Since deposition of LB in the cortex occurs particularly in patients with advanced PD who are also cognitively impaired, it was perhaps natural to ascribe the dementia of advanced PD to these changes in the cortex. However, it must be recognized that almost all demented people with cortical LB also have abundant Alzheimer changes [6]. This overlap of PD and Alzheimer's disease (AD) is of interest, since many patients who are clinically diagnosed in life as having AD, are found in autopsy to have associated LB pathology [7]. Thus, these cases can be regarded as having mixed AD-LB dementia. Accepting this overlap, it is important to stress that even if patients have restricted AD pathology, insufficient by itself to fulfill the arbitrary pathologic criteria for AD, this cannot be taken to mean that these changes will not add to the disease burden and contribute to the cognitive impairment if other pathological changes are present.

Patients with PD dementia are treated with cholinesterase inhibitors [8, 9], and this treatment is as efficacious in this condition as it is in AD. Presumably, the effect is related in both diseases to loss of cholinergic neurons in the nucleus basalis of Meynert [10].

It is therefore quite likely that PD dementia is a complex entity (table 1). Patients with PD dementia always have mixed pathology, with LB adding to AD-like changes. In addition, PD patients, frequently elderly, are never immune to other diseases, including vascular diseases. These vascular changes may affect the brain, and it is illogical to assume that such vascular changes, if they occur, will not add to the load of pathology in both the motor and the cognitive domains.

While it is likely that vascular lesions may be underrecognized in patients with dementia [11, 12], only a few studies have attempted to study the contribution of vascular brain lesions to the progression of PD. In terms of motor impairment, even after excluding cases with 'vascular parkinsonism', Papapetropoulos et al. [13] found that PD patients with coexistent ischemic heart disease, minor strokes or diabetes mellitus had significantly more severe motor impairment and suggested that timely treatment of vascular risk factors may slow down the development of motor impairment. It is unclear, however, whether these patients with vascular risk factors will respond as well to the treatment with dopaminergic drugs. Vascular parkinsonism itself is heterogeneous in terms of its pathogenesis and in its response to therapy [14]. In fact, those PD patients of Papapetropoulos et al. [13] with coexistent vascular disease needed higher doses of dopaminergic medication. Thus, vascular disease was found to be an aggravating factor of the motor manifestations of PD.

The coincidence of PD and vascular disease demands attention because of the report that PD patients may be at a higher risk for stroke and ischemic heart disease [15].

Multiple brain pathologies are the rule rather than the exception in the brains of elderly individuals. Schneider et al. [16] have demonstrated in an autopsy study that patients with multiple coexistent brain diseases were almost three times more likely to exhibit dementia. In that study, multiple pathologies included AD, vascular brain disease and (less commonly) PD.

The mechanism through which vascular disease is associated with dementia in general is not well understood, and is probably heterogeneous. One possibility is the occurrence of leukoaraiosis. While the relationship of white matter changes in AD and vascular dementia has been studied extensively, the existence of white matter changes to PD has received much less attention. In a carefully performed study, Beyer et al. [17] were able to demonstrate that PD patients with dementia had significantly more white matter hyperintensities in the deep white matter and in the periventricular white matter, as seen on MRI. Had those patients not had parkinsonism, they would have been diagnosed possibly with Binswanger's disease (BD), a common brain vasculopathy. However, BD is also associated with motor abnormalities, particularly gait impairment [18]. It is, therefore, difficult to diagnose BD in a patient with advanced PD who also has cognitive impairment, unless relying on brain imaging.

Hughes et al. [19] reported autopsy data of PD patients, and found 'incidental' vascular brain lesions in the brain in very few (3/100). Moreover, it is quite likely that in that study vascular lesions could have been overlooked since only macroscopic evidence of vascular lesions was used. However, the slices used were too thick to identify small lacunes. Additionally, no attention has been paid to white matter lesions (frequently vascular in origin), and the intracerebral blood vessels themselves have not been examined systematically. Several other studies confirmed the high frequency of coexistent cerebrovascular lesions in a series of PD patients. While these lesions have been reported to be predominantly minor, the actual extent of cerebrovascular lesions might have been larger. Again, relatively thick brain slices are very likely to miss small lacunes, and data on white matter lesions and on microangiopathy have not been reported. In any case, it is important to stress that even small lesions can affect cognitive function in people with an underlying neurodegenerative brain disease [20]. Small lacunes, particularly in the basal ganglia, may affect extrapyramidal function [21, 22] and result in parkinsonism, but may also contribute to cognitive decline.

It is clear that attempts to localize brain areas related to cognition have, in general, failed, as demonstrated by many observations on people with small lacunes or microinfarcts. It is quite likely that in many cases the anatomic damage is considerably more diffuse than shown by imaging. On a functional level, almost no attention is given to blood-brain barrier dysfunction, although it is quite likely that it is significantly impaired in patients with small vessel brain disease. Blood-brain barrier dysfunction, as a vascular disorder, may thus be potentially important in causing widespread brain dysfunction, including cognitive impairment, which will not even be reflected by state-of-the-art imaging methods or even neuropathology.

Yet another issue to be considered is the role of hyperhomocysteinemia. High serum homocysteine levels are suspected to be involved in both neurodegenerative and vascular diseases, although none is proven. It is also not clear whether homocysteine itself is toxic or whether homocysteine is a marker of another toxic or neuroprotective mediator, e.g. uric acid [23]. Hyperhomocysteinemia is associated with increased white matter changes in patients with small vessel disease [24]. These considerations are particularly relevant to PD, because treatment with levodopa causes elevation of serum homocysteine levels (unless COMT inhibitors are used simultaneously) [25]. Some data suggest that hyperhomocysteinemia is a risk factor for coronary artery disease in PD patients [26], and thus potentially for cerebrovascular disease as well. In patients suffering from PD, those with hyperhomocysteinemia are more likely to be depressed (and depression is a risk factor for dementia), and have lower neuropsychometric scores [27].

Post-hoc analysis of a prospective controlled study [28] showed that PD patients who were hyperhomocysteinemic at baseline were more likely to deteriorate in the cognitive domain over the next 6 months than those who were normohomocysteinemic at baseline (both groups being treated with placebo only), although in the parallel rivastigmine-treated arms patients did not show this effect, and in fact patients had a tendency for cognitive improvement regardless of baseline homocysteine levels.

Previous studies on a limited number of patients reached conflicting results on the possible contribution of vascular changes to cognition in patients with PD [28–30].

Thus in conclusion, older people frequently suffer from multiple pathologies. Even if any of these pathologies seem minor, they could well have a disproportionate impact on motor and cognitive function. In PD patients, additional vascular lesions may enhance motor disability and make it more resistant to therapy. Similarly, such vascular changes may have deleterious mental effects. Brain imaging may provide important information about cerebral lesions, but it also provides only a partial reflection of the extent of brain damage. While sophisticated methods are available to demonstrate white matter changes in the brain, clinical evaluation of blood-brain barrier integrity and dysfunction is not easy to measure in vivo.

These conclusions have important treatment implications. Attempts to control vascular risk factors such as hypertension, dyslipidemia, obesity and insulin resistance should be maximized in PD patients [31]. While the involvement of homocysteine in neurodegeneration is still being investigated, the possibility of levodopa-induced hyperhomocysteinemia should be considered, since patients can be protected by COMT inhibitors or B vitamins.

References

1 Klein C: Implications of genetics on the diagnosis and care of patients with Parkinson disease. Arch Neurol 2006;63:328–334.
2 Del Tredici K, Rub U, De Vos RA, Bohl JR, Braak H: Where does Parkinson disease pathology begin in the brain? J Neuropathol Exp Neurol 2002;61 413–426.
3 Korczyn AD, Gurevich T: Parkinson's disease: before the motor symptoms and beyond. J Neurol Sci, accepted.
4 Butler TC, van den Hout A, Matthews FE, et al: Dementia and survival in Parkinson disease: a 12-year population study. Neurology 2008;70:1017–1022.
5 Korczyn AD: Dementia in Parkinson's disease. J Neurol 2001;248(suppl 3):1–4.

6 Bower JH, Dickson DW, Taylor L, Maraganore DM, Rocca WA: Clinical correlates of the pathology underlying parkinsonism: a population perspective. Mov Disord 2002; 17:910–916.
7 Weiner MF, Risser RC, Cullum CM, et al: Alzheimer's disease and its Lewy body variant: a clinical analysis of postmortem verified cases. Am J Psychiatry 1996;153:1269–1273.
8 Giladi N, Shabtai H, Gurevich T, Benbunan B, Anca M, Korczyn AD: Rivastigmine (Exelon) for dementia in patients with Parkinson's disease. Acta Neurol Scand 2003;108: 368–373.
9 Emre M, Aarsland D, Albanese A, et al: Rivastigmine for dementia associated with Parkinson's disease. N Engl J Med 2004;351: 2509–2518.
10 Whitehouse PJ, Hedreen JC, White CI, Price DI: Basal forebrain neurons in the dementia of Parkinson disease. Ann Neurol 1983;13: 243–248.
11 Korczyn AD: Mixed dementia – the most common cause of dementia. Ann NY Acad Sci 2002;977:129–134.
12 Schneider JA, Troncoso JC, Zonderman AB, Resnick SM, Crain B, Pletnikova O, O'Brien RJJ: Effect of infarcts on dementia in the Baltimore longitudinal Study of aging. Ann Neurol 2008;64:168–176.
13 Papapetropoulos S, Argyriou AA, Ellul J: Clinical characteristics of late-onset Parkinson disease. Arch Neurol 2003;60:1815–1816.
14 Balash Y, Korczyn AD: Vascular parkinsonism; in Koller WC, Melamed E (eds): Handbook of Clinical Neurology. Parkinson's Disease and Related Disorders. Part 2. Amsterdam, Elsevier, 2007, pp 417–425.
15 Ben-Shlomo Y, Whitehead AS, Smith GD: Parkinson's, Alzheimer's, and motor neurone disease. BMJ 1996;312:724.
16 Schneider JA, Arvanitakis Z, Bang W, Bennett DA: Mixed brain pathologies account for most dementia cases in community-dwelling older persons. Neurology 2007;69: 2197–2204.
17 Beyer MK, Larsen JP, Aarsland D: Gray matter atrophy in Parkinson disease with dementia and dementia with Lewy bodies. Neurology 2007;69:747–754.
18 Thompson PD, Marsden CD: Gait disorder of subcortical arteriosclerotic encephalopathy: Binswanger's disease. Mov Disord 1987; 2:1–8.
19 Hughes AJ, Daniel SE, Lees AJ: Improved accuracy of clinical diagnosis of Lewy body Parkinson's disease. Neurology 2001;57: 1497–1499.
20 Snowdon DA, Greiner LH, Mortimer JA, et al: Brain infarction and the clinical expression of Alzheimer disease. The Nun Study. JAMA 1997;277:813–817.
21 Groswasser IR, Bornstein NM, Korczyn AD: Parkinsonism in patients with lacunar infarcts of the basal ganglia. Eur Neurol 1995; 35:46–49.
22 Tolosa ES, Santamaria J: Parkinsonism and basal ganglia infarcts. Neurology 984;34: 1516.
23 Annanmaki T, Pessala-Driver A, Hokkanen L, Murros K: Uric acid associates with cognition in Parkinson's disease. Parkinsonism Relat Disord 2008;14:576–578.
24 Sachdev P, Parslow R, Salonikas C, et al: Homocysteine and the brain in midadult life: evidence for an increased risk of leukoaraiosis in men. Arch Neurol 2004;61:1369–1376.
25 Korczyn AD: Catechol-O-methyl transferase inhibitors in the treatment of Parkinson's disease; in Galvez-Jimenez N (ed): Scientific Basis for the Treatment of Parkinson's Disease. London, Taylor and Francis, 2005, pp 145–150.
26 O'Suilleabhain PE, Sung V, Hernandez SV, Lacritz L, et al: Elevated plasma homocysteine level in patients with Parkinson disease: motor, affective, and cognitive associations. Arch Neurol 2004;61:865–868.
27 Rogers JD, Sanchez-Saffon A, Frol AB, Diaz-Arrastia R: Elevated plasma homocysteine levels in patients treated with levodopa: association with vascular disease. Arch Neurol 2003;60:59–64.
28 Barone P, Burn DJ, van Laar T, Hsu C, Poewe W, Lane RM: Rivastigmine versus placebo in hyperhomocysteinemic Parkinson's disease dementia patients. Mov Disord 2008;23: 1532–1540.
29 Slawek J, Wieczorek D, Derejko M, Dubaniewicz M, Brockuis B, Sitek E, Wilczewska L, Roszman A, Lass P: The influence of vascular risk factors and white matter hyperintensities on the degree of cognitive impairment in Parkinson's disease. Neurol Neurochir Pol 2008;42:505–512.
30 Haugarvoll K, Aarsland D, Wentzel-Larsen T, Larsen JP: The influence of cerebrovascular risk factors on incident dementia in patients with Parkinson's Disease. Acta Neurol Scand 2005;112:386–339.
31 Rektor I, Goldemund D, Sheardova K, Rektorova I, Michalkova Z, Dufek M: Vascular pathology in patients with idiopathic Parkinson's Disease. Parkinsonism Relat Disord 2009;15:24–29.

Imaging, Biomarkers, Genetics and Diagnostic Markers

Neurodegenerative Diseases

Neurodegenerative Dis 2010;7:131–135
DOI: 10.1159/000289222

Published online: March 3, 2010

Early Detection of Alzheimer's Disease with PET Imaging

V. Berti[a, d] R.S. Osorio[a, b] L. Mosconi[a] Y. Li[a] S. De Santi[a] M.J. de Leon[a, c]

[a]Department of Psychiatry, Center for Brain Health, [b]Departments of Pathology and Psychiatry, Alzheimer's Disease Center, New York University School of Medicine, New York, N.Y., and [c]Nathan Kline Institute, Orangeburg, N.Y., USA; [d]Nuclear Medicine Unit, Clinical Pathophysiology Department, University of Florence, Florence, Italy

Key Words
Alzheimer's disease biomarkers · PET neuroimaging · Early diagnostic tools · Amyloid lesions

Abstract
Preclinical diagnosis of Alzheimer's disease (AD) is one of the major challenges for the prevention of AD. AD biomarkers are needed not only to reveal preclinical pathologic changes, but also to monitor progression and therapeutics. PET neuroimaging can reliably assess aspects of the molecular biology and neuropathology of AD. The aim of this article is to review the use of FDG-PET and amyloid PET imaging in the early detection of AD.

Introduction

Alzheimer's disease (AD) is the most common form of dementia and is characterized by progressive impairments in cognitive function and behavior [1]. The provisional diagnosis of AD is based on clinical history, neurological/psychiatric examinations, cognitive testing and neuroimaging, while a definitive diagnosis requires the postmortem observation of specific pathological lesions: intracellular neurofibrillary tangles (NFT), amyloid-β (Aβ) plaques, synapse/neuronal loss and atrophy [2].

Some of these lesions begin to form 20–30 years before the disease becomes clinically evident [3], indicating the possibility for developing early and sensitive biomarkers of the disease. As a matter of fact, the need for biomarkers in AD is real, in particular to reveal preclinical pathological alterations, to monitor objectively and accurately disease progression, and eventually to evaluate the response to therapy [4].

Several neuroimaging modalities show promising results as early diagnostic tools for AD. These include MRI for structural assessment, and PET imaging for both glucose metabolism and for Aβ and possibly NFT binding.

MRI imaging plays an important and routine role in the differential diagnosis of AD from some other dementias (vascular dementia) [5]. Several studies have shown that medial temporal lobes (MTL) atrophy is an early sign of AD and predicts conversion to dementia in normal subjects [5]. However, functional imaging, especially 2-[^{18}F]fluoro-2-deoxy-D-glucose (FDG) PET, has played the leading role in the early detection of AD. FDG-PET provides qualitative and quantitative estimates of the cerebral metabolic rate of glucose (CMRglc), an index of synaptic functioning and density [6, 7]. The major limitation of this highly sensitive modality (FDG-PET sensitivity in

KARGER
Fax +41 61 306 12 34
E-Mail karger@karger.ch
www.karger.com

Accessible online at:
www.karger.com/ndd

Prof. Mony de Leon
Center for Brain Health, Department of Psychiatry, NYU School of Medicine
550 First Avenue
New York, NY 10016 (USA)
E-Mail mony.deleon@nyumc.org

Table 1. CMRglc reductions in AD and 'high-risk' populations compared to normal controls

Population	CMRglc findings	Percentage reduction vs. controls
AD patients	Regional CMRglc reductions in MTL, PTC, PCC and FC, and WB hypometabolism [9, 13–16]	WB: 28–29% MTL: 20–30% PCC: 18–22% PC: 15–40% FC: 22–24%
Asymptomatic FAD mutations carriers	Hypometabolism in MTL, PTC, PCC and FC [17]	MTL: 12% PCC: 21%
Asymptomatic ApoE4 carriers	Hypometabolism in MTL, PTC, PCC and FC, occipital cortex, and thalamus [18, 19]	PCC: 10.5% PTC: 10% FC: 9.8%
Asymptomatic patients with a maternal family history of AD	Hypometabolism in MTL, PCC/precuneus, IP and FC [21]	MTL: 15% PCC: 22% IP: 12% FC: 10%
MCI	Hypometabolism in MTL, PCC and PTC in amnestic MCI [20] Nonamnestic MCI show either absence of cortical hypometabolism or CMRglc reductions in ACC and PTC [20, 22]	MTL: 8.6% IP: 8.9%
SMC	Hypometabolism in the PHG, PTC, inferior frontal cortex and thalamus [19]	PHG: 18% PTC: 16%

ACC = Anterior cingulate cortex; PC = parietal cortex; IP = inferior parietal lobe; PHG = parahippocampal gyrus; WB = whole brain.

histopathologically confirmed AD is 94%) [8] is its lack of disease specificity (73%), as reductions in CMRglc are often found in other dementias [9]. A new and effective strategy is to use amyloid PET radiotracers to target the amyloid lesions of AD [10, 11]. This approach increases specificity and improves diagnostic accuracy, particularly if combined with FDG [12].

FDG-PET Imaging

FDG-PET studies in AD demonstrate consistent and progressive CMRglc reductions, whose extent and topography correlate with symptom type and severity [13]. Virtually all FDG-PET studies report that, compared to age-matched healthy normal controls, AD patients show both widespread global metabolic impairment and regional metabolic reductions involving MTL, parietotemporal (PTC) and posterior cingulate cortices (PCC) [9, 13–15] (table 1). The frontal cortex (FC) is also involved in more advanced AD stages [9, 16]. This pattern is seen in contrast to relative preservation of primary motor/visual areas, cerebellum, thalamus and basal ganglia (fig. 1).

Importantly, CMRglc reductions have been observed with FDG-PET before the onset of AD symptoms, highlighting the importance of PET as a tool for early detection and estimation of increased risk for future dementia.

So far, research in the early diagnosis of AD has focused on individuals from 'high-risk' populations who are more likely to develop the disease as compared to 'low-risk' subjects. These 'high-risk' populations include carriers of any of the autosomal dominant mutations for early-onset familial AD (FAD) [17], carriers of an apolipoprotein E4 (ApoE4) allele [18, 19], individuals with subjective memory complaints (SMC) or mild cognitive impairment (MCI) [9, 19, 20], and individuals with a family history of AD, particularly when the mothers are affected [21].

Most of the studies show AD-like CMRglc reductions in these at-risk groups, intermediate between controls and AD patients, years prior to clinical decline (table 1).

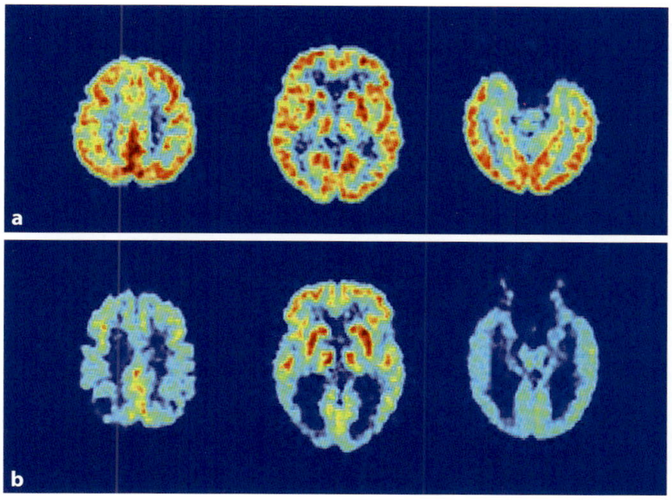

Fig. 1. FDG-PET scans from two representative subjects: normal subject (**a**) and AD subject (**b**). PET scans are displayed in the axial plane, from the top to the bottom of the brain, at the level of the centrum-semiovale (left), basal ganglia (center), and MTL (right). Note the hypometabolism involving parietotemporal regions, posterior cingulate/precuneus, medial temporal cortex, and to a lesser extent FC in the AD patient as compared to the normal subject.

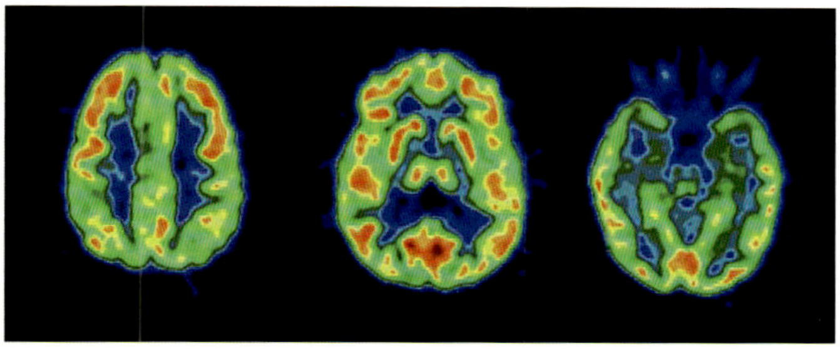

Fig. 2. FDG-PET scan from a representative MCI subject. PET scan is displayed in the axial plane, from the top to the bottom of the brain, at the level of the centrum-semiovale (left), basal ganglia (center), and MTL (right). Note the moderate hypometabolism involving posterior cingulate/precuneus, parietal and medial temporal cortices.

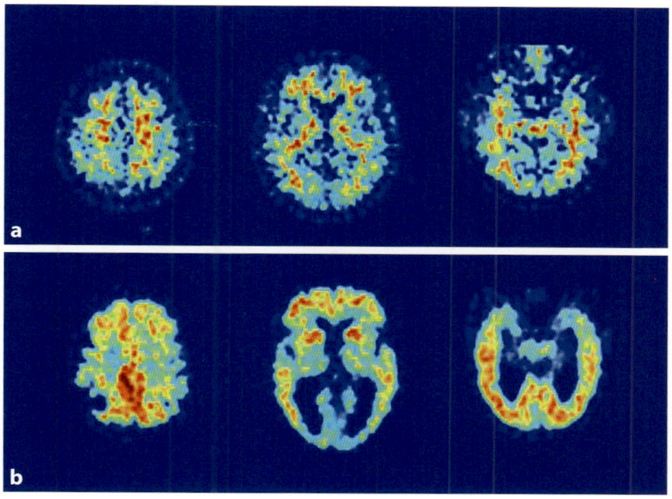

Fig. 3. PIB-PET scans from two representative subjects: normal subject (**a**) and AD subject (**b**). PET scans are displayed in the axial plane, from the top to the bottom of the brain, at the level of the centrum-semiovale (left), basal ganglia (center), and MTL (right). Note that in the normal subject PIB is distributed only in the white matter, reflecting nonspecific uptake, and in the AD patient PIB uptake is present in several cortical regions, such as frontal, parietal, posterior cingulate/precuneus and lateral temporal cortices, and in basal ganglia.

For example, MCI conversion studies report a predictive pattern of CMRglc reductions involving the regions typically hypometabolic in AD, such as MTL, PCC and PTC. These patterns are not present in 'stable' MCI (fig. 2) [20, 22]. Likewise, in cognitively normal subjects, a pattern of MTL hypometabolism with subsequent cortical reductions was demonstrated to precede and predict decline to MCI and postmortem verified AD [23, 24]. However, CMRglc reductions are less effective in predicting decline in SMC and nonamnestic MCI, two subtypes whose outcome appears to be more heterogeneous, reflecting other dementia and psychiatric disorders [19, 22].

Amyloid PET Imaging

The development of amyloid imaging ligands has greatly advanced our understanding of the pathophysiology of AD. Among Aβ PET tracers, the best known is N-methyl-[^{11}C]-2-(4^{0}-methylaminophenyl)-6-hydroxybenzothiazole, also known as Pittsburgh Compound-B (PIB) [10]. PIB-PET studies demonstrate significant PIB retention in AD patients as compared to controls, mostly evident in the middle and prefrontal cortex, PTC, PCC/precuneus, occipital lobes, thalamus and striatum [10, 25] (fig. 3). About 50% of amnestic MCI patients are PIB positive, and PIB retention is found also in as many as 22% of normal elderly [26]. These findings, when considered together with pathology reports that PIB may not be specific for dense classical Aβ plaques [27], suggest that PIB-PET may be difficult to interpret in nonsymptomatic subjects.

Table 2. PIB-PET imaging studies in AD and 'high-risk' populations compared to normal controls

Risk factor	PIB-PET findings	PIB uptake values
AD patients	Increased PIB uptake in middle and lateral FC, PC, LTC, PCC/precuneus, OC, thalamus and striatum [10, 25]	FC: 1.8 PC: 1.9 LTC: 1.7 PCC: 1.9 OC: 1.7 Striatum: 1.6
FAD mutation carriers	Increased PIB uptake in striatum, FC, LTC [28]	Striatum: 2.0 FC: 1.6 LTC: 1.4
ApoE4	Increased PIB uptake in FC, PCC/precuneus, LTC, PC, basal ganglia [29]	FC: 1.4 PCC: 1.5 LTC: 1.4 PC: 1.4 Striatum: 1.4
MCI	54% with increased PIB uptake in FC, ACC, IP, PCC/precuneus [30]; 46% with PIB uptake in the normal range [30]	In the PIB-positive group: FC: 1.6 ACC: 1.6 IP: 1.6 PCC: 1.8

PIB uptake values: cerebral-to-cerebellar PIB standardized uptake ratios.
LTC = Lateral temporal cortex; OC = occipital cortex.

Several PIB studies examined 'high-risk' populations in order to identify AD neuropathological changes prior to the development of dementia symptoms (table 2). Both asymptomatic FAD mutation carriers [28] and ApoE4 carriers [29] showed increased PIB uptake than controls. PIB-PET studies in MCI patients showed a subset with high PIB retention and a subset with low PIB retention [30]. In longitudinal studies, MCI patients who later converted to AD showed higher PIB uptake than nonconverters and, interestingly, none of the PIB-negative MCI converted to AD [30], suggesting the possibility for PIB-PET to predict the future conversion to AD. However, prediction studies among at risk and nonsymptomatic normal elderly have not been reported.

Interestingly, our recent data [12] show that MCI patients are identified by PIB-PET with 75% accuracy from controls. However, only 54% of the PIB+ MCI patients also showed FDG reductions, reflecting a dissociation between fibrillar amyloid load and CMRglc reductions. The greatest improvement in diagnostic accuracy comes from the combination of the two modalities with the accuracy raised to 90% in the identification of MCI patients, suggesting that PIB alone may not be sufficient in the determination of risk among at-risk subjects, and a combination with a complementary modality, such ad FDG-PET, is necessary. Longitudinal studies are needed to assess whether risk of decline is higher in MCI patients with both fibrillar amyloid deposits and CMRglc reductions, compared to either deficit alone.

Another amyloid PET imaging tracer, 2-(1-96-(2-^{18}F-fluoroethyl)(methyl)amino)2-naphthyl)ethyldene) malononitrile (^{18}F-FDDNP) has been studied to a lesser extent in AD. FDDNP is a fluorinated radiotracer that binds with high specificity to both Aβ fibrils and NFTs [11]. ^{18}F-FDDNP binding was elevated in AD and MCI patients as compared with healthy elderly, and showed uptake in the MTL, yielding 100% diagnostic separation between AD and controls, and 95% between MCI and controls [11].

The capacity of ^{18}F-FDDNP to bind to NFT in addition to Aβ could be a potential early diagnostic advantage as it may reveal early NFT pathology [31]. It is known that NFT pathology appears in the MTL in early stages of AD [3], and an increased NFT load is highly correlated with memory impairment, while amyloid deposits are not [32]. However, further studies are needed to assess the extent to which ^{18}F-FDDNP helps establish early diagnosis and increase diagnostic specificity. Limitations regarding this tracer have been published [32].

Conclusion

The search for sensitive and specific biomarkers for AD has been a challenge. Several FDG-PET studies have shown that hypometabolism in the MTL and cortical areas could be useful as an imaging biomarker for asymptomatic 'high-risk' populations. There remains a great need to increase the preclinical diagnostic accuracy, and the combination of FDG-PET with amyloid PET imaging has proven an effective strategy in the identification of AD and MCI. Future studies targeting normal elderly with various risk factors for AD are warranted.

Acknowledgement

Supported by a grant from the Alzheimer's Disease Research Unit CIEN Foundation – Reina Sofia Foundation, Madrid, Spain.

References

1 Cummings JL: Toward a molecular neuropsychiatry of neurodegenerative diseases. Ann Neurol 2003;54:147–154.

2 Mirra SS, Heyman A, McKeel D, Sumi SM, Crain BJ, Brownlee LM, et al: The consortium to establish a registry for Alzheimer's disease (CERAD). II. Standardization of the neuropathologic assessment of Alzheimer's disease. Neurology 1991;41:479–486.

3 Braak H, Braak E: Neuropathological stageing of Alzheimer related changes. Acta Neuropathologica 1991;82:239–259.

4 Berg D: Biomarkers for the early detection of Parkinson's and Alzheimer's disease. Neurodegener Dis 2008;5:133–136.

5 Rusinek H, De Santi S, Frid D, Tsui W, Tarshish C, Convit A, et al: Regional brain atrophy rate predicts future cognitive decline: 6-year longitudinal MR imaging study of normal aging. Radiology 2003;229:691–696.

6 Rocher AB, Chapon F, Blaizot X, Baron JC, Chavoix C: Resting-state brain glucose utilization as measured by PET is directly related to regional synaptophysin levels: a study in baboons. Neuroimage 2004;20:1894–1898.

7 Pellerin L, Magistretti PJ: Glutamate uptake into astrocytes stimulates aerobic glycolysis: a mechanism coupling neuronal activity to glucose utilization. PNAS 1994;91:10625–10629.

8 Silverman DH, Small GW, Chang CY, Lu CS, Kung De Aburto MA, Chen W, et al: Positron emission tomography in evaluation of dementia: regional brain metabolism and long-term outcome. JAMA 2001;286:2120–2127.

9 Mosconi L, Tsui WH, Herholz K, Pupi A, Drzezga A, Lucignani G, et al: Multicenter standardized 18F-FDG PET diagnosis of mild cognitive impairment, Alzheimer's disease, and other dementias. J Nucl Med 2008; 49:390–398.

10 Klunk WE, Engler H, Nordberg A, Yanming W, Blomqvist G, Holt DP, et al: Imaging brain amyloid in Alzheimer's disease with Pittsburgh Compound-B. Ann Neurol 2004; 55:306–319.

11 Small GW, Kepe V, Ercoli LM, Siddarth P, Bookheimer SY, Miller KJ, et al: PET of brain amyloid and tau in mild cognitive impairment. N Engl J Med 2006;355:2652–2663.

12 Li Y, Rinne JO, Mosconi L, Pirraglia E, Rusinek H, DeSanti S: Regional analysis of FDG and PIB-PET images in normal aging, mild cognitive impairment, and Alzheimer's disease. Eur J Nucl Med Mol Imaging 2008; 35:2169–2181.

13 Mosconi L: Brain glucose metabolism in the early and specific diagnosis of Alzheimer's disease. Eur J Nucl Med 2005;32:486–510.

14 Mosconi L, De Santi S, Li Y, Li J, Zhan J, Tsui WH, et al: Visual rating of medial temporal lobe metabolism in mild cognitive impairment and Alzheimer's disease using FDG-PET. Eur J Nucl Med 2006;33:210–221.

15 Minoshima S, Giordani B, Berent S, Frey KA, Foster NL, Kuhl DE: Metabolic reduction in the posterior cingulate cortex in very early Alzheimer's disease. Ann Neurol 1997;42: 85–94.

16 Foster NL, Chase TN, Mansi L, Brooks R, Fedio P, Patronas NJ, et al: Cortical abnormalities in Alzheimer's disease. Ann Neurol 1984;16:649–654.

17 Mosconi L, Sorbi S, de Leon MJ, Li Y, Nacmias B, Bessi V, et al: Hypometabolism exceeds atrophy in presymptomatic early-onset familial Alzheimer's disease. J Nucl Med 2006:47:1778–1786.

18 Reiman EM, Chen K, Alexander GE, Caselli RJ, Bandy D, Osborne D, et al: Functional brain abnormalities in young adults at genetic risk for late-onset Alzheimer's dementia. PNAS 2004;101:284–289.

19 Mosconi L, De Santi S, Brys M, Tsui WH, Pirraglia E, Glodzik-Sobanska L, et al: Hypometabolism and altered cerebrospinal fluid markers in normal apolipoprotein E E4 carriers with subjective memory complaints. Biol Psychiatry 2008 15;63:609–618.

20 Drzezga A, Lautenschlager N, Siebner H, Riemenschneider M, Willoch F, Minoshima S, et al: Cerebral metabolic changes accompanying conversion of mild cognitive impairment into Alzheimer's disease: a PET follow-up study. Eur J Nucl Med 2003;30: 1104–1113.

21 Mosconi L, Brys M, Switalski R, Mistur R, Glodzik-Sobanska L, Pirraglia E, et al: Maternal family history of Alzheimer's disease predisposes to reduced brain glucose metabolism. PNAS 2007;104:19067–19072.

22 Anchisi D, Borroni B, Franceschi M, Kerrouche N, Kalbe E, Beuthien-Beumann B, et al: Heterogeneity of brain glucose metabolism in mild cognitive impairment and clinical progression to Alzheimer disease. Arch Neurol 2005;62:1728–1733.

23 de Leon MJ, Convit A, Wolf OT, Tarshish CY, DeSanti S, Rusinek H, et al: Prediction of cognitive decline in normal elderly subjects with 2-[(18)F]fluoro-2-deoxy-D-glucose/positron-emission tomography (FDG/PET). PNAS 2001;98:10966–10971.

24 Mosconi L, Mistur R, Switalski R, Tsui WH, Glodzik L, Li Y, et al: FDG-PET changes in brain glucose metabolism from normal cognition to pathologically verified Alzheimer's disease. Eur J Nucl Med Mol Imaging 2009; 36:811–822.

25 Kemppainen N, Aalto S, Wilson I, Nagren K, Helin S, Bruck A, et al: Voxel-based analysis of PET amyloid ligand [11C]PIB uptake in Alzheimer disease. Neurology 2006;67: 1575–1580.

26 Mintun MAM, LaRossa GN, Sheline YIM, Dence CSM, Lee SYP, Mach RHP, et al: [11C]PIB in a nondemented population: potential antecedent marker of Alzheimer disease. Neurology 2006;67:446–452.

27 Lockhart A, Lamb JR, Osredkar T, et al: PIB is a non-specific imaging marker of amyloid-beta (Aβ) peptide-related cerebral amyloidosis. Brain 2007;130 2607–2615.

28 Klunk WE, Price JC, Mathis CA, Tsopelas ND, Lopresti BJ, Ziolko SK, et al: Amyloid deposition begins in the striatum of presenilin-1 mutation carriers from two unrelated pedigrees. J Neurosci 2007;27:6174–6184.

29 Reiman EM, Chen K, Liu X, Bandy D, Yu M, Lee W, et al: Fibrillar amyloid-beta burden in cognitively normal people at 3 levels of genetic risk for Alzheimer's disease. PNAS 2009;106:6820–6825.

30 Wolk DA, Price JC, Saxton JA, Snitz BE, James JA, Lopez OL, et al: Amyloid imaging in mild cognitive impairment subtypes. Ann Neurol 2009;65:557–568.

31 de Leon MJ, Mosconi L, Logan J: Seeing what Alzheimer saw. Nat Med 2007;13:129–131.

32 Powell MR, Smith GE, Knopman DS, Parisi JE, Boeve BF, Petersen RC, et al: Cognitive measures predict pathologic Alzheimer disease. Arch Neurol 2006;63:865–868.

Imaging, Biomarkers, Genetics and Diagnostic Markers

Neuro-degenerative Diseases

Neurodegenerative Dis 2010;7:136–138
DOI: 10.1159/000289223

Published online: March 3, 2010

Amyloid Imaging in Early Detection of Alzheimer's Disease

Agneta Nordberg

Division of Alzheimer Neurobiology, Geriatric Clinic, Karolinska University Hospital Huddinge, Karolinska Institutet, Stockholm, Sweden

Key Words

Alzheimer's disease · Amyloid imaging · Positron emission tomography · Pittsburgh compound B · Mild cognitive impairment · Early diagnostic markers · CSF biomarkers

Abstract

Amyloid imaging has provided evidence for early detection of amyloid (Aβ) load in prodromal Alzheimer's disease (AD). Several amyloid tracers have been developed for studies with positron emission tomography (PET). Early detection of at-risk subjects will be important in the future for a successful treatment of AD. The high Aβ load in the brain measured by PET in patients with mild cognitive impairment that later will convert to AD suggests early, significant, ongoing pathological processes prior to cognitive impairment. PET Aβ imaging will also be used for discrimination of AD from other dementia disorders, as well for the evaluation of anti-Aβ drugs.

Introduction

Alzheimer's disease (AD) is characterized by a complex pathology where the presence of amyloid plaques and neurofibrillary tangles have been considered the histopathological hallmarks since Dr. Alois Alzheimer described them more than 100 years ago.

There has recently been a rapid development of molecular imaging techniques in neurodegenerative disorders. The introduction of different positron emission tomography (PET) tracers for in vivo amyloid imaging in AD has provided tools to image amyloid in the living brain and thus increased our understanding of the complex disease processes of AD [1–3]. The in vivo amyloid (Aβ) imaging technology may contribute to the further understanding of Aβ protein aggregation and plaque formation. The accumulation of Aβ peptide in the brain seems to start preferentially in neocortical areas years before cognitive problems appear in AD subjects. The critical role of different forms of Aβ, soluble Aβ oligomers and fibrillar Aβ deposits is still not fully known [4]. A great challenge is to try to detect Aβ in early stages of AD, even in prodromal AD, and to determine which Aβ form should be targeted for drug therapy in AD. This is of special interest when development of anti-amyloid therapies is in progress.

Amyloid Imaging in AD

The development of small molecules for amyloid imaging PET studies has so far been very promising, and several PET tracers (both ^{11}C-labelled and ^{18}F-labelled) have been used for amyloid imaging by PET in AD patients and other forms of dementia (table 1). The Pittsburgh compound B (PIB) amyloid PET ligand has so far

KARGER

Fax +41 61 306 12 34
E-Mail karger@karger.ch
www.karger.com

1660–2854/10/0073–0136$26.00/0

Accessible online at:
www.karger.com/ndd

Prof. Agneta Nordberg
Division of Alzheimer Neurobiology, Karolinska Institutet
Karolinska University Hospital Huddinge, Novum 5th floor
SE–141 86 Stockholm (Sweden)
Tel. +46 8 5858 5467, Fax +46 8 5858 5470, E-Mail Agneta.K.Nordberg@ki.se

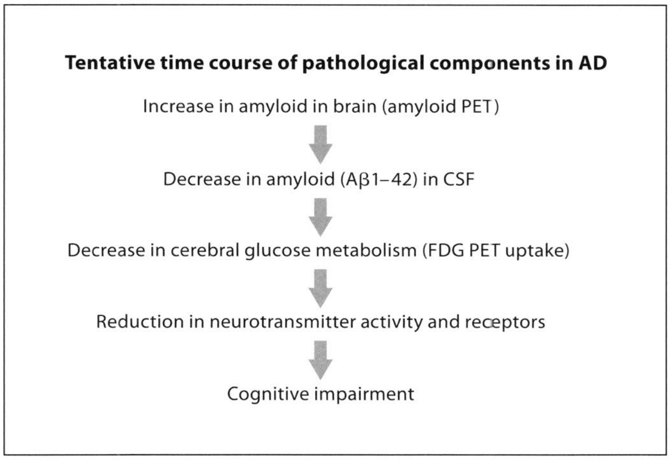

Fig. 1. Measurable changes in pathological components in AD evolution.

been the most studied among the amyloid ligands. A robust difference in ^{11}C-PIB retention has been observed in mainly cortical, but also subcortical brain regions of AD patients compared to age-matched controls [2, 3, 5]. Some difference in brain specificity as well as sensitivity has been observed between the PET amyloid ligands. Thus ^{18}F-FDDNP has shown a different regional retention in AD brains compared to ^{11}C-PIB [6], which might at least partly be explained by a 10 times lower binding affinity [7]. It is also important to verify amyloid PET imaging in vivo with amyloid measurement at autopsy. A significant correlation has been reported between in vivo PIB brain retention and Aβ levels and ^{3}H-PIB binding in autopsy and biopsy tissue [8–10].

Correlation of Amyloid Imaging with Other Structural and Functional Parameters and CSF Biomarkers

Stable PIB retention was observed at 2-year follow-up scans with ^{11}C-PIB in 16 AD patients, while the patients showed decline in cerebral glucose metabolism (^{18}F-FDG uptake) and cognitive performance [11]. A significant decrease in brain volume with no change in PIB retention was recently reported in a 1-year follow-up study in AD and patients with mild cognitive impairment (MCI) [12]. We recently performed a 5-year follow-up study with ^{11}C-PIB in 9 AD patients. No significant change was observed in mean ^{11}C-PIB retention of the group, although some

Table 1. Different amyloid PET ligands studied in AD patients

^{18}F-FDDNP
^{11}C-PIB
^{11}C-SB-13
^{11}C-BF-227
^{18}F-BAY94-9172
^{18}F-AV-144
^{11}C-AZD2184

individual changes were observed in separate AD patients [Kadir et al., submitted].

PIB studies in MCI patients have shown ^{11}C-PIB retention intermediate between AD and controls [13–16]. A bimodal distribution with high ^{11}C-PIB retention in 11 MCI patients was observed, while there was a low PIB retention in 10 MCI patients [15]. After 2 years' follow-up, 7 MCI patients with high PIB retentions had converted to AD but none of the MCI patients with low PIB retention had [15]. Okello et al. [16] recently reported similar high conversion of MCI patients with high PIB retention after 3 years' follow-up (82%).

A significant correlation has been observed between CSF Aβ1–42 and PIB retention in MCI and AD patients [15, 17]. Both Aβ PET imaging as well as CSF Aβ seem to be able to detect early changes in progression of AD compared to PET cerebral glucose metabolism imaging, atrophy measurement by MRI or cognitive testing (fig. 1).

Studies in patients at risk for developing AD will provide further understanding of the evolution of amyloid in the brain and its relation to functional changes including cognition.

Amyloid Imaging in Subjects at Risk and in Healthy Subjects

In subjects at risk for developing AD, amyloid imaging represents an important study. Early amyloid deposition in the brain has been observed by PIB PET in presenilin 1 (PS1) mutation carriers [18]. A somewhat higher PIB retention has been observed in the striatum of PS1 carriers compared to sporadic AD [19, 20]. A high PIB retention has also been observed in some elderly with normal cognition [13, 21]. It is important to clinically follow these healthy subjects and investigate whether they will convert to AD.

Amyloid Imaging in Non-AD Dementia Disorders

PET studies in patients with frontotemporal dementia and Parkinson's disease have shown mainly negative PIB scans, while positive PIB PET scans have been observed in the brains of patients with Lewy body dementia [for review, see 2, 3].

Amyloid Imaging in Evaluation of Antiamyloid Therapy

Aβ imaging will be very important for the evaluation of new antiamyloid therapies in AD. An important question is whether ongoing immunization therapy trials will show reduction in amyloid load in the brain by PET imaging. In a recent study, phenserine with properties to influence the synthesis of Aβ was tested in a group of AD patients. PIB PET imaging was used as an outcome measurement together with cerebral glucose metabolism, cognitive testing and CSF biomarkers [20]. In AD patients, reciprocal changes were observed with a decrease in PIB brain retention and an increase in CSF Aβ40 following 6 months of treatment with phenserine [21].

Aβ imaging will probably be useful as an outcome measure for evaluation of antiamyloid therapy. Emerging new data are expected from molecular amyloid imaging as well as from other pathological features including tau phosphorylation, microglia activation and inflammatory processes in AD.

Acknowledgements

We are very grateful for the financial support from the Swedish Research Council (project No. 05817), Stone's Foundation, Alzheimer Foundation in Sweden, Brain Foundation, Foundations for Old Servants, Swedish Brain Power, Knut and Alice Wallenberg Foundation, the EC-FP6-Project Dime, LSHB-CT-2005-512146, and QLK6-CT-2000-00502.

References

1 Nordberg A: PET imaging of amyloid in Alzheimer's disease. Lancet Neurol 2004;3:519–527.
2 Jagust W: Mapping brain β-amyloid. Curr Opin Neurol 2009;22:356–361.
3 Nordberg A: Amyloid imaging in Alzheimer's disease. Neuropsychologia 2008;46:1636–1641.
4 Walsh DM, Selkoe DJ: A beta oligomers – a decade of discovery. J Neurochem 2007;101:1172–1184.
5 Klunk WE, Engler H, Nordberg A, et al: Imaging brain amyloid in Alzheimer's disease using the novel PET tracer, PIB. Ann Neurol 2004;55:306–319.
6 Tolbom N, Yaqub M, van der Flier WM, et al: Detection of Alzheimer pathology in vivo using both ^{11}C-PIB and ^{18}F-FDDNP PET. J Nucl Med 2009;50:191–197.
7 Thompson PW, Ye L, Morgenstern JL, et al: Interaction of the amyloid imaging tracer FDDNP with hallmark Alzheimer's disease pathologies. J Neurochem 2009;109:623–630.
8 Ikonomovic MD, Klunk WE, Abrahamson EE, et al: Postmortem correlates of in vivo PIB-PET amyloid imaging in a typical case of Alzheimer's disease. Brain 2008;63:621–631.
9 Leinonen V, Alafuzoff I, Aalto S, et al: Assessment of β amyloid in a frontal cortical brain biopsy specimen and by positron emission tomography with carbon 11-labeled Pittsburgh compound B. Arch Neurol 2008;65:1304–1309.
10 Svedberg MM, Hall H, Hellström-Lindahl E, et al: [(11)C]PIB-amyloid binding and levels of Abeta40 and Abeta42 in postmortem brain tissue from Alzheimer patients. Neurochem Int 2009;54:347–357.
11 Engler H, Forsberg A, Almqvist O, et al: Two-year follow-up for amyloid deposition in patients with Alzheimer's disease. Brain 2006;129:2856–2866.
12 Jack CR, Lowe VJ, Weigand SD, et al: Serial PIB and MRI in normal, mild cognitive impairment and Alzheimer's disease-implications for sequence of pathological events in Alzheimer's disease. Brain 2009;132:1355–1365.
13 Rowe CC, Ng S, Ackersmann U, et al: Imaging beta-amyloid burden in aging and dementia. Neurology 2007;68:1718–1725.
14 Price JC, Klunk WE, Lopresti BJ, et al: Kinetic modeling of amyloid binding in humans using PET imaging and Pittsburgh compound B. J Cereb Blood Flow Metab 2005;25:1528–1547.
15 Forsberg A, Engler H, Almkvist O, et al: PET imaging of amyloid deposition in patients with mild cognitive impairment. Neurobiol Aging 2008;29:1456–1465.
16 Okello A, Koivunen BM, Edison P, et al: Conversion of amyloid positive and negative MCI to AD over 3 years: an 11C-PIB PET study. Neurology 2009;73:754–760.
17 Fagan AM, Head D, Shah AR, et al: Decreased cerebrospinal fluid Aβ42 correlates with brain atrophy in cognitively normal elderly. Ann Neurol 2009;65:176–183.
18 Klunk WE, Price JC, Mathis CA, et al: Amyloid deposition begins in the striatum of presenilin-1 mutation carriers from two unrelated pedigrees. J Neurosci 2007;27:6174–6184.
19 Schöll M, Almkvist O, Axelman K, et al: Glucose metabolism and PIB binding in carriers of His163Tyr presenilin 1 mutation. Neurobiol Aging, in press.
20 Pike KE, Savage G, Villemagne VL, et al: β-Amyloid imaging in memory in non-demented individuals: evidence for preclinical Alzheimer's disease. Brain 2007;130:2837–2844.
21 Kadir A, Andreasen N, Almkvist O, et al: Effect of phenserine on brain functional activity and amyloid in AD. Ann Neurol 2008;63:621–631.

Neurodegenerative Diseases

Neurodegenerative Dis 2010;7:139–142
DOI: 10.1159/000289224

Published online: March 3, 2010

Inability of Plasma and Urine F2A-Isoprostane Levels to Differentiate Mild Cognitive Impairment from Alzheimer's Disease

Elliott J. Mufson[a] Sue Leurgans[b]

[a]Department of Neurological Sciences, and [b]Rush Alzheimer's Disease Center, Rush University Medical Center, Chicago, Ill., USA

Key Words
Alzheimer's disease biomarkers · Isoprostane · Mild cognitive impairment · Oxidative stress

Abstract
Background: Oxidative stress has been implicated in the pathogenesis of Alzheimer's disease (AD). The pathobiological changes related to AD occur long before the overt clinical symptoms. The plasma lipid peroxidation enzyme F2-isoprostane has been suggested as a biomarker to detect the progression from mild cognitive impairment (MCI) to AD. ***Objective:*** To test whether plasma and urine F2-isoprostane was diagnostic for dementia in living people. ***Methods:*** Plasma and urine were collected from 222 Religious Orders Study participants with a clinical diagnosis of no cognitive impairment, MCI or AD at time of fluid collection. Isoprostane levels were determined using gas chromatography/mass spectroscopy. ***Results:*** Plasma and urine F2-isoprostane levels did not differ between the three clinical groups. Postmortem neuropathologic diagnosis of subjects who died during the course of the study was not associated with baseline blood or plasma F2-isoprostane levels. ***Conclusions:*** In living people, plasma or urine isoprostane levels were not sensitive enough to discriminate between individuals with a clinical diagnosis of no cognitive impairment, MCI or AD.

Introduction

Increases in brain markers of oxidation and reduced activities of antioxidant enzymes implicate oxidative damage in the pathobiology of Alzheimer's disease (AD). Isoprostanes which arise from free radical-mediated peroxidation of polyunsaturated fatty acids were elevated in brain tissue and cerebral spinal fluid (CSF) obtained at autopsy in advanced and early AD [1–7], as well as in CSF harvested intra vitam from sporadic and familial AD [6, 8]. Since obtaining CSF via a spinal tap can be stressful and not easily obtained in most clinics, investigators have quantified isoprostanes in plasma and urine with studies showing increased [6] or no change [6, 7] in early and late stage AD. To assist in resolving this issue, we measured plasma and urine F2-isoprostane levels from a cohort of living people with a clinical diagnosis of no cognitive impairment (NCI), mild cognitive impairment (MCI) or AD.

Subjects and Methods

Subjects
In 2003, plasma and urine samples were obtained antemortem from participants in the Religious Orders Study, a longitudinal clinical-pathological study of aging and AD [1, 9]. Clinical diagnoses of AD dementia, MCI and NCI at the time of sample collection are based upon evaluation closest to fluid collection using previously described criteria [9]. At baseline, 167 (75%) of the subjects were clinically classified as NCI, 34 (15%) as MCI, and 21

KARGER
Fax +41 61 306 12 34
E-Mail karger@karger.ch
www.karger.com

1660–2854/10/0073–0139$26.00/0

Accessible online at:
www.karger.com/ndd

Prof. Elliott J. Mufson, PhD
Rush University Medical Center
1735 W. Harrison Street, Suite 300
Chicago, IL 60612 (USA)
Tel. +1 312 563 3558, Fax +1 312 563 3571, E-Mail emufson@rush.edu

Table 1. Clinical characteristics of living subjects

Characteristic	Baseline clinical diagnosis				Comparison by diagnosis group, p
	NCI (n = 167)	MCI (n = 34)	AD (n = 21)	total (n = 222)	
Males	44 (26%)	8 (24%)	7 (33%)	59 (27%)	0.720[a]
Years of education[b]	17.7 ± 3.0	17.6 ± 3.1	18.3 ± 3.4	17.8 ± 3.0	0.141[c]
ApoE ε4 alleles	39 (24%)	12 (35%)	10 (48%)	61 (28%)	0.044[a]
Age at blood draw, years[b]	79.8 ± 6.3	83.5 ± 5.9	86.3 ± 7.0	80.9 ± 6.6	<0.0001[c]
MMSE at blood draw[b]	29.0 ± 1.3	27.4 ± 2.2	16.1 ± 7.7	27.6 ± 4.6	<0.0001[c]
Global cognitive score[b]	0.4 ± 0.5	−0.3 ± 0.5	−2.0 ± 0.9	0.1 ± 0.9	<0.0001[c]
Subjects on statins	50 (30%)	10 (29%)	3 (14%)	63 (28%)	0.32[a]
Urine isoprostane, ng/mg creatinine[d, e]	2.8 ± 126%	2.6 ± 170%	3.9 ± 105%	2.8 ± 132%	0.246[c]
Plasma isoprostane, pg/ml[d, e]	107 ± 73%	111 ± 87%	138 ± 70%	109 ± 75%	0.250[c]

MMSE = Mini-Mental State Exam.
[a] χ^2 test; [b] Mean ± SD; [c] Kruskal-Wallis test; [d] ANOVA; [e] GM ± GCV.

(9%) as AD. Subjects who died during the course of the study received a consensus conference final clinical diagnosis and their brains were neuropathologically examined according to CERAD [10], NIA-Reagan criteria [11] and Braak scoring [12]. ApoE genotyping was performed as previously reported [13].

Isoprostane Levels

Plasma and urine were cooled to 4°C, spun within 15 min, aliquoted as 960 μl plasma with 40 μl 20× protease inhibitor solution (Complete; Roche, Indianapolis, Ind., USA), and stored at −80°C until measurement [2–5, 13]. Levels of isoprostane iPα-VI (F2A) were determined by gas chromatography/mass spectroscopy [2–5, 13]. The inter-and intra-assay variability of the assays was approximately 5%.

Statistical Analysis

Since F2-isoprostane levels displayed a skewed distribution, the data are presented as the geometric means (GM) and geometric coefficients of variation (GCV), which are presented as GM± (GCV; percentage difference from the mean) [14]. F2-isoprostane, neuropathologic and demographic data were compared using analysis of variance (ANOVA) or Kruskal-Wallis test, gender distribution by a χ^2 test, and association of plasma with urine F2-isoprostane levels by the Spearman's rank correlation coefficient. Ordinal logistic regression examined the relationship between F2-isoprostane and neuropathologic data. Statistical significance was set at $\alpha = 0.05$.

Results

At baseline, the mean age of the NCI (79.6 years) subjects was significantly less than that of both MCI (83.5 years) and AD (86.3 years) subjects (Kruskal-Wallis, $p < 0.0001$). Mini-Mental State Exam scores differed significantly among the groups (Kruskal-Wallis, $p < 0.001$); post-hoc testing showed that the means for the NCI (28.9) and MCI (27.4) groups did not differ significantly from each other, but both were significantly higher than that of the AD (16.2) group (table 1). ApoE ε4 allele status differed significantly between the three clinical groups ($\chi^2 = 6.25$; $p = 0.044$; table 1). Plasma F2-isoprostane levels were not associated with age, education, sex or use of statins ($p > 0.15$); urine levels were higher for males ($p = 0.026$, Spearman correlation) and those on statins had lower urine isoprostane levels ($p = 0.0244$). F2-isoprostane levels were determined for 134 (74%) NCI, 32 (18%) MCI and 14 (8%) AD cases. Plasma F2-isoprostane was not measured in 33 (22%) NCI, 2 (6%) MCI, and 7 (33%) AD subjects. The overall GM ± GCV for plasma F2-isoprostane was 107 pg/ml ± 73%, and 2.80 ng/mg ± 132% for urine creatinine. Plasma and urine F2-isoprostane levels were not correlated (Spearman correlation, 0.67, $p < 0.0001$) and did not differ among the three clinical groups at the time of specimen draw. Mean urine levels were 2.8 ng/mg creatinine for NCI, 2.6 ng/mg creatinine for MCI and 3.7 ng/mg creatinine for AD, and plasma F2-isoprostane levels were 107 pg/ml for NCI, 111 pg/ml for MCI and 138 pg/ml for AD.

A consensus postmortem clinical evaluation of the 63 deceased subjects revealed 22 as NCI (2 were MCI at baseline; 20 were NCI), 15 as MCI (6 were NCI at baseline; 9 were MCI) and 26 as AD (14 were AD at baseline, 5 were MCI and 7 were NCI; table 2). Although these clinical groups did not differ in Braak staging, by NIA-Reagan diagnosis the AD group was neuropathologically more

Table 2. Neuropathological characteristics of deceased subjects

Neuropathology	Consensus postmortem clinical diagnosis				Comparison by diagnosis group	Pairwise comparisons
	NCI (n = 22)	MCI (n = 15)	dementia (n = 26)	total (n = 63)		
Distribution of Braak scores						
0	1	0	0	1	p = 0.291[a]	–
I/II	6	3	2	11		
III/IV	14	9	17	40		
V	1	3	7	11		
Distribution of NIA Reagan diagnosis (likelihood of AD)						
No AD	0	0	0	0	p = 0.004[a]	NCI < AD
Low	13	9	6	28		
Intermediate	9	4	15	28		
High	0	2	5	7		
Distribution of Modified CERAD diagnosis						
No	7	7	3	17	p = 0.008[a]	(NCI, MCI) < AD
Possible	3	2	3	8		
Probable	11	4	10	25		
Definite	1	2	10	13		

[a] Kruskal-Wallis test.

advanced compared to NCI (ANOVA, $p = 0.004$), whereas using CERAD criteria the AD group was more advanced neuropathologically than both NCI and MCI subjects (ANOVA, $p = 0.0008$; table 2). Postmortem neuropathology was not associated with plasma F2-isoprostane levels based upon ordinal logistic regression models.

Discussion

Despite differences in ages between the NCI, MCI and AD subjects examined at time of specimen collection, we found no difference in plasma and urine F2A-isoprostane levels, consistent with other reports [6, 15]. By contrast, others report elevated brain, CSF and plasma F2-isoprostane levels in MCI and AD [6], suggesting that F2-isoprostane levels could act as a biomarker for AD. The inconsistency in using peripheral compared to CSF F2-isoprostane level as a biomarker for AD remains to be determined. Since every cell produces F2-isoprostane, peripheral production unrelated to a particular neurodegenerative disease may easily confound the usefulness of plasma and urine F2-isoprostane levels as a biomarker for AD. Moreover, F2-isoprostane quantification is sensitive to various confounding variables including diet, exercise, body mass index and other diseases associated with lipid peroxidation [16]. These factors as well as methods of measurement vary across studies and could possibly underlie the inconsistency in peripheral F2-isoprostane measurements. However, a comparative study using a variety of analytic measures of plasma and urine F2-isoprostane failed to reproducibly demonstrate an increase in isoprostane levels in AD versus controls [6].

Although we found that postmortem neuropathologic diagnosis of subjects who died since entering the study was not associated with baseline plasma F2-isoprostane levels, brain F2-isoprostane levels correlate with reduction in brain weight and Braak staging [13, 17]. These findings suggest that brain, but not peripheral F2-isoprostane levels more accurately reflect the burden of underlying AD pathology rather than clinical status. Despite these neuropathological observations, as first reported by Montine et al. [18], plasma F2-isoprostane levels do not appear to be a sensitive biomarker for the clinical progression of AD.

Acknowledgements

We thank Dr. D. Pratico for performing the F2-isoprostane analysis at the University of Pennsylvania. We are indebted to the support of the participants in the Religious Orders Study; for a list of participating groups see the website http://www.rush.edu/rumc/page-R12394.html. Supported by PO1AG14449, PO1AG09466 and P50AG10161.

References

1 Counts SE, Nadeem M, Lad SP, Wuu J, Mufson EJ: Differential expression of synaptic proteins in the frontal and temporal cortex of elderly subjects with mild cognitive impairment. J Neuropathol Exp Neurol 2006; 65:592–601.

2 Praticò D, MY Lee V, Trojanowski JQ, Rokach J, Fitzgerald GA: Increased F2-isoprostanes in Alzheimer's disease: evidence for enhanced lipid peroxidation in vivo. FASEB J 1998;12:1777–1783.

3 Praticò D, Iuliano L, Amerio G, Tang LX, Rokach J, Sabatino G, Violi F: Down's syndrome is associated with increased 8,12-iso-iPF2alpha-VI levels: evidence for enhanced lipid peroxidation in vivo. Ann Neurol 2000;48: 795–798.

4 Praticò D, Clark CM, Liun F, Rokach J, Lee VY, Trojanowski JQ: Increase of brain oxidative stress in mild cognitive impairment: a possible predictor of Alzheimer disease. Arch Neurol 2002;59:972–976.

5 Praticò D, Clark CM, Lee VM, Trojanowski JQ, Rokach J, FitzGerald GA: Increased 8,12-iso-iPF2alpha-VI in Alzheimer's disease: correlation of a noninvasive index of lipid peroxidation with disease severity. Ann Neurol 2000;48:809–812.

6 Montine TJ, Montine KS, McMahan W, Markesbery WR, Quinn JF, Morrow JD: F2-isoprostanes in Alzheimer and other neurodegenerative diseases. Antioxid Redox Signal 2005;7:269–275.

7 Irizarry MC, Yao Y, Hyman BT, Growdon JH, Praticò D: Plasma F2A isoprostane levels in Alzheimer's and Parkinson's disease. Neurodegener Dis 2007;4:403–405.

8 Ringman JM, Younkin SG, Pratico D, Seltzer W, Cole GM, Geschwind DH, Rodriguez-Agudelo Y, Schaffer B, Fein J, Sokolow S, Rosario ER, Gylys KH, Varpetian A, Medina LD, Cummings JL: Biochemical markers in persons with preclinical familial Alzheimer disease. Neurology 2008;71:85–92.

9 Bennett DA, Wilson RS, Schneider JA, Evans DA, Beckett LA, Aggarwal NT, Barnes LL, Fox JH, Bach J: Natural history of mild cognitive impairment in older persons. Neurology 2002;59:198–205.

10 Mirra SS, Heyman A, McKeel D Sumi SM, Crain BJ, Brownlee LM, Vogel FS, Hughes JP, van Belle G, Berg L: The consortium to establish a registry for Alzheimer's disease (CERAD). II. Standardization of the neuropathologic assessment of Alzheimer's disease. Neurology 1991;41:479–486.

11 National Institute on Aging and Reagan Institute working group on diagnosis criteria for the neuropathological assessment of Alzheimer's disease: consensus recommendations for the postmortem diagnosis of AD. Neurobiol Aging 1997;18:S1–S2.

12 Braak H, Braak E: Neuropathological stageing of Alzheimer-related changes. Acta Neuropathol 1991;82:239–259.

13 Forman MS, Mufson EJ, Leurgans S, Praticò D, Joyce S, Leight S, Lee VM, Trojanowski JQ: Cortical biochemistry in MCI and Alzheimer disease: lack of correlation with clinical diagnosis. Neurology 2007;68:757–763.

14 Kirkwood TB: Geometric mean and measures of dispersion. Biometrics 1979;35:908–909.

15 Feillet-Coudray C, Tourtauchaux R, Niculescu M, Rock E, Tauveron I, Alexandre-Gouabau MC, Rayssiguier Y, Jalenques I, Mazur A: Plasma levels of 8-epiPGF2alpha, an in vivo marker of oxidative stress, are not affected by aging or Alzheimer's disease. Free Radic Biol Med 1999;27:463–469.

16 Basu S, Helmersson J: Factors regulating isoprostane formation in vivo. Antioxid Redox Signal 2005;7:221–235.

17 Montine TJ, Markesbery WR, Zackert W, Sanchez SC, Roberts LJ 2nd, Morrow JD: The magnitude of brain lipid peroxidation correlates with the extent of degeneration but not with density of neuritic plaques or neurofibrillary tangles or with APOE genotype in Alzheimer's disease patients. Am J Pathol 1999;155:863–868.

18 Montine TJ, Quinn JF, Milatovic D, Silbert LC, Dang T, Sanchez S, Terry E, Roberts LJ 2nd, Kaye JA, Morrow JD: Peripheral F2-isoprostanes and F4-neuroprostanes are not increased in Alzheimer's disease. Ann Neurol 2002;52:175–179.

Imaging, Biomarkers, Genetics and Diagnostic Markers

Neurodegenerative Diseases

Neurodegenerative Dis 2010;7:143–147
DOI: 10.1159/000289225

Published online: March 3, 2010

Increased CD44 Gene Expression in Lymphocytes Derived from Alzheimer Disease Patients

D. Uberti[a] G. Cenini[a] S.A. Bonini[a] M. Barcikowska[b] M. Styczynska[b] A. Szybinska[c] M. Memo[a]

[a]Department of Biomedical Sciences and Biotechnologies, University of Brescia, Brescia, Italy; [b]Medical Research Centre, Polish Academy of Science, and [c]Laboratory of Neurodegeneration International Institute of Molecular and Cell Biology, Warsaw, Poland

Key Words

Lymphocyte · Unfolded p53 isoform · CD44 gene · Peripheral marker

Abstract

In this study, we demonstrated for the first time an increased CD44 gene expression in lymphocytes derived from Alzheimer's disease (AD) patients in comparison with healthy subjects. CD44 is a surface antigen expressed by cells of the immune and central nervous system as well as in a variety of other tissues. Functioning as adhesion molecule, CD44 is furthermore involved in driving immune response into infected tissues, including the CNS. We also found that lymphocytes of the same patients expressed significant levels of unfolded p53 isoform, confirming what we already demonstrated in fibroblasts and lymphocytes derived from other cohorts of AD patients. A correlation between p53 and CD44 expression has been well demonstrated in cancer cells, suggesting that CD44 could be a target gene of mutant p53, or either mutant p53 could lack its ability to negatively regulate CD44 expression. The contemporaneous increased expression of unfolded p53 and CD44 in AD lymphocytes may suggest that these two molecules cross-talk together participating in peripheral immune response during the development of the disease.

Introduction

Early diagnosis of Alzheimer's disease (AD) is an important first step in the management of this disease. The prediction of the incipient disease allows an earlier pharmacological approach. In this context, identification of new putative biomarkers [1] can increase the accuracy of clinical diagnosis but, more importantly, it makes earlier diagnosis possible. In the last 20 years, independent scientific groups have looked for biological and biochemical alterations in peripheral tissues of AD patients, because of their easy accessibility. The concept of peripheral biomarker implies the involvement of many cell phenotypes in the disease and suggests that AD can be considered as a systemic disease. The major difficulty in the universal acceptance of a peripheral biomarker for CNS disease is its relevance in the pathogenesis of the

KARGER

Fax +41 61 306 12 34
E-Mail karger@karger.ch
www.karger.com

1660–2854/10/0073–0143$26.00/0

Accessible online at:
www.karger.com/ndd

Maurizio Memo, PhD
Department of Biomedical Sciences and Biotechnologies
Viale Europa 11
IT–25124 Brescia (Italy)
Tel. +39 030 371 7516, Fax +39 030 371 7409, E-Mail memo@med.unibs.it

illness. The study of accredited biomarkers found in CSF has failed when the same were looked for in periphery, suggesting that if metabolic and biochemical alterations occur in peripheral cells, they do not necessarily mirror events occurring in the AD brain. Our research group disclosed some years ago an anomalous conformational altered (unfolded) p53 isoform in fibroblasts and lymphocytes of AD [2, 3]. This marker apparently was very far from the known mechanisms involved in the pathogenesis of the disease. This opened two questions: (a) what is the significance of the expression of a conformational 'mutant-like' p53 isoform, and (b) secondarily, why is this isoform found exclusively in AD patients? Crystallographic studies on p53 tertiary structure have been often correlated with its gene mutations. Structural studies have allowed classification of p53 mutant protein into two large categories: (a) mutations which interfere with DNA sequence binding, and (b) mutations that determine an important conformational alteration. Interestingly, exposure of wild-type p53 to metal chelators such as EDTA, oxidant compounds [4–6], or synthetic nitric oxide donors (such as S nitro-N-acetylpenicilamine and S-nitrosoglutathione) [7] resulted in a rapid switch from wild-type to the unfolded 'mutant-like' form, suggesting that conformational changes can be also the result of posttranscriptional modifications. In addition, we demonstrated that the exposure to nanomolar concentrations of β-amyloid peptides 1–40 induced the expression of a mutant-like p53 isoform in different cellular models [8, 9]. It is noteworthy that mutant p53 was found to acquire new transcriptional functions [10–14]. Whether unfolded p53 found in AD is endowed with such functional activity is not known. Anyway, learning from the cancer field, some genes, which correlated with mutant p53, may have relevance in the pathogenesis of AD. Genes such as IGF1R, IL6 and CD44 [15–17] attracted our attention because of their observed role in the immune system. In fact, in recent years the relevance of immune response in AD has been revised [18–20], suggesting a surveillance role of the immune system before disease onset, rather than a harmful event. Schwartz's group has obtained a large body of evidence suggesting that under normal conditions CNS immune surveillance, primarily mediated by T lymphocytes recognizing CNS antigens, is important for maintaining cognitive abilities and the capacity for neuronal cell renewal in adulthood [21–23]. In this regard, we took into consideration the CD44 gene for its role in driving immune response in infected tissues, including the CNS. The aim of this study was (a) to measure CD44 mRNA expression in immortalized lymphocytes derived from AD patients and (b) to investigate whether or not it correlated with p53 conformational status.

Table 1. Demographic and clinical details of all subjects (mean ± SD)

	AD	Controls
Males/females	11/5	4/15
Age, years	65 ± 5.5	76 ± 14
LOI, months	55 ± 31	
MMSE	12 ± 10	28 ± 2.6

LOI = Length of illness; MMSE = Mini-Mental State Examination.

Methods

Subjects

Sporadic AD patients and healthy subjects were enrolled at the Department of Neurology, MSWiA Hospital, Warsaw, Poland. The demographic and clinical information is reported in table 1. Control subjects were individuals with no clinical signs of neurological or psychiatric diseases. All these subjects were examined by a senior neurologist or geriatrician, and diagnosis of dementia was made according to DSM-IV and the NINCDS-ADRDA criteria. Dementia was diagnosed based upon interview, objective and neurological examination, cognitive evaluation, and laboratory and radiological (CT scan) investigation. Cognitive status was quantified using the Mini-Mental State Examination.

Quantitative Real-Time PCR

Real-time PCR was performed according to Ferrari-Toninelli et al. [24]. The oligonucleotide sequences of the primers used are as follows for CD44: forward primer 5′-TTC ATC CTC GGG TGT GCT AT-3′, reverse primer 5′-GTA CAC CCC AAC CTC AGT GG-3′. The PCR program was initiated by 10 min at 95°C before 40 cycles, each for 15 s at 95°C and 1 min at 60°C.

Immunoprecipitation Analysis

p53 conformational state was analyzed by immunoprecipitation as previously detailed [2]. Briefly, 100 μg of protein extracts was used for immunoprecipitation experiments performed with 1 μg of the conformation-specific antibodies PAb1620 (wild-type specific) or PAb240 (mutant specific).

Statistical Evaluation

Results are given as mean ± standard error mean values. Statistical significance of differences was determined by t test. Significance was accepted at $p < 0.05$.

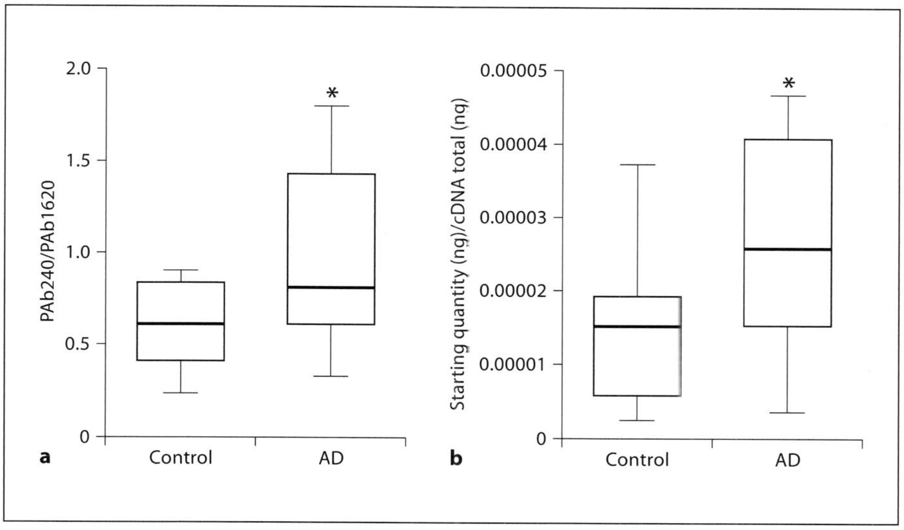

Fig. 1. a p53 conformational state in control and AD lymphocytes. The graph shows the ratio between the intensity of PAb240 and PAb1620 immunoreactive bands obtained from controls (n = 19) and AD (n = 16) lymphocytes. Data are expressed as mean ± SD. * $p < 0.001$. **b** CD44 gene expression in lymphocytes derived from 16 AD patients and 19 healthy subjects. Data represent starting quantity over total cDNA of each sample and are expressed as mean ± SD. * $p < 0.01$.

Results and Discussion

p53 conformational state in lymphocytes derived from AD and non-AD subjects was studied by the immunoprecipitation technique using two conformational-specific antibodies, PAb1620 and PAb240, which discriminate folded versus unfolded p53 tertiary structure [8]. In particular, the PAb1620 epitope is exposed in the wild-type p53 form that is competent for DNA binding and depends on the tertiary folding of the protein. In contrast, the PAb240 epitope is cryptic in the protein that is competent for DNA binding but is exposed by denaturation. Immunoprecipitates were then analyzed by Western blot analysis with a rabbit polyclonal p53 antibody. Data were expressed as the ratio of PAb240/PAb1620. A statistically significant unfolded p53 increase was found in AD patients in comparison to control subjects (fig. 1a). These data confirmed what we already found in another cohort of patients [3].

The new result of the present study is the expression of CD44 mRNA in AD patients (fig. 1b). CD44 has been extensively studied in the lymphoid compartment as a molecule involved in the development and differentiation of T and B cells and an activation marker increased on cell surface following stimulation by antigen and mitogen [25]. Furthermore, CD44 exerts an important role in addressing lymphocytes in infected tissues, including the CNS [26]. Increased expression of CD44 variant 6 on monocyte surface has been found to correlate with the development of encephalitis in HIV-1-infected macaques [27]. The same authors, in a longitudinal analysis of monocyte cell surface markers demonstrated that as early as 28 days after the inoculation, CD44v6 staining was able to distinguish pathological from control cases, suggesting that monocyte surface markers may serve as a marker for CNS disease. cDNA samples derived from 16 AD patients and 19 control subjects were processed for real-time PCR analysis using specific primers for CD44 standard transcript A statistically significant enhancement of CD44 mRNA was found in AD in comparison to control subjects (fig. 1b).

CD44 values in both AD and control were highly widespread, probably because its activation depends on different factors. In this regard, it has also been reported that CD44 expression correlates with T memory lymphocytes, and CD44-positive T lymphocytes correlate with aging [28, 29]. In the present study, only the standard isoform of CD44 was evaluated. In fact, nine variants (v2–v10) of the protein have been identified [30]. These variants differ from the standard CD44 molecule in that they contain additional peptide domains inserted into the extracellular portion of transmembrane protein. In contrast to standard CD44, which is almost ubiquitously expressed, the variety of CD44 isoforms (CD44v) has a much more restricted distribution. For example, CD44v6 is expressed on activated lymphocytes and macrophages [30]. This suggests the need to further investigate the coexpression of CD44v protein on mononuclear cell surface, and especially variant 6.

CD44 is also studied as a tumor marker. Numerous studies correlated increased CD44 expression with tumor growth and metastatic potential of tumor cells [31–33]. In addition, in many tumor tissue samples the expression of CD44 correlates with high expression of p53. Godar et al. [34] demonstrated that high levels of CD44 in breast cancer samples correlated with mutant p53, and they concluded that wild-type p53 negatively regulates CD44 expression. On the other hand, another study demonstrated that mutant p53 in lymphoblastoid cells induced the activation of CD44 gene, indicating CD44 as a target gene of mutant p53 [17]. Whether or not CD44 is a target gene of unfolded p53 is now matter of investigation. The correlation between CD44 and unfolded p53 in AD can assume an intriguing significance also in the possible role of the immune system in AD pathology. Recent evidence from animal models suggests that the activated microglia that surround senile plaques have been recruited from the blood [35]. Our working hypothesis is that cross-talk between unfolded p53 and CD44 in AD lymphocytes may have relevance in mediating immune response in AD pathology.

References

1 Thal LJ, Kantarci K, Reiman EM, Klunk WE, Weiner MW, Zetterberg H, Galasko D, Pratico D, Griffin S, Schenk D, Siemers E: The role of biomarkers in clinical trials for Alzheimer disease. Alzheimer Dis Assoc Disord 2006;20:6–15.

2 Uberti D, Lanni C, Carsana T, Francisconi S, Missale C, Racchi M, Govoni S, Memo M: Identification of a mutant-like conformation of p53 in fibroblasts from sporadic Alzheimer's disease patients. Neurobiol Aging 2006;27:1193–1201.

3 Lanni C, Racchi M, Mazzini G, Ranzenigo A, Polotti R, Sinforiani E, Olivari L, Barcikowska M, Styczynska M, Kuznicki J, Szybinska A, Govoni S, Memo M, Uberti D: Conformationally altered p53: a novel Alzheimer's disease marker? Mol Psychiatry 2008;13:641–647.

4 Hainaut P, Mann K: Zinc binding and redox control of p53 structure and function. Antioxid Redox Signal 2001;3:611–623.

5 Meplan C, Richard MJ, Hainaut P: Redox signalling and transition metals in the control of the p53 pathway. Biochem Pharmacol 2000;59:25–33.

6 Rainwater R, Parks D, Anderson ME, Tegtmeyer P, Mann K: Role of cysteine residues in regulation of p53 function. Mol Cell Biol 1995;15:3892–3903.

7 Calmels S, Hainaut P, Ohshima H: Nitric oxide induces conformational and functional modifications of wild-type p53 tumor suppressor protein. Cancer Res 1997;57:3365–3369.

8 Uberti D, Cenini G, Olivari L, Ferrari-Toninelli G, Porrello E, Cecchi C, Pensalfini A, Liguri G, Govoni S, Racchi M, Maurizio M: Over-expression of amyloid precursor protein in HEK cells alters p53 conformational state and protects against doxorubicin. J Neurochem 2007;103:322–333.

9 Lanni C, Uberti D, Racchi M, Govoni S, Memo M: Unfolded p53: a potential biomarker for Alzheimer's disease. J Alzheimers Dis 2007;12:93–99.

10 Zalcenstein A, Weisz L, Stambolsky P, Bar J, Rotter V, Oren M: Repression of the msp/mst-1 gene contributes to the antiapoptotic gain of function of mutant p53. Oncogene 2006;25:359–369.

11 Strano S, Dell'Orso S, Di Agostino S, Fontemaggi G, Sacchi A, Blandino G: Mutant p53: an oncogenic transcription factor. Oncogene 2007;26:2212–2219.

12 Strano S, Munarriz E, Rossi M, Cristofanelli B, Shaul Y, Castagnoli L, Levine AJ, Sacchi A, Cesareni G, Oren M, Blandino G: Physical and functional interaction between p53 mutants and different isoforms of p73. J Biol Chem 2000;275:29503–29512.

13 Weisz L, Zalcenstein A, Stambolsky P, Cohen Y, Goldfinger N, Oren M, Rotter V: Transactivation of the egr1 gene contributes to mutant p53 gain of function. Cancer Res 2004;64:8318–8327.

14 Di Agostino S, Strano S, Emiliozzi V, Zerbini V, Mottolese M, Sacchi A, Blandino G, Piaggio G: Gain of function of mutant p53: The mutant p53/nf-y protein complex reveals an aberrant transcriptional mechanism of cell cycle regulation. Cancer Cell 2006;10:191–202.

15 Werner H, Karnieli E, Rauscher FJ, LeRoith D: Wild-type and mutant p53 differentially regulate transcription of the insulin-like growth factor I receptor gene. Proc Natl Acad Sci USA 1996;93:8318–8323.

16 Margulies L, Sehgal PB: Modulation of the human interleukin-6 promoter (IL-6) and transcription factor C/EBP beta (NF-IL6) activity by p53 species. J Biol Chem 1993;268:15096–15100.

17 Zschenker O, Borgmann K, Streichert T, Meier I, Wrona A, Dikomey E: Lymphoblastoid cell lines differing in p53 status show clear differences in basal gene expression with minor changes after irradiation. Radiother Oncol 2006;80:236–249.

18 Bonotis K, Krikki E, Holeva V, Aggouridaki C, Costa V, Baloyannis S: Systemic immune aberrations in Alzheimer's disease patients. J Neuroimmunol 2008;193:183–187.

19 Speciale L, Calabrese E, Saresella M, Tinelli C, Mariani C, Sanvito L, Longhi R, Ferrante P: Lymphocyte subset patterns and cytokine production in Alzheimer's disease patients. Neurobiol Aging 2007;28:1163–1169.

20 Xue SR, Xu DH, Yang XX, Dong WL: Alterations in lymphocyte subset patterns and co-stimulatory molecules in patients with Alzheimer disease. Chin Med J (Engl) 2009;122:1469–1472.

21 Ziv Y, Ron N, Butovsky O, Landa G, Sudai E, Greenberg N, Cohen H, Kipnis J, Schwartz M: Immune cells contribute to the maintenance of neurogenesis and spatial learning abilities in adulthood. Nat Neurosci 2006;9:268–275.

22 Kipnis J, Cohen H, Cardon M, Ziv Y, Schwartz M: T cell deficiency leads to cognitive dysfunction: implications for therapeutic vaccination for schizophrenia and other psychiatric conditions. Proc Natl Acad Sci USA 2004;101:8180–8185.

23 Schwartz M, Ziv Y: Immunity to self and self-maintenance: a unified theory of brain pathologies. Trends Immunol 2008;29:211–219.

24 Ferrari-Toninelli G, Bonini SA, Bettinsoli P, Uberti D, Memo M: Microtubule stabilizing effect of notch activation in primary cortical neurons. Neuroscience 2008;154:946–952.

25 Zarcone D, De Rossi G, Tenca C, Marroni P, Mauro FR, Cerruti GM, Albi N, Fiorucci S, Velardi A, Grossi CE: Functional and clinical relevance of CD44 variant isoform expression on B-cell chronic lymphocytic leukemia cells. Haematologica 1998;83:1088–1098.

26 Goodison S, Urquidi V, Tarin D: CD44 cell adhesion molecules. Mol Pathol 1999;52:189–196.

27 Marcondes MC, Lanigan CM, Burdo TH, Watry DD, Fox HS: Increased expression of monocyte CD44v6 correlates with the development of encephalitis in rhesus macaques infected with simian immunodeficiency virus. J Infect Dis 2008;197:1567–1576.
28 Ernst DN, Weigle WO, McQuitty DN, Rothermel AL, Hobbs MV: Stimulation of murine T cell subsets with anti-CD3 antibody. Age-related defects in the expression of early activation molecules. J Immunol 1989;142: 1413–1421.
29 Rigolio R, Perseghin P, Jonsson S, Petersson J, Cavaletti G, Cilio CM: A new device to study ex-vivo the effects of extracorporeal photochemotherapy on the immune system. J Photochem Photobiol B 2007;88:68–75.
30 Screaton GR, Bell MV, Jackson DG, Cornelis FB, Gerth U, Bell JI: Genomic structure of DNA encoding the lymphocyte homing receptor CD44 reveals at least 12 alternatively spliced exons. Proc Natl Acad Sci USA 1992; 89:12160–12164.
31 Zolota V, Tsamandas AC, Melachrinou M, Batistatou A, Scopa C: Expression of CD44 protein in renal cell carcinomas: association with p53 expression. Urol Oncol 2002;7:13–17.
32 Zavrides HN, Zizi-Sermpetzoglou A, Panousopoulos D, Athanasas G, Elemenoglou I, Peros G: Prognostic evaluation of CD44 expression in correlation with Bcl-2 and p53 in colorectal cancer. Folia Histochem Cytobiol 2005;43:31–36.
33 Evan GI: The ever-lengthening arm of p53. Cancer Cell 2008;14:108–110.
34 Godar S, Ince TA, Bell GW, Feldser D, Donaher JL, Bergh J, Liu A, Miu K, Watnick RS, Reinhardt F, McAllister SS, Jacks T, Weinberg RA: Growth-inhibitory and tumor-suppressive functions of p53 depend on its repression of CD44 expression. Cell 2008; 134:62–73.
35 Simard AR, Soulet D, Gowing G, Julien JP, Rivest S: Bone marrow-derived microglia play a critical role in restricting senile plaque formation in Alzheimer's disease. Neuron 2006;49:489–502.

Imaging, Biomarkers, Genetics and Diagnostic Markers

Neuro-degenerative Diseases

Neurodegenerative Dis 2010;7:148–152
DOI: 10.1159/000289226

Published online: March 3, 2010

Human Analogue of the Morris Water Maze for Testing Subjects at Risk of Alzheimer's Disease

J. Laczó[a] R. Andel[c] M. Vyhnalek[a] K. Vlcek[b] H. Magerova[a] A. Varjassyova[a] M. Tolar[d] J. Hort[a]

[a]Department of Neurology, Charles University, and [b]Department of Neurophysiology of Memory, Czech Academy of Sciences, Prague, Czech Republic; [c]School of Aging Studies, University of South Florida, Tampa, Fla., and [d]Department of Neurology, Yale University School of Medicine, New Haven, Conn., USA

Key Words
Alzheimer's disease · Mild cognitive impairment · Spatial memory · Water maze task · Apolipoprotein E

Abstract
Background: Patients with Alzheimer's disease (AD) and amnestic mild cognitive impairment (MCI) have difficulties with spatial orientation. ***Objective:*** To test hypothesis that spatial navigation is impaired early in MCI patients representing the presymptomatic stage of AD. ***Methods:*** We tested patients with probable AD (n = 21), MCI, further classified according to Petersen's criteria as amnestic MCI (aMCI) single domain (n = 11), aMCI multiple domain (n = 31), or nonamnestic MCI (n = 7). The aMCI group was also stratified using cued recall according to Dubois' criteria into memory impairment of the hippocampal type (n = 10) and isolated memory retrieval impairment-nonhippocampal (n = 32) and also according to ApoE4 status into E4+ (n = 12) and E4– (n = 30). These patients and controls (n = 28) were tested in the human variant of the Morris water maze. Depending on the subtest, the subjects could use the egocentric or allocentric (hippocampus-dependent) navigation. ***Results:*** The AD and aMCI multiple domain groups were impaired in all subtests. The aMCI single domain group was impaired in allocentric subtests. The hippocampal MCI group performed poorer than the nonhippocampal MCI group and similarly to the AD group. The ApoE4+ group was as bad as the AD group when compared with the E4– group. ***Conclusion:*** aMCI subjects represent a very heterogeneous population, and spatial memory or cued recall examination can add more value to aMCI classification. ApoE4+ patients are more impaired than ApoE4– patients.

Introduction

Spatial navigation is believed to be impaired early, but has been little studied in Alzheimer's disease (AD) and mild cognitive impairment (MCI) [1, 2]. The well-separable modes of spatial navigation include egocentric and allocentric navigation. Egocentric navigation uses information about distances and angles from the subject positions. Allocentric navigation is hippocampus dependent and uses a flexible representation of a distal landmarks ensemble independent of actual subject positions. At the Department of Physiology of the Czech Academy of Sci-

KARGER
Fax +41 61 306 12 34
E-Mail karger@karger.ch
www.karger.com

1660–2854/10/0073–0148$26.00/0

Accessible online at:
www.karger.com/ndd

Dr. Jakub Hort
Charles University, 2nd Medical School, Department of Neurology
Memory Disorders Clinic, V Uvalu 84
CZ–15006 Prague (Czech Republic)
Tel. +420 224 436 816, Fax +420 224 436 820, E-Mail jakub.hort@seznam.cz

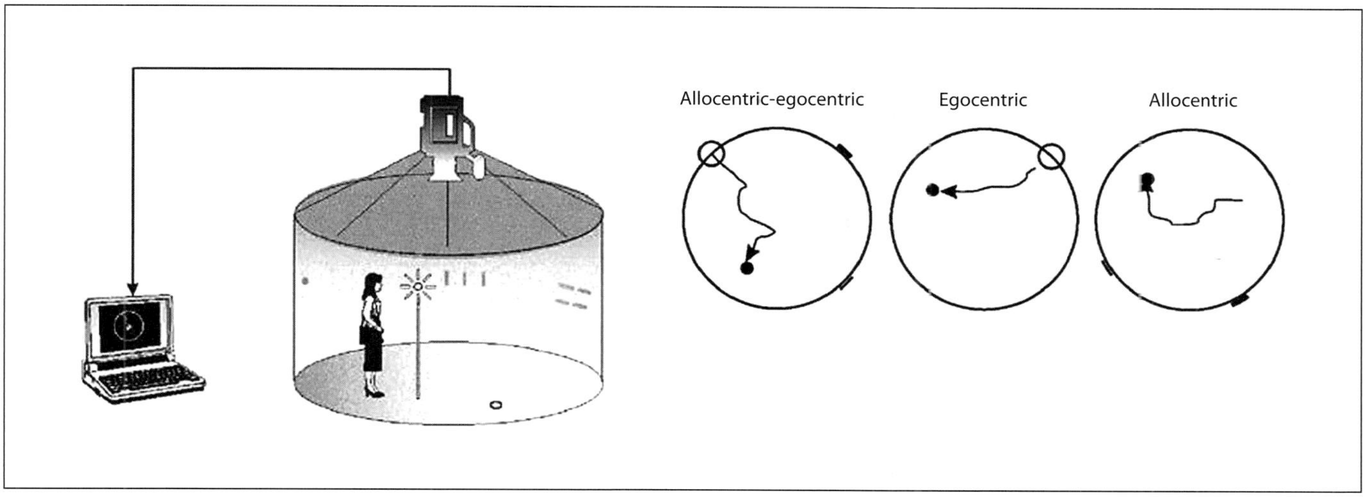

Fig. 1. The BVA – spatial navigation experimental room setting.

ences, a variant of Morris water maze for humans was invented [3] called the Blue Velvet Arena (BVA). Our aim was to test three hypotheses: (a) differences between aMCI patients according to Petersen's concept, (b) differences between aMCI patients according to Dubois' concept, and (c) differences between E4+ and E4– aMCI patients.

Subjects and Methods

Subjects

All subjects were examined by MRI, neurological and medical evaluation, semi-structured interview and extensive neuropsychological testing. Subjects were excluded if they scored more than 5 points on the Global Deterioration Scale or more than 4 points on the Hachinski scale.

Patients were classified into three groups. (1) Mild to moderate AD group (n = 21). They fulfilled DSM-IV criteria for dementia and NINCDS-ADRDA criteria for probable AD. (2) Patients with MCI (n = 49). They fulfilled Petersen's criteria [4], and were subclassified into following groups: naMCI (n = 7) with impairment only in the nonmemory domain, and aMCI with score lower than 1.5 SE only in memory tests, aMCIsd (n = 11) or in multiple domains – aMCImd (n = 31). The aMCI group was also stratified, using the cued recall procedure in Grober and Buschke's test according to Dubois' criteria [5], as memory impairment of the hippocampal type – HaMCI (n = 10) and isolated retrieval impairment – NHaMCI (n = 32). The aMCI group was also stratified according to ApoE4 status, where blood samples were collected to determine ApoE genotype, into ApoE4+ (n = 12) and E4– (n = 30) groups. (3) Volunteers with no memory impairment who served as controls (n = 28).

Grober and Buschke's Test

This verbal memory test consists of 16 items presented on four individual cards (four items per card), where a semantic cue is given and the subject is asked to identify the picture on the card. Then the card is removed and immediate recall is tested by again providing the cue and asking to recall the item. After all four cards have been presented, the subject has to recall as many of the items as possible without any cues. When the patient cannot recall any additional items, appropriate cues for the remaining items are provided. This test takes advantage of the finding that subjects with frontal lobe impairment benefit from strategies that facilitate the retrieval of information (e.g. reminder cues), whereas patients with HaMCI show significantly less benefit from these strategies.

Testing Apparatus

The BVA (fig. 1) is a circular tent 2.9 m in diameter made of a 2.8-meter-high dark blue velvet curtain. Position of an infrared LED diode is recorded by a computerized tracking system connected to a TV camera fixed above the centre of the arena. Two signs on the arena wall are used as navigational cues. Unless they are turned on, the signs are invisible to the subject. The different sign is used as a start location. In the computer version, a map view of the arena was projected on a computer screen and the subject moved the cursor with a mouse.

The Hidden Goal Task

This task is to locate an invisible goal. It separates the allocentric from the egocentric way of navigation by providing either the start position and/or two navigational cues to the subject. The Hidden Goal Task includes the computer and the real space version in four phases. Each phase of the test consists of 8 trials with the start-cue-goal configuration in eight different rotations. The subject is shown the correct position of the goal at the beginning of the test and after the each trial. In the real version, correct location of the goal is marked by a laser pointer

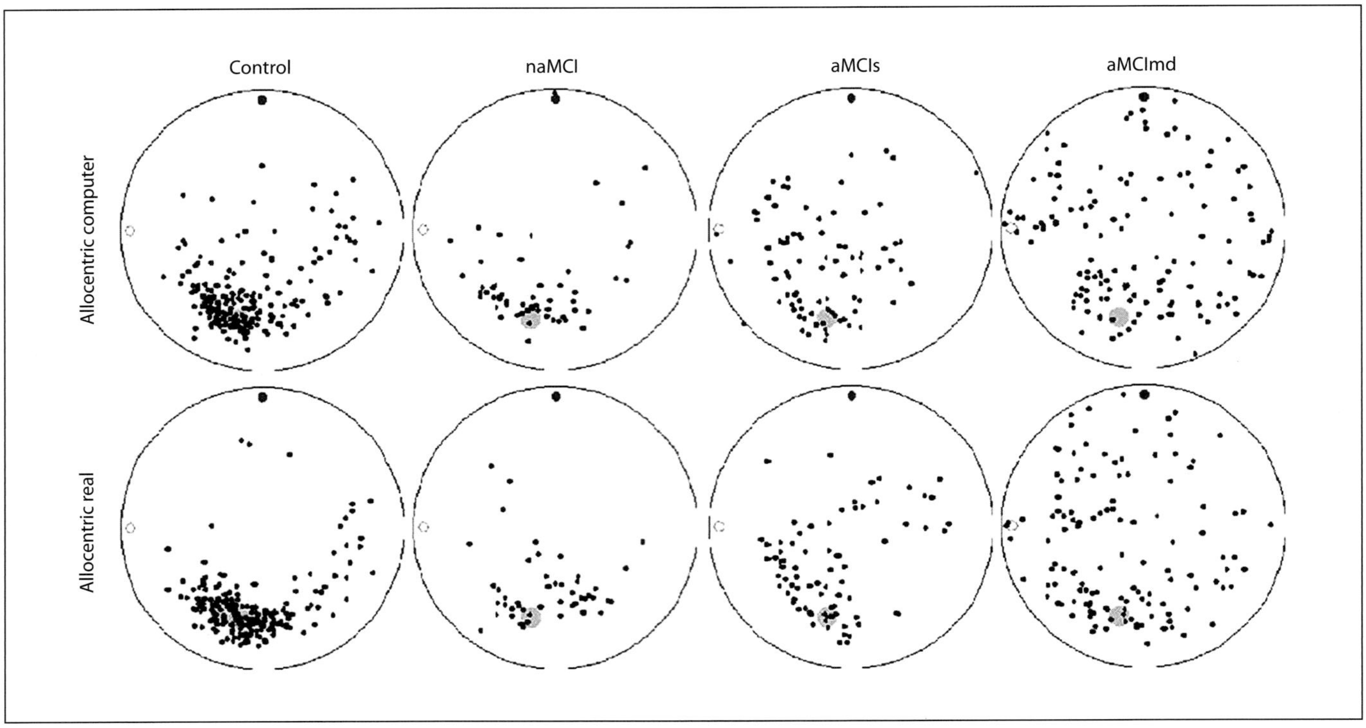

Fig. 2. Hit pattern in the allocentric subtest.

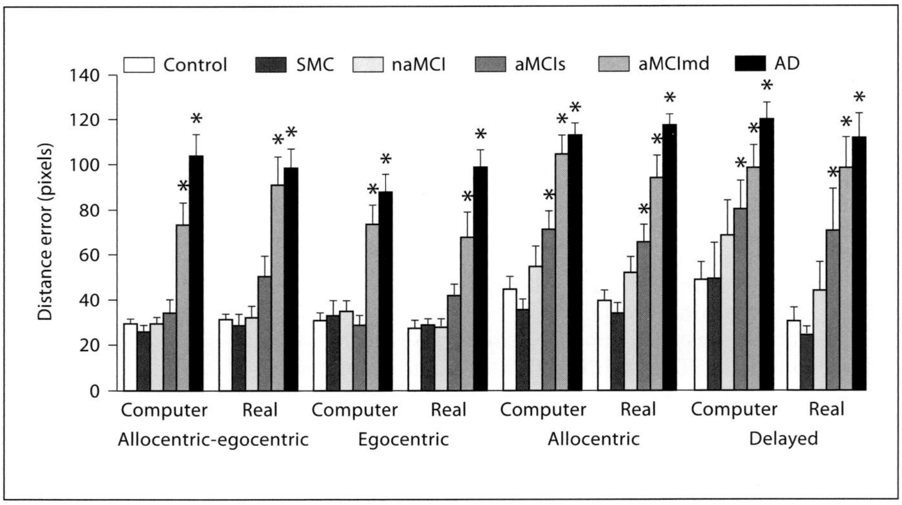

Fig. 3. Between-group differences according to Petersen's concept. SMC = Subjective memory complaints.

projecting a small red circle on the arena floor. The subject is instructed to remember the goal location relative to the start position and/or the orientation cues on the wall. In phase 1 (allocentric + egocentric), both the start-goal relationship and the relative positions of the two orientation cues can be used to locate the goal for eight trials. In phase 2 (egocentric), only the start position can be used to locate the goal. In phase 3 (allocentric), only the two orientation cues can be used for navigation. This time, each trial starts from a different start location relative to the goal. In the last phase (allocentric delayed), the effect of the 30-min time delay is measured. Performance on each trial is measured by the distance error between the subject's choice and the actual goal location.

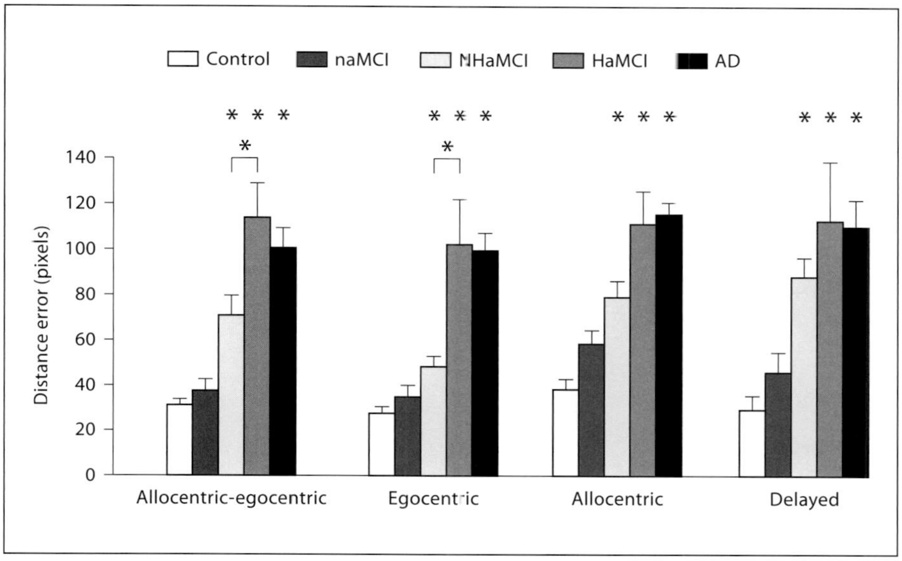

Fig. 4. Between-group differences according to Dubois' concept.

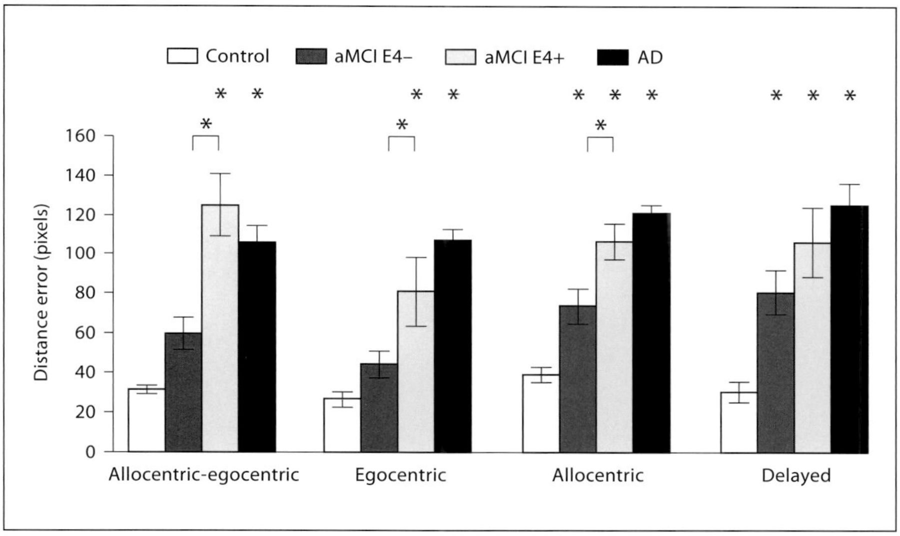

Fig. 5. Between-group differences according to ApoE4 status.

Results

The AD and aMCImd groups were impaired in all subtests ($p < 0.001$). The aMCIsd group was impaired in the allocentric and delayed subtests ($p < 0.022$). No differences were found in the performance of the naMCI group (all $p < 0.127$; fig. 2, 3). There were substantial differences between the HaMCI and NHaMCI groups. The HaMCI group performed worse than the NHaMCI group in the allocentric-egocentric and egocentric subtests ($p < 0.004$), and in the allocentric subtest the difference approached statistical significance ($p = 0.069$; fig. 4). The HaMCI group was impaired in all spatial navigation subtests (all $p < 0.001$) and did not differ from the AD group in any subtests (fig. 4). The impairment in the NHaMCI group was not as severe as in the previous groups ($p < 0.05$), and this group outperformed the AD group in all subtests ($p < 0.003$) except the delayed one ($p = 0.225$). The aMCI E4+ group performed worse than the aMCI E4– group in all subtests ($p < 0.002$; fig. 5). The aMCI E4+ group performed worse than the control group in all subtests (all $p < 0.001$) and was similar to the AD group (all $p < 0.001$). The aMCI E4– group was impaired only in the allocentric and delayed subtests ($p = 0.002$; fig. 5).

Conclusions

We have found that aMCI patients form a very heterogeneous population, where spatial memory or cued recall examination can add more value to aMCI classification. The differences in spatial navigation observed in the aMCI subgroups in relation to ApoE4 status are in agreement with results yielded in animal research [6] and with controversial results yielded in bapineuzumab or rosiglitazone clinical trials. As our method has been found helpful in the diagnosis of MCI patients [7, 8] we are developing computer tests which can be used in a broader clinical setting.

Acknowledgements

Supported by the Grant Agency of the Czech Republic grants 309/09/1053 and 309/09/0286.

References

1 Mapstone M, Steffenella TM, Duffy CJ: A visuospatial variant of mild cognitive impairment: getting lost between aging and AD. Neurology 2003;60:802–808.

2 Monacelli AM, Cushman LA, Kavcic V, Duffy CJ: Spatial disorientation in Alzheimer's disease: the remembrance of things passed. Neurology 2003;61:1491–1497.

3 Kalova E, Vlcek K, Jarolimova E, Bures J: Allothetic orientation and sequential ordering of places is impaired in early stages of Alzheimer's disease: corresponding results in real space tests and computer tests. Behav Brain Res 2005;159:175–186.

4 Petersen RC: Mild cognitive impairment as a diagnostic entity. J Intern Med 2004;256:183–194.

5 Dubois B, Albert ML: Amnestic MCI or prodromal Alzheimer's disease? Lancet Neurol 2004;3:246–248.

6 Raber J, Wong D, Yu G-Q, Buttini M, Mahley RW, Pitas RE, Mucke L: Alzheimer's disease: apolipoprotein E and cognitive performance. Nature 2000;404:352–354.

7 Hort J, Laczó J, Vyhnálek M, Bojar M, Bures J, Vlcek K: Spatial navigation deficit in amnestic mild cognitive impairment. Proc Natl Acad Sci USA 2007;104:4042–4047.

8 Laczó J, Andel R, Vlček K, Maťoška V, Vyhnálek M, Tolar M, Bojar M, Hort J: Spatial navigation and APOE in amnestic mild cognitive impairment. Submitted to Neurology.

Neuro-degenerative Diseases

Neurodegenerative Dis 2010;7:153–159
DOI: 10.1159/000289227

Published online: March 3, 2010

Social Odor Recognition: A Novel Behavioral Model for Cognitive Dysfunction in Parkinson's Disease

Michael M. Monaghan Lauren Leddy Mei-Li Amy Sung Kristin Albinson Katie Kubek Menelas N. Pangalos Peter H. Reinhart Margaret M. Zaleska Thomas A. Comery

Discovery Neuroscience, Pfizer Global Research and Development, Princeton, N.J., USA

Key Words
Olfaction · Memory · MPTP · Parkinson's disease

Abstract
Background: Parkinson's disease (PD) is a progressive neurodegenerative condition characterized by an increasing loss of dopaminergic neurons resulting in motor dysfunction. However, cognitive impairments in PD patients are a common clinical feature that has gained increased attention. ***Objective:*** The purpose of the current study was to evaluate the effects of an MPTP-induced dopaminergic lesion in mice on social odor recognition (SOR) memory. ***Methods:*** Mice were acutely treated with MPTP and evaluated for memory impairments in the SOR assay and characterized using biochemical and immunohistochemical methods approximately 2 weeks later. ***Results:*** Here we demonstrate that SOR memory is sensitive to MPTP treatment and that it correlates with multiple measures of nigrostriatal integrity. MPTP treatment of C57BL/6N mice produced a profound decrease in dopamine levels, dopamine transporter binding and tyrosine hydroxylase immunoreactivity in the striatum. These impairments in stratial dopaminergic function were blocked by pretreatment with the MAO-B inhibitor deprenyl. Changes in the dopaminergic system parallel those observed in SOR with MPTP treatment impairing recognition memory in the absence of a deficit in odor discrimination during learning. Deprenyl pretreatment blocked the MPTP-induced impairment of SOR memory. ***Conclusion:*** The use of the SOR memory model may provide a preclinical method for evaluating cognitive therapies for PD.

Introduction

Parkinson's disease (PD) is defined by a cluster of motor deficits such as tremor, rigidity and bradykinesia emanating from a loss of dopaminergic neurons in the substantia nigra. In addition to these core symptoms, PD patients suffer from autonomic impairments as well as psychological disturbances that include cognitive dysfunction, particularly in the domains of executive function, working memory, attention and verbal fluency [1]. Functional neuroimaging analyses during cognitive assessment tasks in PD patients suggest that abnormal striatal function may underlie some of these cognitive deficits [reviewed in 2]. The occurrence of cognitive dysfunc-

KARGER
Fax +41 61 306 12 34
E-Mail karger@karger.ch
www.karger.com

1660–2854/10/0073–0153$26.00/0

Accessible online at:
www.karger.com/ndd

Michael M. Monaghan
Discovery Neuroscience
Pfizer Global Research and Development, CN8000
Princeton NJ 08534 (USA)
Tel. +1 732 274 4159, Fax +1 732 274 4755, E-Mail monaghm@wyeth.com

tion in this population is often evident at the time of diagnosis and frequently progresses in the later stages of the disease to dementia, a major debilitating factor severely affecting the patient's quality of life [3, 4]. Thus, restoring cognitive function remains a critical unmet need for PD patients.

In humans and non-human primates, the systemic administration of the neurotoxin MPTP recapitulates many of the cardinal clinical features of PD including tremor, akinesia, postural instability and the loss of dopaminergic neurons of the nigrostriatal pathway [5]. In non-human primate, chronic MPTP treatment can lead to deficits in attention and executive function at the onset of motor impairments, suggesting that this model may also have utility for evaluating PD-associated cognitive impairments [6, 7]. For practical reasons, most MPTP studies use the mouse model, which also displays a relatively selective loss of dopaminergic neurons in the substantia nigra. An extensive literature assessing the functional consequence of an MPTP lesion has been focused on motor impairments, while there are very little data available demonstrating cognitive effects [8]. In addition, most cognitive assays in mice have been developed to measure hippocampal function involving some form of spatial information, a brain region not particularly germane to PD.

The purpose of the current study was to evaluate the effects of an MPTP-induced lesion in mice on social odor recognition (SOR) memory. Interestingly, olfactory dysfunction is one of the early indicators of PD [9]. In this study, we employed a recent variant of the SOR memory assay, which was used to demonstrate alcohol-induced memory loss in rats [10]. This procedure uses objects that were imbued with male conspecific odors, a very salient and ethologically relevant stimulus for male mice. Our results show that MPTP-induced loss of nigrostriatal terminals produces a loss in recognition memory in mice.

Materials and Methods

Subjects

Male, 10-week-old C57BL/6N (Taconic) and CD-1 (Charles River) mice were group housed by strain for all pharmacological treatments, then housed singly for all behavioral experiments and maintained on food and water ad libitum with 12-hour light/dark cycle. Animal protocols were performed in accordance with NIH's Guide for the Care and Use of Laboratory Animals, and approved by Wyeth's IACUC.

Pharmacological Treatments

Mice (C57BL/6N) were injected with deprenyl (Sigma M003) 10 mg/kg or vehicle (i.p.) followed by 4 consecutive injections of MPTP (Sigma M0896) 20 mg/kg (i.p.) every 2 h. The sequence of behavioral testing began approximately 1 week (5–9 days) after MPTP treatment, with SOR habituation, training and testing occurring over the following 8 days, followed by an open field activity assessment a day later. The study was concluded by the collection of tissue the next day, approximately 2 weeks after MPTP treatment. The mice were sacrificed and their brains harvested in one of two ways, depending on outcome assessment. For determination of dopamine (DA) content and DA transporter (DAT) binding, fresh striatal tissue was dissected, whereas for immunohistochemical analyses, brains were removed and processed following transcardial perfusion. Details of immunohistochemical procedures including quantitative analysis of DAT density and DA concentration in the striatum were previously reported [11].

SOR Assay

Habituation, training and testing occurred in the subject's home cage (HC). Mice were individually housed with 5 spherical wooden beads, approximately 2.5 cm in diameter (Woodworks LTC, Fort Worth, Tex., USA) for a 6-day habituation period to familiarize animals with the beads and saturate the wooden beads with individual mouse odors. Beads were removed from each cage and sealed in individual plastic bags 30 min prior to training. Behavioral assessment and pharmacological treatment were done only in the C57BL/6N mouse strain. The CD-1 strain of mouse was selected for donors of novel odors because C57BL/6J mice have been reported to have difficulties discriminating odor cues between males of their own strain [12]. All the wooden beads used were laden with odors from individual mice, as described above, and were used as objects that were either from their HC, or from cages of one of two CD-1 male mice (N1 and N2). Training consisted of three, 1-min trials separated by a 1-min intertrial interval. During these trials, each animal was presented with three of their own HC beads and one novel odor bead (N1), which was taken from a cage of the first CD-1 mouse (N1). Beads were removed from the HC during each intertrial interval. Exploration time of each bead was hand recorded by an experimenter, who was blind to the treatment. Exploration time was defined as the amount of time the animal was actively sniffing a bead in close proximity (<5 mm). Other behaviors such as gnawing and pushing the bead were not scored as exploratory time. This training period was considered to be a series of learning trials in which the animal becomes familiar with the novel odor bead. Immediately following training, used beads were removed and discarded. Twenty-four hours later, animals were subjected to a 1-min test trial in which animals were presented with two HC beads saturated with their own odor (HC), one bead from the CD-1 mouse experienced the previous day (N1, which should now be familiar) and one completely novel bead from a new, never experienced, CD-1 mouse (N2). Time spent exploring each bead was again hand recorded by an experimenter blind to experimental group. Increased exploration of the N2 bead over the N1 bead suggests memory of the N1 bead acquired from training. Positioning of beads during the training trials was identical across the 3 trials but randomized for every animal. The positioning of beads during the testing phase was randomized with respect to the bead position on the training trials and across subjects.

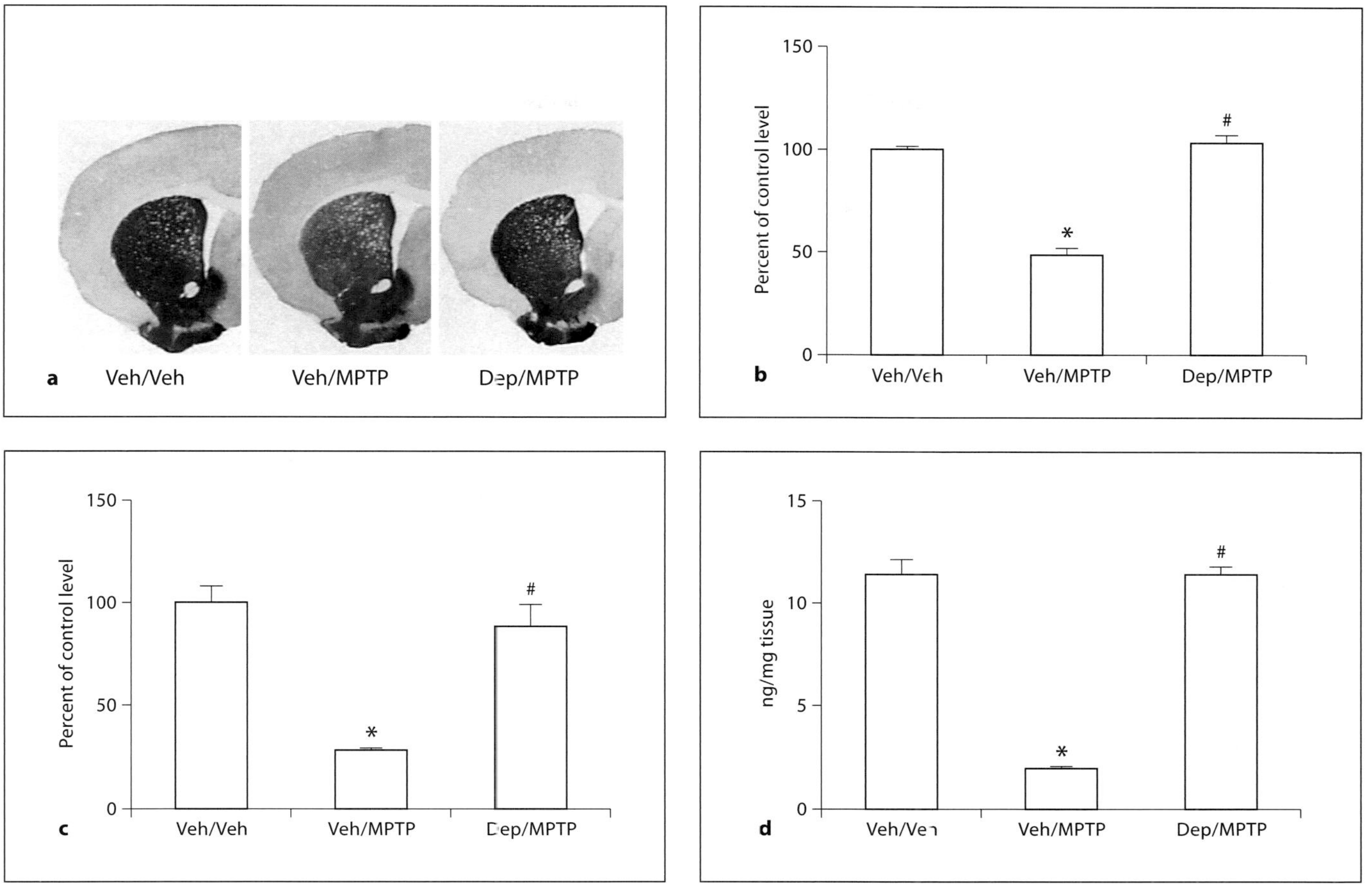

Fig. 1. Multiple measurements assessing the integrity of dopaminergic terminals in the striatum of control, MPTP- and deprenyl/MPTP-treated C57BL/6N mice sacrificed after behavioral studies. **a** Representative micrographs of TH staining of coronal brain sections (single hemisphere) for each treatment group. **b** Quantitative measurement of intensity of TH immunoreactivity in the dorsal striatum indicating a significant reduction in the MPTP-treated mice which was blocked by deprenyl pretreatment. **c** Quantitative measurement of DATs located on nigrostriatal terminals using a radioligand binding of $[^3H]$ MFZ 2–12 showing significant reduction following MPTP treatment which was blocked by deprenyl pretreatment. **d** Measurements of striatal DA (ng/mg tissue) levels in homogenized striatal tissue using HPLC indicated significant reduction in the MPTP-treated subjects which was similarly blocked with deprenyl pretreatment (data presented as means ± SEM, n = 7–9; * $p < 0.0001$, Veh/Veh vs. Veh/MPTP; # $p < 0.0001$, Veh/MPTP vs. Dep/MPTP).

A two-way ANOVA statistical test was performed on all training exploration times, measuring the amount of exploration of each bead averaged over the 3 trials for each mouse, and all testing phase exploration times measuring the percentage of time exploring each bead over the 1-min trial for each mouse. Animals were excluded from analysis if they did not explore for at least 5 s during training or at least 2 s during testing phase.

Open Field Activity Assessment
Individual mice were placed in a novel environment for 30 min, and distance traveled was assessed using automated monitoring equipment (Ethovision, Noldus). A one-way ANOVA statistical test was performed on total distance traveled.

Results

Multiple methods were used to assess dopaminergic innervation of the striatum, namely (1) the intensity of tyrosine hydroxylase (TH) immunoreactivity; (2) DAT binding site density, and (3) DA concentration. All the above outcomes were evaluated immediately following the final day of behavioral testing, ~2 weeks after MPTP treatment. Data from all three measures indicated that MPTP treatment produced a significant loss of dopaminergic terminals in the striatum. Optical density mea-

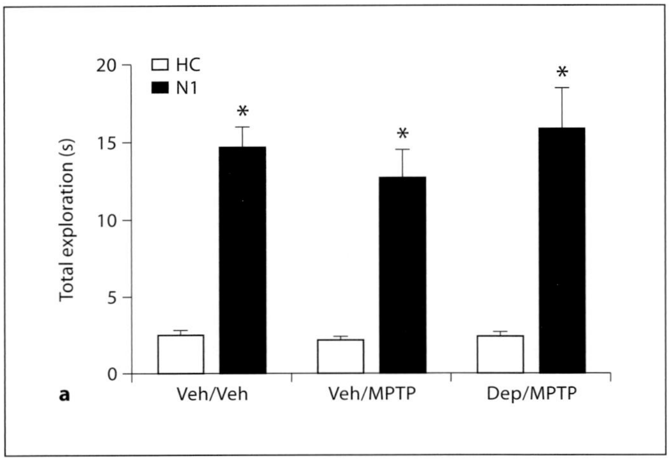

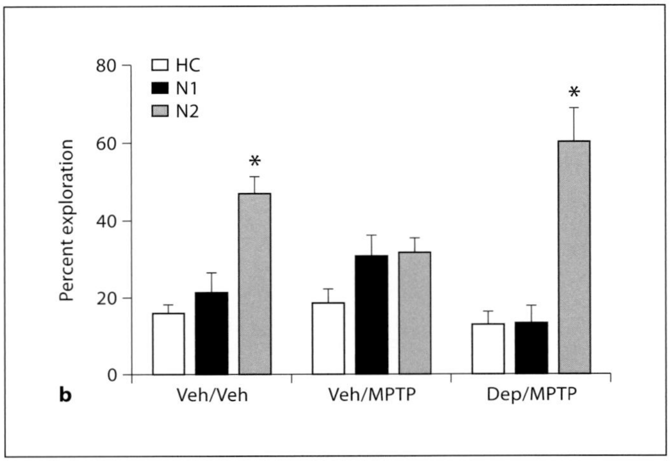

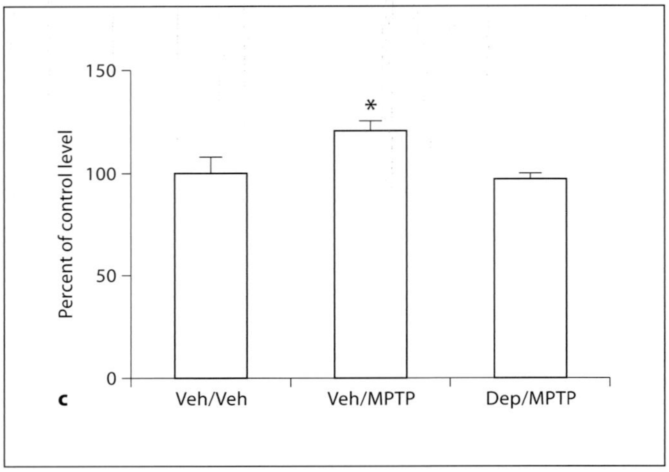

Fig. 2. Assessment of social odor training (**a**), recognition memory (**b**) and open field activity (**c**) of control, MPTP- and deprenyl/MPTP-treated mice. **a** All treatment groups explored the novel scented bead (N1) significantly (* $p < 0.0001$) more than the beads from their HCs. **b** In testing, vehicle and deprenyl/MPTP groups explored N2 significantly more than N1, the odor that was explored on the previous day (N2 vs. N1, $p < 0.0001$). MPTP-treated subjects did not differentiate N2 from N1. **c** MPTP-treated mice traveled a significantly ($p < 0.01$) greater distance in novel environment in 30 min than both the control and deprenyl/MPTP-treated groups (data presented as means ± SEM, n = 11–13).

surement of TH immunoreactivity (fig. 1b), DAT binding density (fig. 1c) and DA concentration (fig. 1d) were 48, 28 and 17% of control levels, respectively. Pretreatment with deprenyl (10 mg/kg) completely blocked the MPTP-induced loss of nigrostriatal terminals as indicated by all three indices of nigrostriatal integrity (fig. 1).

In the SOR assay, the time spent exploring the three familiar HC beads during the training phase were averaged and compared with the time spent exploring the N1 bead. Animals in all three treatment groups, vehicle/vehicle, vehicle/MPTP and deprenyl/MPTP, demonstrated clear preference for the N1 bead, as indicated by significantly greater exploration time ($p < 0.0001$; fig. 2a). There were no significant differences in exploring N1 between the treatment groups.

In the testing phase, a bead from an unfamiliar mouse was introduced, such that there were two familiar HC beads, an N1 bead with a CD-1 mouse odor previously experienced during training, and a bead with the odor from a second unfamiliar CD-1 mouse, N2. The vehicle-treated group explored N2 significantly more than both N1 and the HC beads ($p < 0.0001$). The MPTP-treated group displayed equal exploration of the N1 and the N2 bead ($p < 0.94$). Mice treated with deprenyl prior to MPTP treatment, preferentially explored N2 compared to both N1 and the familiar HC beads, similar to the pattern observed in the vehicle-treated group ($p < 0.0001$; fig. 2b). The total mean exploration time of all the beads in the testing phase for the vehicle (7.5 s, ± 1.6 SEM), MPTP (7.1 s, ± 1.0 SEM) and deprenyl/MPTP groups (8.0 s, ± 1.5 SEM) was not significantly different.

General locomotor activity was evaluated to determine if MPTP treatment produced some generalized debilitative effect that would affect the animal's ability to investigate the wooden beads. MPTP-treated subjects showed no evidence of gross motor impairment, as determined by total distance traveled, despite the profound loss of DA in the striatum. Instead, MPTP treatment resulted in 21% increase in distance traveled compared to vehicle-treated mice ($p < 0.001$), which was not present in mice treated with deprenyl and MPTP (fig. 2c).

Discussion

Social recognition memory in rodents is demonstrated when a subject spends more time investigating unfamiliar conspecifics than familiar ones. Social memory is mediated mainly by olfactory cues [13] and has been demonstrated to decline with advancing age [14]. In this procedure, social recognition is entirely mediated by olfactory cues in that there was no exposure to the mice themselves but, rather, to their scents that were transferred to wooden beads. Vehicle-treated mice demonstrated an intact social odor memory in the testing phase by preferentially exploring the wooden bead with the novel scent (N2) over the bead they explored briefly the previous day (N1). In contrast, MPTP-treated subjects demonstrated a loss of recognition memory when they failed to preferentially explore a bead with a novel scent (N2) over a bead with an odor they became familiar with on the previous day (N1). Deprenyl pretreatment blocked the loss of recognition memory by preventing the loss of dopaminergic terminals in the striatum.

These results were consistent with other findings that showed a cognitive impairment in delayed alternation task of spatial learning [15], associative olfactory memory test [16] and social recognition task [17] in MPTP-treated mice. Using an identical MPTP dosing regimen and the same strain of mouse, a loss of associative olfactory memory was first detected 30 days after treatment, not at an earlier 7-day period, and in the absence of any effect on odor discrimination or motor function. Similarly, we report an SOR memory impairment 2 weeks following MPTP treatment with no clear motor impairment as demonstrated by an increase in distanced traveled in the open field, which has been reported by others [15]. Relatedly, Dluzen and Kreutzberg [17] reported diminished social recognition at 5–10 days after a modest dose of MPTP; however, without a significant loss of DA in the striatum or other brain regions, which is in contrast to our study and the literature cited above [15, 16]. Surprisingly, L-DOPA treatment, just prior to memory assessment, completely restored normal social recognition memory in the absence of a dopaminergic deficit. Significant reductions in norepinephrine concentrations in both the hippocampus and olfactory bulb were detected in MPTP-treated mice but neither of these deficits were mitigated with L-DOPA, if anything, these deficits were exacerbated, possibly challenging the role of this neurotransmitter system in mediating this apparent memory impairment. Thus, it is difficult to conclude from this study the neuronal substrate or neurotransmitter system underlying this memory deficit. In attempting to reconcile the findings of this study with what we report here, there are also important distinctions to consider which include, among others, the strain of mouse used and the social stimulus to be recalled. They used a male CD-1 strain of mouse that has been shown to be particularly resistant to MPTP-induced dopaminergic neurotoxicity [18]. Furthermore, MPTP effects on other neurotransmitter systems, particularly the noradrenergic system, are not as well documented in the C57BL/6N mouse but have been reported [19] and warrant further investigation. The social stimulus used by these investigators involved multiple exposures to an ovariectomized female mouse which, unlike our stimuli, is multifaceted, interactive and may introduce additional behavioral systems (sexual), which complicates direct comparison with our study. In conclusion, an investigation into the effects of MPTP on nondopaminergic systems in the olfactory bulb and other regions are necessary to confirm the role of the nigrostriatal system mediating the loss in social recognition memory reported in this study.

The olfactory bulb in rodents contains a population of dopaminergic interneurons, periglomerular cells, as well as dopaminergic receptors on olfactory receptor neurons that are important in processing odor information [20]. Furthermore, manipulation of dopaminergic function, through genetic deletion of native DATs or D2 receptors, or pharmacological blockade of D2 receptors, impairs olfactory discrimination [21, 22]. While MPTP treatment predominantly affects the dopaminergic cells that make up the nigrostriatal pathway, there have been reports of other dopaminergic neurons damaged by this treatment [23], which potentially may lead to impaired olfactory function through the loss of dopaminergic neurons in the olfactory bulb. While we did not evaluate the effect on dopaminergic neurons in the olfactory bulb, Mitsumoto et al. [24], using an identical MPTP dosing regimen with the same strain of mouse, reported a modest loss (16%) of protein levels of TH, a rate-limiting enzyme of DA synthesis, and perhaps more critically, no significant loss of DA concentration in the olfactory bulb. The resistance of dopaminergic periglomerular cells to MPTP treatment was attributed to absence of detectable levels of dopaminergic transporters, one of the transport mechanisms through which the neurotoxin MPP+ gains access to the cell. Furthermore, MPTP-treated mice preferentially explored the novel odor (N1) over the familiar odors (HC) on the training day, demonstrating that they were able to discriminate odors. The lack of evidence demonstrating MPTP-induced dopaminergic changes in the olfactory bulb and clear evidence of olfactory discrimination during the training phase of this experiment suggest that the lack of preference for N2 over N1 in MPTP-treated subjects during the testing phase is not a result of sensory impairments.

As was expected, MPTP treatment induced a significant loss of dopaminergic terminals in the striatum indicated by a reduction in TH staining, DAT binding density and the concentration of DA. Deprenyl, a MAO-B inhibitor, which blocks the conversion of MPTP to the active neurotoxic agent MPP+, completely prevented the loss of DA terminals in the striatum. Together, these data suggest that the loss of nigrostriatal terminals was responsible for the impairment of recognition memory in MPTP-treated mice. However, given the limited scope of this paper, we cannot exclude the possibility that MPTP treatment produced neuronal loss in other brain regions, particularly mesolimbic projections, which may have contributed to this cognitive deficit [16, 19, 23].

Therapeutic approaches to the treatment of cognitive deficits associated with PD are likely to be administered at a time when the cognitive and motoric dysfunction and neuronal degeneration are already present. As such, the evaluation of novel cognitive therapies in the SOR model would most frequently occur after the MPTP lesion has been established. However, in situations where pharmacological treatment overlaps the production of the MPTP lesion the potential confounds this procedure presents must be addressed to appropriately interpret any SOR findings. Of specific concern would be evidence that the pharmacological treatment is not interfering with the development of the lesion, either by blocking the conversion of MPTP to MPP+ or its uptake into neurons through MAO-B or DAT inhibition.

In summary, using a relatively simple procedure, we demonstrated a loss of SOR memory in MPTP-treated mice. Additional studies are required to precisely determine the neural substrates that underlie this form of memory and its relevance to PD. Nevertheless, this preclinical model may provide the tools for understanding memory impairments in PD and contribute to the development of new therapies for the treatment of this disease.

Acknowledgement

The authors would like to thank Dr. Timothy Schallert for introducing us to the SOR procedure, his insights, guidance and sharing of unpublished data.

References

1 Zgaljardic DJ, Borod JC, Foldi NS, Mattis P: A review of the cognitive and behavioral sequelae of Parkinson's disease: relationship to frontalstriatal circuitry. Cogn Behav Neurol 2003;16:193–210.

2 Grahn JA, Parkinson JA, Owen AM: The cognitive functions of the caudate nucleus. Prog Neurobiol 2008;86:141–155.

3 Muslimovic D, Post B, Speelman JD, Schmand B: Cognitive profiles of patients with newly diagnosed Parkinson's disease. Neurology 2005;65:1239–1245.

4 Schrag A, Jahanshahi M, Quinn N: What contributes to quality of life in patients with Parkinson's disease? J Neurol Neurosurg Psychiatry 2000;69:308–312.

5 Bove J, Prou D, Perier C, Przedborski S: Toxin-induced models of Parkinson's disease. NeuroRx 2005;2:484–494.

6 Schneider JS, Kovelowski CJ: Chronic exposure to low doses of MPTP. I. Cognitive deficits in motor asymptomatic monkeys. Brain Res 1990;519:122–128.

7 Decamp E, Schneider JS: Attention and executive function deficits in chronic low-dose MPTP-treated non-human primates. Eur J Neurosci 2004;20:1371–1378.

8 Sedelis M, Schwarting RK, Huston JP: Behavioral phenotyping of the MPTP mouse model of Parkinson's disease. Behav Brain Res 2001;125:109–125.

9 Liberini P, Parola S, Spano PF, Antonini L: Olfaction in Parkinson's disease: methods of assessment and clinical relevance. J Neurol 2000;247:88–96.

10 Spinetta MJ, Woodlee MT, Feinberg LM, Stroud C, Schallert K, Cormack LK, Schallert T: Alcohol-induced retrograde memory impairment in rats: prevention by caffeine. Psychopharmacology 2008;201:361–371.

11 Arias RL, Sung M-L A, Vasylyev D, Zhang M-Y, Albinson K, Kubek K, Kagen N, Beyer C, Lin Q, Dwyer JM, Zaleska MM, Bowlby MR, Dunlop J, Monaghan M: Amiloride is neuroprotective in an MPTP model of Parkinson's disease. Neurobiol Dis 2008;31:334–341.

12 Arakawa H, Arakawa K, Blanchard DC, Blanchard RJ: Scent marking behavior in male C57/BL/6J mice: sexual and developmental determination. Behav Brain Res 2007;182:73–79.

13 Sawyer TF, Hengehold AK, Perez WA: Chemosensory and hormonal mediation of social memory in male rats. Behav Neurosci 1984;98:908–913.

14 Terranova JP, Perio A, Worms P, Le Fur G, Soubrie P: Social olfactory recognition in rodents: deterioration with age, cerebral ischaemia and septal lesion. Behav Pharmacol 1994;5:90–98.

15 Tanila H, Bjorklund M, Riekkinen P: Cognitive changes in mice following moderate MPTP exposure. Brain Res Bull 1998;45:577–582.
16 Vuckovic MG, Wood RI, Holschneider DP, Abernathy A, Togasaki DM, Smith A, Petzinger GM, Jakowec MW: Memory, mood, dopamine, and serotonin in the 1-methyl-4-phenyl-1,2,3,6-tetrahydropyridine-lesioned mouse model of basal ganglia injury. Neurobiol Dis 2008;32:319–327.
17 Dluzen DE, Kreutzberg JD: 1-Methyl-4-phenyl-1,2,3,6-tetrahydropyridine (MPTP) disrupts social memory/recognition processes in the male mouse. Brain Res 1993;609:98–102.
18 Sonsalla PK, Heikkila RE: Neurotoxic effects of 1-methyl-4-phenyl-1,2,3,6-tetrahydropyridine (MPTP) and methamphetamine in several strains of mice. Prog Neuropsychopharmacol Biol Psychiatry 1988;12:345–354.
19 Seniuk NA, Tatton WG, Greenwood CE: Dose-dependent destruction of the coeruleus-cortical and nigral-striatal projections by MPTP. Brain Res 1990;527:7–20.
20 Brunig I, Sommers M, Hatt H, Bormann J: Dopamine receptor subtypes modulate olfactory bulb gamma-aminobutyric acid type A receptors. Proc Natl Acad Sci 1999;96:2456–2460.
21 Tillerson JL, Caudle WM, Parent JM, Gong C, Schallert T, Miller GW: Olfactory discrimination deficits in mice lacking the dopaminergic transporter or D2 dopamine receptor. Behav Brain Res 2006;172:97–105.
22 Wilson DA, Sullivan RM: The D2 antagonist spiperone mimics the effects of olfactory deprivation on mitral/tufted cell odor response patterns. J Neurosci 1995;15:5574–5581.
23 German DC, Nelson EL, Liang C-L, Speciale SG, Sinton CM, Sonsalla PK: The neurotoxin MPTP causes degeneration of specific nucleus A8, A9 and A10 dopaminergic neurons in the mouse. Neurodegeneration 1996;5:299–312.
24 Mitsumoto Y, Mori A, Ohashi S, Nakai M, Moriizumi T: Differential effects of 1-methyl-4-phenyl-1,2,3,6-tetrahydropyridine in the olfactory bulb and the striatum in mice. Neurosci Res 2005;51:111–115.

Imaging, Biomarkers, Genetics and Diagnostic Markers

Neuro-degenerative Diseases

Neurodegenerative Dis 2010;7:160–162
DOI: 10.1159/000289228

Published online: March 3, 2010

Cognitive Event-Related Potentials and Oscillations in the Subthalamic Nucleus

Ivan Rektor Marek Baláž Martina Bočková

First Department of Neurology, Masaryk University, St. Anne's Hospital, Brno, Czech Republic

Key Words
Cognitive activities · Subthalamic nucleus · Basal ganglia · P3-like potential · Event-related desynchronization/synchronization

Abstract
Background: The cognitive role of the subthalamic nucleus (STN) remains largely unknown. ***Methods/Results:*** A modified protocol with a dual task elicited local field event-related potentials (ERPs) within the STN. No generators of ERPs were elicited by the standard oddball protocol in the STN (at variance with recordings from the putamen, caudate and pallidum). Repetitive transcranial magnetic stimulation (rTMS) over the right inferior frontal cortex caused a shortening of latencies of ERPs in standard and dual protocols. No changes were observable after the rTMS over the dorsolateral prefrontal cortex and sham stimulation. In the STN, only the tasks with an increased demand on executive functions produced the α-/β-event-related desynchronization/synchronization in visuomotor tasks with single letters writing. ***Conclusion:*** Our results indicate a specific, task-related involvement of the STN in the cognitive activities. Cognitive processing in the STN is possibly processed via hyperdirect cortico-STN pathway. Certain effects of deep brain stimulation surgery on cognitive performance could be explained by a direct effect on 'cognitive' parts of the STN.

According to our earlier studies based on intracerebral recordings of cognitive event-related potentials (ERPs) in epilepsy surgery candidates, the cognitive activities in the basal ganglia (BG) are organized in some way other than the well-known organization of the cortico-BG-thalamo-cortical circuits [1]. We report the results of three substudies here. In the first two, the auditory oddball ERPs were recorded from the area of the subthalamic nucleus (STN). Finally, a cognitive event-related desynchronization/synchronization (ERD/S) study in α- and β-frequency bands was performed.

Methods

Recordings were obtained from patients with Parkinson's disease from externalized four-contact deep brain stimulation (DBS) electrodes implanted in the STN. Usually, two of the four contacts of each electrode (0.5-mm intercontact distance and 1.5 mm electrode contact width) were positioned inside the STN according to clinical effect, perioperative microrecording and stimulation.

The recording of bioelectrical activity was performed during the interoperative period (before battery implantation). Recordings were performed using the 8-channel Nihon Kohden Neuropack 4200EP/EMG device, and later using the 32-channel EEG system TruScan Alien. The signal was filtered in the range 1–200 Hz, time base 1,200 ms; a biauricular reference electrode was used. The sampling rate was 256 Hz.

In 10 patients, involvement of STN in executive functions was tested by an auditory oddball paradigm [2]. Tones were delivered through earphones, at a 2-Hz frequency: frequent tones were delivered at 1,000 Hz and 70 dB, for 0.1 s; rare (target) tones were

KARGER
Fax +41 61 306 12 34
E-Mail karger@karger.ch
www.karger.com

1660–2854/10/0073–0160$26.00/0

Accessible online at:
www.karger.com/ndd

Prof. Dr. Ivan Rektor, CSc
First Department of Neurology, Masaryk University
St. Anne's Hospital, Pekarska 53
CZ–656 91 Brno (Czech Republic)
Tel. +420 543 182 623, Fax +420 543 182 624, E-Mail irektor@med.muni.cz

Table 1. ERD (%) in α- and β-frequency ranges during performance of the four tasks of the experimental protocol

Subject No.	ERD			
	task 1	task 2	task 3	task 4
1	0	0	–40%, IF 12–16 Hz bilaterally	NA
2	0	0	0	–60%, IF 14–20 Hz bilaterally
3	0	0	0	–50%, IF 10–14 Hz bilaterally
4	0	0	–40%, IF 10–14 Hz right side	–30%, IF 14–18 Hz right side
5	0	0	–50%, IF 8–18 Hz bilaterally	–60%, IF 14–18 Hz bilaterally

IF = Individual frequency; 0 = no significant changes.

delivered at 2,000 Hz and 70 dB, for 0.1 s. The tones were randomly generated at a 5:1 ratio.

The subjects were instructed to recognize the target tones and to silently count them in the standard protocol.

A modified paradigm increased demands on executive functions. The tasks consisted of silently changing a date upon each target presentation. The subjects were given a two-item date which included the day of the week and the ordinal date (e.g. Monday the 19th). The date had to be updated after each target stimulus [2].

We found a local source, a steep rise in amplitude, in the ERPs (P3-like potential) recorded during the dual task protocol within the STN in 8 of the 14 electrodes. In the remaining 6 electrodes, there were no ERP generators present. The occurrence of generator activity in STN was significant ($p < 0.0001$; test of homogeneity of binomial distribution). We did not observe a voltage change in the ERPs recorded during the standard protocol. ERP latencies were significantly longer in the modified protocol in the contacts with the best motor response (Wilcoxon matched pairs test).

In the second study, we raised the question whether the STN connections with cortical structures influence its participation in cognitive functions and examined two possible candidates for such a cooperation – the dorsolateral prefrontal cortex (DLPFC) and the inferior frontal cortex (IFC).

The repetitive transcranial magnetic stimulation (rTMS) modifies the cortical excitability. One rTMS session (600 pulses) of 1-Hz stimulation was delivered to each patient over the right IFC (BA 44) or over the right DLPFC (BA 9, 46). The DLPFC has been associated with executive functions and with higher cognitive functions, while the IFC was shown to be important for the executive functions as well. The direct connection between the IFC and the STN – the 'hyperdirect' pathway and its putative influence on motor aspects of STN activity has been described earlier.

The ERPs were recorded using the same method and technique as described above. rTMS over the right IFC caused a statistically significant shortening of latencies of ERPs in both protocols in all patients. No such changes were observable either after the sham rTMS of IFC or after the active rTMS of the DLPFC area. There was again a voltage change present in the STN with a modified protocol.

The aim of this work was to examine the involvement of the STN in the neurocognitive networks in four visuomotor cognitive tasks with single letters writing. The α- and β-ERD/S was used as the method of the EEG signal analysis. The ERD of the α- and β-bands is interpreted as a correlate of an activated cortical area, and the ERS correlate of a cortical deactivation.

The EEG signal was recorded from the STN in 5 patients. The used experimental protocol was previously tested in a SEEG study in epilepsy surgery patients and showed a specific activation of the prefrontal and lateral temporal neocortex [3]. The letters of the alphabet, presented in a random order on a monitor, served as the visual stimuli. The duration of the stimulus exposure was 200 ms, of the interstimulus interval 16 s; the mean number of trials was 50. Subjects performed four visuomotor cognitive tasks: (1) single letter counting, (2) copying, (3) writing another letter (planning, inhibition of automatic responses) and (4) writing another letter inversed (planning, inhibition of automatic responses, mental inversion). Data were first segmented according to the stimulation trigger onset. The individual frequency windows were determined in the α-band (7–14 Hz) and the β-band (16–30 Hz) using time frequency analysis (TFA). The trials were processed by a complex demodulation technique to ascertain the envelope of power in the individual frequency bands and averaged. A decrease in band power indicates induced (nonphase-locked, noncoherent) ERD, and an increase in band power indicates event-related synchronization ERS. The significance of the differences between the mean power observed during the baseline and that measured inside evaluated interval was expressed as a probability value (p) using a nonparametric Wilcoxon rank sum (signed rank) test for paired samples.

Results

The α- and β-ERD were expressed during the two more complex tasks with increased demand on the executive functions: task 3 (in 3 of 5 subjects) and task 4 (in 4 of 5 subjects; table 1). No significant changes were detected during the first two tasks.

The results demonstrated specific and selective activation in the STN evoked by complex cognitive tasks.

Discussion

The role of the BG in cognitive processing is largely unknown. An integrative role of the BG, with subsequent modulation of cortical cognitive processing has been suggested [1]. In some cases, direct connections with the cortex that bypass the circuitries might underlie the processing of specific cognitive functions. This might be the case of STN. The standard oddball ERP (P3-like potentials) was recorded in the putamen, caudate and pallidum [1] but not in the STN. STN seems to be specifically involved in the processing of some cognitive activities, e.g. of the executive functions. A modified protocol with a dual task elicited local-field ERPs within the STN. rTMS 1 Hz over the right IFC caused a significant shortening of latencies of ERPs in both protocols. No such changes were observable either after the sham rTMS or after the active rTMS over the DLPFC. In the STN, only the tasks with an increased demand on executive functions produced the α- and β-ERD/S. ERD/S was tested in visuomotor tasks with single letters writing. Our results indicate a specific, task-related involvement of the STN in the cognitive activities. Cognitive processing in the STN is possibly processed via a hyperdirect pathway. These findings are more intriguing if we consider that our target was either directly in the motor part of the STN or in its immediate vicinity, according to the perioperation microrecording results and the effect of the DBS procedure on the motor performance of the patients. The neuronal pools involved in cognitive activities may be located in close vicinity to, or even overlap with, the neurons active in motor functions. Certain effects of DBS surgery on cognitive performance could be explained by a direct effect on 'cognitive' parts of the STN.

Acknowledgement

Supported by MŠMT ČR research project No. MSM 0021622404.

References

1 Rektor I, Bareš M, Brázdil M, Kaňovský P, Rektorová I, Sochůrková D, Kubová D, Kuba R, Daniel P: Cognitive and movement-related potentials recorded in the human basal ganglia. Mov Disord 2005;20:562–568.
2 Baláž M, Rektor I, Pulkrábek J: Participation of the subthalamic nucleus in executive functions: an intracerebral recording study. Mov Disord 2008;23:553–557.
3 Bočková M, Chládek J, Jurák P, Halámek J, Rektor I: Executive functions processed in the frontal and lateral temporal cortices: intracerebral study. Clin Neurophysiol 2007; 118:2625–2636.

Imaging, Biomarkers, Genetics and Diagnostic Markers

Neuro-degenerative Diseases

Neurodegenerative Dis 2010;7:163–166
DOI: 10.1159/000289229

Published online: March 3, 2010

Oophorectomy, Menopause, Estrogen, and Cognitive Aging: The Timing Hypothesis

Walter A. Rocca[a, b] Brandon R. Grossardt[c] Lynne T. Shuster[d]

[a]Division of Epidemiology, Department of Health Sciences Research, [b]Department of Neurology, [c]Division of Biomedical Statistics and Informatics, Department of Health Sciences Research, and [d]Women's Health Clinic, Department of Internal Medicine, College of Medicine, Mayo Clinic, Rochester, Minn., USA

Key Words

Oophorectomy · Menopause · Estrogen · Neuroprotection · Dementia · Cognitive impairment · Timing hypothesis

Abstract

Background: The concept of neuroprotective effects of estrogen in women remains controversial. ***Objective:*** To explore the timing hypothesis in relation to cognitive aging and dementia. ***Methods:*** We reviewed existing literature, conducted some reanalyses, and combined results graphically. ***Results:*** Current evidence suggests that estrogen may have either protective effects or harmful effects on the brain depending on age, type of menopause (natural versus surgical), or stage of menopause. The comparison of women with ovarian conservation versus women who underwent bilateral oophorectomy provided evidence for a sizeable neuroprotective effect of estrogen in women in the premenopausal years (most commonly before age 50 years). Several case-control studies and cohort studies also showed a neuroprotective effect in women who received estrogen treatment in the early postmenopausal phase (most commonly at ages 50–60 years). However, recent clinical trials showed that women who initiated estrogen treatment in the late postmenopausal phase (ages 65–79 years) experienced an increased risk of dementia and cognitive decline. ***Conclusion:*** The neuroprotective effects of estrogen depend on age, type of menopause, and stage of menopause (timing hypothesis).

Introduction

The concept of neuroprotective effects of estrogen in women remains controversial because these effects may vary with the timing of treatment [1, 2]. Thus, we combined findings from both observational studies and clinical trials to explore the timing hypothesis in relation to cognitive aging and dementia. This article is a review of existing literature and includes some reanalysis of published data and the graphic combination of results. Figures 1 and 2 illustrate the existing evidence in support of a neuroprotective effect of estrogen in women.

Evidence of Neuroprotective Effects of Estrogen in Animal Experiments

Most experiments involved the removal of the ovaries and subsequent administration of estrogen in female animals. These experiments suggested several mechanisms

KARGER

Fax +41 61 306 12 34
E-Mail karger@karger.ch
www.karger.com

Accessible online at:
www.karger.com/ndd

Walter A. Rocca, MD, MPH
Division of Epidemiology, Department of Health Sciences Research
Mayo Clinic, 200 First Street SW
Rochester, MN 55905 (USA)
Tel. +1 507 284 3568, Fax +1 507 284 1516, E-Mail rocca@mayo.edu

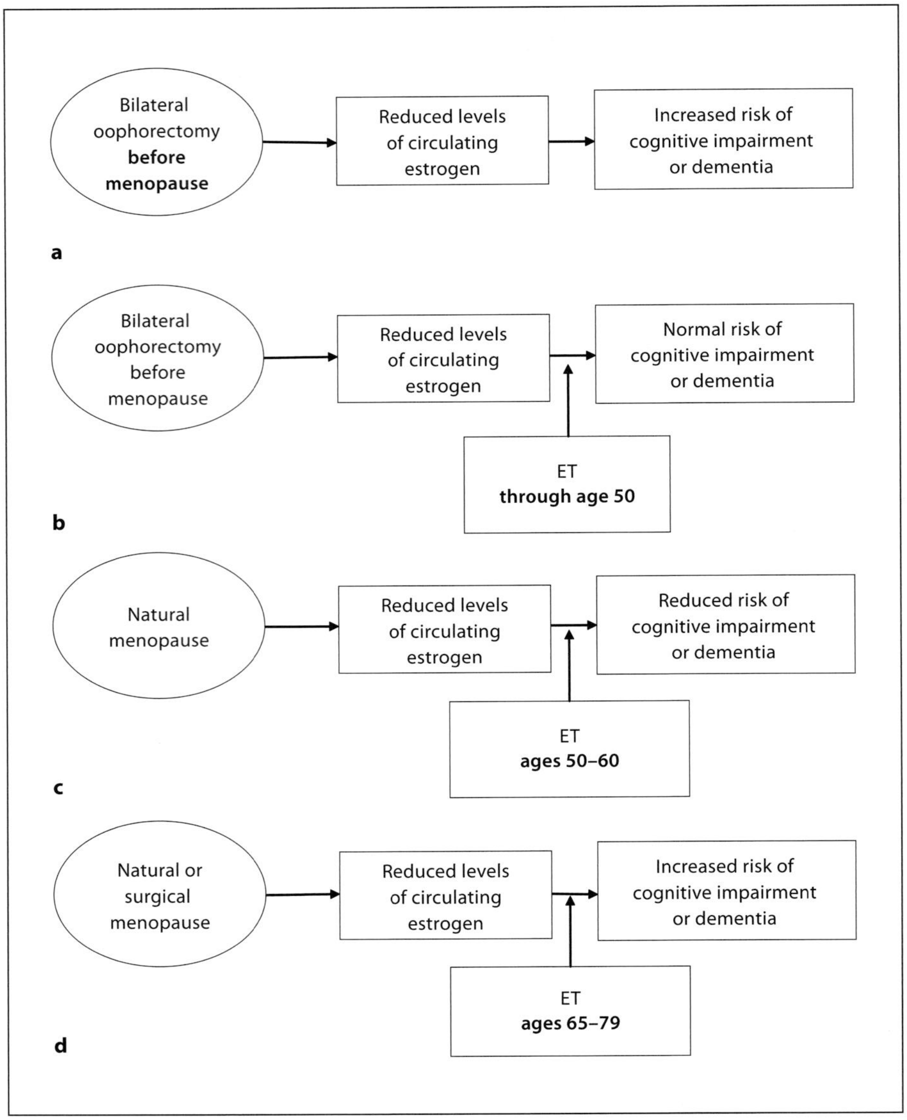

Fig. 1. Four possible clinical situations relevant to the timing hypothesis of estrogen neuroprotection. **a** Women who underwent bilateral oophorectomy early in life experienced premature estrogen deficiency and increased risk of cognitive impairment or dementia. **b** Women who underwent bilateral oophorectomy and were treated with estrogen through age 50 years or later had the same risk of cognitive impairment or dementia as the general population. **c** Women who underwent natural menopause and were treated with estrogen in the early postmenopausal phase (most commonly at ages 50–60 years) had a reduced risk of cognitive impairment or dementia. **d** Women who underwent natural menopause or surgical menopause (hysterectomy with or without bilateral oophorectomy) and initiated estrogen treatment (ET) at ages 65–79 years had an increased risk of cognitive impairment and dementia. The apparent paradox of these four clinical situations is resolved by postulating an interaction between timing and ET (timing hypothesis).

of action. (1) Estrogen improves synapse formation on dendritic spines in hippocampi of ovariectomized rats [3, 4]. (2) Estrogen may improve cerebral blood flow and glucose metabolism, and it may act as an antioxidant [3–5]. (3) Estrogen increases choline acetyltransferase activity in the basal forebrains and hippocampi of ovariectomized rats [5, 6]. (4) Estrogen reduces the deposition of β-amyloid in the brain, whereas progesterone has the opposite effect [7]. (5) Estrogen prevents mitochondrial damage [8]. Thus, there is strong and consistent evidence of neuroprotective effects of estrogen in animal models [2, 9].

Evidence of Neuroprotective Effects of Estrogen in Women before the Age of Natural Menopause

Important observations on the effects of estrogen in younger women come from studies of women who underwent bilateral oophorectomy before reaching natural menopause. The hormonal changes occurring after bilateral oophorectomy in premenopausal women are different from those occurring during natural menopause or after bilateral oophorectomy in women who already experienced natural menopause. In particular, bilateral oophorectomy before menopause causes an abrupt deficiency of estrogen as well as a deficiency of

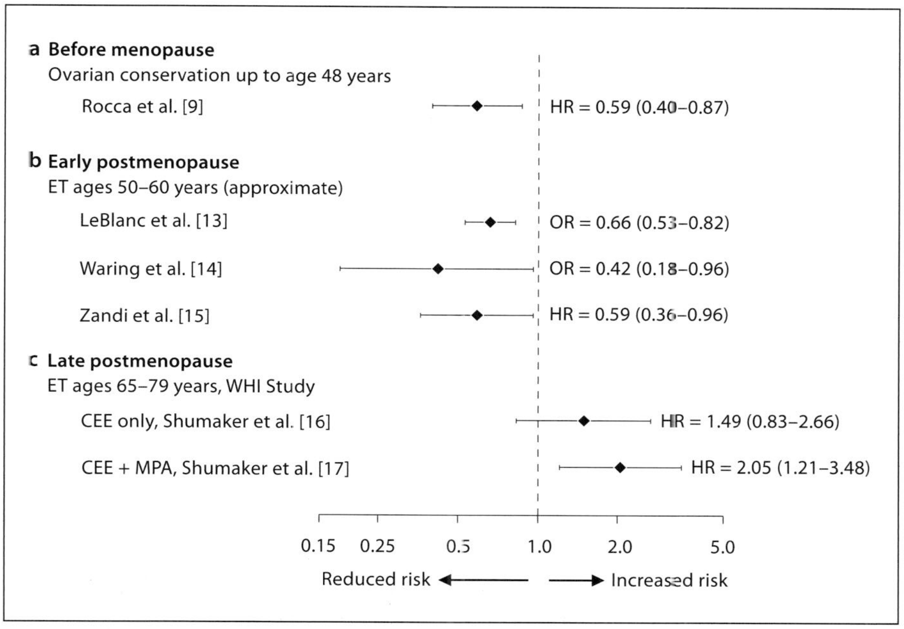

Fig. 2. The effect of estrogen on the risk of cognitive decline or dementia varies with age, type of menopause, and stage of menopause (relative risk estimated by an odds ratio or a hazard ratio and 95% confidence intervals; logarithmic scale). **a** Women with ovarian conservation before menopause (most commonly before age 50 years) have a reduced long-term risk of cognitive decline or dementia compared to women who underwent bilateral oophorectomy. **b** Treatment with estrogen in the early postmenopausal phase (most commonly at ages 50–60 years) is associated with a reduced long-term risk of cognitive decline or dementia. **c** Initiation of ET in the late postmenopausal phase (ages 65–79 years) is associated with an increased risk of cognitive impairment or dementia. CEE = Conjugated equine estrogen; HR = hazard ratio; MPA = medroxyprogesterone acetate; OR = odds ratio.

progesterone and testosterone, and a disruption of the hypothalamic-pituitary-ovarian axis [8]. The disruption of the axis is associated with an abrupt increase in gonadotropins (luteinizing hormone and follicle-stimulating hormone).

The available scientific evidence on cognitive sequelae of bilateral oophorectomy is limited [9, 10]. However, the recent Mayo Clinic cohort study showed an almost doubled long-term risk of cognitive impairment or dementia in women who underwent oophorectomy before menopause (fig. 1a) [9]. The study also showed a trend of increasing risk of cognitive impairment and dementia with younger age at time of oophorectomy [9]. It remains uncertain whether the harmful effects of bilateral oophorectomy are mediated entirely by estrogen deficiency or also by other hormonal mechanisms [8, 11]. However, women who underwent bilateral oophorectomy before age 49 years, but received estrogen treatment (ET) through age 50 years or longer, did not experience an increased risk of cognitive impairment or dementia (fig. 1b) [9].

The only experimental evidence specific for ET after bilateral oophorectomy in women comes from the clinical trials of Sherwin and colleagues involving small groups of women with short-term treatment and minimal follow-up (2–3 months). These short-term trials consistently suggested a neuroprotective effect of estrogen when initiated after oophorectomy [12].

Evidence of Neuroprotective Effects of Estrogen in Women in the Early Postmenopausal Phase

Case-control and cohort studies have consistently shown a protective effect when ET was started in early postmenopause (most commonly at ages 50–60 years; fig. 1c) [13–15]. These observational findings have been criticized because they could be the result of confounding. It is argued that other factors such as higher socioeconomic status, higher education, or better general health may be the real causes of neuroprotection and that ET is only a surrogate marker. However, it is also possible that the observational findings are not due to confounding and that the contradiction between observational studies and clinical trials is due to timing differences.

Evidence of Deleterious Effects of Estrogen Initiated in the Late Postmenopausal Phase

The Women's Health Initiative (WHI) clinical trials showed an increased risk of dementia or mild cognitive impairment among women who initiated treatment with estrogen alone or in combination with progestin at ages 65–79 years (fig. 1d) [16, 17]. However, these trials focused on the effects of ET initiated many years after the onset of natural menopause, and the discrepancy between the WHI results and observational data may be explained by the timing of initiation of estrogen [1, 2]. Indeed, the effects of estrogen on the brain are probably preventive, and when vascular or degenerative lesions have occurred, estrogen cannot reverse the lesions.

The results from the WHI clinical trials have been inappropriately extrapolated from women in the late postmenopausal phase to younger women in the early postmenopausal phase, and to much younger women who underwent bilateral oophorectomy before menopause. Thus, after publication of the WHI results, many women discontinued ET or avoided starting ET at all ages, including women who underwent bilateral oophorectomy before age 50 years [18–20].

Conclusions

A combination of current scientific evidence from animal studies and from both observational studies and clinical trials suggests that estrogen is neuroprotective; however, the neuroprotective effects are dependent on age, type of menopause, and stage of menopause. The apparent contradiction of results from observational studies versus results from clinical trials may be explained by the timing hypothesis (fig. 2).

Acknowledgments

This research was supported by the National Institute of Neurological Disorders and Stroke (grant R01 NS033978) and the National Institute of Arthritis and Musculoskeletal and Skin Diseases (grant R01 AR030582).

References

1 Manson JE, Bassuk SS, Harman SM, Brinton EA, Cedars MI, Lobo R, Merriam GR, Miller VM, Naftolin F, Santoro N: Postmenopausal hormone therapy: new questions and the case for new clinical trials. Menopause 2006; 13:139–147.

2 Siegfried T: Neuroscience: it's all in the timing. Nature 2007;445:359–361.

3 McEwen BS, Alves SE: Estrogen actions in the central nervous system. Endocr Rev 1999;20:279–307.

4 Monk D, Brodaty H: Use of estrogens for the prevention and treatment of Alzheimer's disease. Dement Geriatr Cogn Disord 2000; 11:1–10.

5 Gibbs RB, Aggarwal P: Estrogen and basal forebrain cholinergic neurons: implications for brain aging and Alzheimer's disease-related cognitive decline. Horm Behav 1998; 34:98–111.

6 Markowska AL, Savonenko AV: Effectiveness of estrogen replacement in restoration of cognitive function after long-term estrogen withdrawal in aging rats. J Neurosci 2002;22:10985–10995.

7 Huang J, Guan H, Booze RM, Eckman CB, Hersh LB: Estrogen regulates neprilysin activity in rat brain. Neurosci Lett 2004;367: 85–87.

8 Morrison JH, Brinton RD, Schmidt PJ, Gore AC: Estrogen, menopause, and the aging brain: how basic neuroscience can inform hormone therapy in women. J Neurosci 2006;26:10332–10348.

9 Rocca WA, Bower JH, Maraganore DM, Ahlskog JE, Grossardt BR, de Andrade M, Melton LJ 3rd: Increased risk of cognitive impairment or dementia in women who underwent oophorectomy before menopause. Neurology 2007;69:1074–1083.

10 Shuster LT, Gostout BS, Grossardt BR, Rocca WA: Prophylactic oophorectomy in premenopausal women and long-term health. Menopause Int 2008;14:111–116.

11 Rocca WA, Shuster LT, Grossardt BR, Maraganore DM, Gostout BS, Geda YE, Melton LJ 3rd: Long-term effects of bilateral oophorectomy on brain aging: unanswered questions from the Mayo Clinic Cohort Study of Oophorectomy and Aging. Womens Health (Lond Engl) 2009;5:39–48.

12 Lethaby A, Hogervorst E, Richards M, Yesufu A, Yaffe K: Hormone replacement therapy for cognitive function in postmenopausal women. Cochrane Database Syst Rev 2008: CD003122.

13 LeBlanc ES, Janowsky J, Chan BK, Nelson HD: Hormone replacement therapy and cognition: systematic review and meta-analysis. JAMA 2001;285:1489–1499.

14 Waring SC, Rocca WA, Petersen RC, O'Brien PC, Tangalos EG, Kokmen E: Postmenopausal estrogen replacement therapy and risk of AD: a population-based study. Neurology 1999;52:965–970.

15 Zandi PP, Carlson MC, Plassman BL, Welsh-Bohmer KA, Mayer LS, Steffens DC, Breitner JC: Hormone replacement therapy and incidence of Alzheimer disease in older women: the Cache County Study. JAMA 2002;288: 2123–2129.

16 Shumaker SA, Legault C, Kuller L, Rapp SR, Thal L, Lane DS, Fillit H, Stefanick ML, Hendrix SL, Lewis CE, Masaki K, Coker LH: Conjugated equine estrogens and incidence of probable dementia and mild cognitive impairment in postmenopausal women: Women's Health Initiative Memory Study. JAMA 2004;291:2947–2958.

17 Shumaker SA, Legault C, Rapp SR, Thal L, Wallace RB, Ockene JK, Hendrix SL, Jones BN 3rd, Assaf AR, Jackson RD, Kotchen JM, Wassertheil-Smoller S, Wactawski-Wende J: Estrogen plus progestin and the incidence of dementia and mild cognitive impairment in postmenopausal women: the Women's Health Initiative Memory Study: a randomized controlled trial. JAMA 2003;289:2651–2662.

18 Buist DS, Newton KM, Miglioretti DL, Beverly K, Connelly MT, Andrade S, Hartsfield CL, Wei F, Chan KA, Kessler L: Hormone therapy prescribing patterns in the United States. Obstet Gynecol 2004;104:1042–1050.

19 Haas JS, Kaplan CP, Gerstenberger EP, Kerlikowske K: Changes in the use of postmenopausal hormone therapy after the publication of clinical trial results. Ann Intern Med 2004;140:184–188.

20 Hersh AL, Stefanick ML, Stafford RS: National use of postmenopausal hormone therapy: annual trends and response to recent evidence. JAMA 2004;291:47–53.

Imaging, Biomarkers, Genetics and Diagnostic Markers

Neuro-degenerative Diseases

Neurodegenerative Dis 2010;7:167–169
DOI: 10.1159/000289230

Published online: March 3, 2010

Pharmacogenomic Protocols in CNS Disorders and Dementia

Ramón Cacabelos

EuroEspes Biomedical Research Center, Institute for CNS Disorders and Genomic Medicine, EuroEspes Chair of Biotechnology and Genomics, Camilo José Cela University, Bergondo, Coruña, Spain

Key Words
Alzheimer's disease · Biomarkers · Pharmacogenomics · Apolipoprotein E

Abstract
The application of genomic procedures as diagnostic and therapeutic tools is a major challenge for the coming decades. Pharmacogenomic factors may account for 60–90% of drug variability in drug disposition and pharmacodynamics. About 25% of the 100 most prescribed drugs in the USA and the EU are psychotropic drugs, currently used in dementia. Approximately 60–80% of CNS drugs are metabolized via enzymes of the CYP gene superfamily; 18% of neuroleptics are major substrates of CYP1A2 enzymes, 40% of CYP2D6, and 23% of CYP3A4; 24% of antidepressants are major substrates of CYP1A2 enzymes, 5% of CYP2B6, 38% of CYP2C19, 85% of CYP2D6, and 38% of CYP3A4; 7% of benzodiazepines are major substrates of CYP2C19 enzymes, 20% of CYP2D6, and 95% of CYP3A4. About 57.76% of patients with Alzheimer's disease are extensive metabolisers (EMs) for CYP2D6 enzymes, 31.06% are intermediate metabolisers (IMs), 5.28% are poor metabolisers (PMs), and 5.90% are ultrarapid metabolisers (UMs); 73.71% are CYP2C19-EMs, 25.12% IMs, and 1.16% PMs; 60.87% are CYP2C9-EMs, 34.16% IMs, and 4.97% PMs; 82.75% are CYP3A4/5-EMs, 15.88% IMs, and 1.37% UMs. A trigenic cluster integrating CYP2D6+CYP2C19+CYP2C9 polymorphic variants yields 82 different haplotype-like profiles, representing 36 different pharmacogenetic phenotypes in which only 26.51% of patients show a pure 3EM phenotype. These data clearly indicate that the incorporation of pharmacogenomic protocols to dementia research and clinical trials can foster therapeutics optimization by helping to develop cost-effective pharmaceuticals and improve drug efficacy and safety.

Introduction

More than 90% of functional genes of the human genome are expressed in the CNS in a time- and age-dependent manner. About 80% of major CNS disorders are the result of complex interactions between environmental inducers and pathogenomic substrates. For example, 255 genes have been associated with dementia, 205 with schizophrenia, 106 with depression, 107 with anxiety, 103 with stroke, 385 with different types of ataxia, 155 with epilepsia, 83 with meningioma, 105 with glioblastoma, 27 with astrocytoma, 73 with Parkinson's disease, and more than 30 genes with cerebrovascular disorders [1]. The golden rule for most of these complex disorders, includ-

KARGER

Fax +41 61 306 12 34
E-Mail karger@karger.ch
www.karger.com

1660–2854/10/0073–0167$26.00/0

Accessible online at:
www.karger.com/ndd

Prof. Dr. Ramón Cacabelos, EuroEspes Biomedical Research Center
Institute for CNS Disorders and Genomic Medicine
EuroEspes Chair of Biotechnology and Genomics, Camilo José Cela University
ES–15165-Bergondo, Coruña (Spain)
Tel. +34 981 780 505, Fax +34 981 780 511, E-Mail rcacabelos@euroespes.com

ing Alzheimer's disease (AD), is that the higher the number of genes involved in the disease pathogenesis, the earlier the onset of the disease, the faster its clinical course, and the poorer its therapeutic outcome [2].

Important differences have been found between the AD population (n = 1,364) and healthy subjects (n = 3,311) in different biological parameters. Blood pressure values, glucose levels and cholesterol levels are higher in AD than in healthy elderly subjects. Approximately 20% of AD patients are hypertensive, 25% are diabetics, 50% are hypercholesterolemic, and 23% are hypertriglyceridemic. Over 25% of the patients exhibit high GGT activity, 5–10% show anemic conditions, 30–50% show an abnormal cerebrovascular function, and over 60% show frontal, parietal, and temporal qEEG anomalies. Significant differences are currently seen between females and males, indicating the effect of gender on the disease phenotype. All these parameters are highly relevant when treating AD patients as some of them reflect a concomitant pathology which also needs therapeutic consideration.

Determinant Factors for Sensitivity and Specificity of Pharmacogenomic Studies

The pharmacogenomic outcome depends upon many different determinant factors including (a) genomic profile (family history, ethnic background, disease-related genotype, pharmacogenomic genotype, nutrigenomic genotype), (b) disease phenotype (age at onset, disease severity, clinical symptoms), (c) concomitant pathology, (d) genotype-phenotype correlations, (e) nutritional conditions, (f) age and gender, (g) pharmacological profile of the drugs, (h) drug-drug interactions, (i) gene expression profile, (j) transcriptomic cascade, (k) proteomic profile, and (l) metabolomic networking. The dissection and further integration of all these factors is of paramount importance for the assessment of the pharmacogenomic outcome in terms of safety and efficacy [1].

Apolipoprotein E-Related Biomarkers

Functional genomics studies have demonstrated the influence of many genes on AD pathogenesis and phenotype expression. Apolipoprotein E (APOE)-4 may influence AD pathology interacting with amyloid precursor protein metabolism and Aβ accumulation, enhancing hyperphosphorylation of tau protein and neurofibrillary tangle formation, reducing choline acetyltransferase activity, increasing oxidative processes, modifying inflammation-related neuroimmunotrophic activity and glial activation, altering lipid metabolism, lipid transport and membrane biosynthesis in sprouting and synaptic remodeling, and inducing neuronal apoptosis [3].

Different APOE genotypes confer specific phenotypic profiles to AD patients. Some of these profiles may add risk or benefit when the patients are treated with conventional drugs, and in many instances the clinical phenotype demands the administration of additional drugs which increase the complexity of therapeutic protocols. From studies designed to define APOE-related AD phenotypes [4, 5], several conclusions can be drawn: (a) the age at onset is 5–10 years earlier in approximately 80% of AD cases harboring the APOE-4/4 genotype; (b) the serum levels of ApoE are the lowest in APOE-4/4, intermediate in APOE-3/3 and APOE-3/4, and highest in APOE-2/3 and APOE-2/4; (c) serum cholesterol levels are higher in APOE-4/4 than in the other genotypes; (d) HDL cholesterol levels tend to be lower in APOE-3 homozygotes than in APOE-4 allele carriers; (e) LDL cholesterol levels are systematically higher in APOE-4/4 than in any other genotype; (f) triglyceride levels are significantly lower in APOE-4/4; (g) nitric oxide levels are lower in APOE-4/4; (h) the presence of the APOE-4 allele enhances Aβ burden in senile plaques; (i) blood histamine levels are reduced in APOE-4/4 carriers; (j) brain atrophy is increased in APOE-4/4>APOE-3/4>APOE-3/3; (k) brain mapping shows a significant increase in slow wave activity in APOE-4/4; (l) brain hemodynamics is significantly worse in APOE-4/4 than in APOE-3 carriers; (m) lymphocyte apoptosis is enhanced in APOE-4 carriers; (n) cognitive deterioration is faster in APOE-4/4 patients; (o) in 3–8% of AD cases, the presence of some dementia-related metabolic deficits (e.g., iron, folic acid, vitamin B_{12} deficiencies) accumulate in APOE-4 carriers; (p) behavioral disturbances (bizarre behaviors, psychotic symptoms), alterations in circadian rhythm patterns (e.g., sleep disorders), and mood disorders (anxiety, depression) are slightly more frequent in APOE-4 carriers; (q) atherosclerosis is also more frequent in APOE-4 carriers; (r) liver metabolism and transaminase activity also differ in APOE-4/4 with respect to other genotypes; (s) blood pressure (hypertension) and other cardiovascular risk factors also accumulate in APOE-4, and (t) APOE-4/4 are the poorest responders to conventional drugs. These twenty major phenotypic features clearly illustrate the biological disadvantage of APOE-4 homozygotes and the potential consequences these patients may experience when they receive pharmacological treatment [3–5].

CYP-Related Pharmacogenomics

The microsomal, membrane-associated P450 isoforms CYP3A4, CYP2D6, CYP2C9, CYP2C19, CYP2E1 and CYP1A2 are responsible for the oxidative metabolism of more than 90% of marketed drugs. About 60–80% of the psychotropic agents currently used for the treatment of neuropsychiatric disorders are metabolized via enzymes of the CYP family, especially CYP1A2, CYP2B6, CYP2C8/9, CYP2C19, CYP2D6 and CYP3A4. CYP3A4 metabolizes more drug molecules than all other isoforms together. Most of these polymorphisms exhibit geographic and ethnic differences. These differences influence drug metabolism in different ethnic groups in which drug dosage should be adjusted according to their enzymatic capacity, differentiating between normal or extensive metabolisers (EMs), intermediate metabolisers (IMs), poor metabolisers (PMs) and ultrarapid metabolisers (UMs) [1].

In dementia, as in any other CNS disorder, CYP genomics is a highly important issue, since in practice over 90% of patients with dementia are daily consumers of psychotropics. Furthermore, some acetylcholinesterase inhibitors are metabolized via CYP enzymes. CYP2D6, CYP2C19, CYP2C9 and CYP3A4/5 deserve special consideration. The enzymes encoded by these four genes are responsible for over 80% of the drugs currently taken by patients with dementia [1, 2, 5].

In a recent study with 644 AD patients, we found 57.76% CYP2D6-EMs, 31.06% IMs, 5.28% PMs, and 5.90% UMs; 73.71% were CYP2C19-EMs, 25.12% IMs, and 1.16% PMs. CYP2C9 genotypes were as follows: *1/*1-EM 60.87%, *1/*2-IM 23.98%, *1/*3-IM 10.17%, *2/*2-PM 2.54%, *2/*3-PM 2.16%, and *3/*3-PM 0.25%, globally representing 60.87% CYP2C9-EMs, 34.16% IMs, and 4.97% PMs. CYP2C9-Ile359Leu (CYP2C9*3) and CYP2C9-Arg144Cys (CYP2C9*2) variants are associated with warfarin sensitivity. Clustering together CYP2C9 and VKORC1 variants, we can estimate that approximately 30% of the elderly population are sensitive to warfarin anticoagulants. Concerning CYP3A4/5 polymorphisms, 82.75% of AD cases were EMs (CYP3A5*3/*3), 15.88% were IMs (CYP3A5*1/*3), and 1.37% were UMs (CYP3A5*1/*1).

A genetic map integrating the most prevalent CYP2D6+CYP2C19+CYP2C9 polymorphic variants in a trigenic cluster yields 82 different haplotype-like profiles. The most frequent trigenic genotypes in the AD population are *1*1-*1*1-*1*1 (25.70%), *1*1-*1*2-*1*2 (10.66%), *1*1-*1*2-*1*1 (10.45%), *1*4-*1*1-*1*1 (8.09%), *1*4-*1*2-*1*1 (4.91%), *1*4-*1*1-*1*2 (4.65%), and *1*1-*1*3-*1*3 (4.33%). These 82 trigenic genotypes represent 36 different pharmacogenetic phenotypes. According to these trigenic clusters, only 26.51% of the patients show a pure 3EM phenotype, 15.29% are 2EM1IM, 2.04% are pure 3IM, 0% are pure 3PM, and 0% are 1UM2PM (the most deficient phenotype possible).

Approximately 18% of neuroleptics are major substrates of CYP1A2 enzymes, 40% of CYP2D6, and 23% of CYP3A4; 24% of antidepressants are major substrates of CYP1A2 enzymes, 5% of CYP2B6, 38% of CYP2C19, 85% of CYP2D6, and 38% of CYP3A4; 7% of benzodiazepines are major substrates of CYP2C19 enzymes, 20% of CYP2D6, and 95% of CYP3A4 [1].

These data clearly indicate that the incorporation of pharmacogenomic protocols to dementia research and clinical trials can foster therapeutics optimization by helping to develop cost-effective pharmaceuticals and to improve drug efficacy and safety.

References

1 Cacabelos R: Pharmacogenomic biomarkers in neuropsychiatry: The path to personalized medicine in mental disorders; in Ritsner MS (ed): The Handbook of Neuropsychiatric Biomarkers, Endophenotypes and Genes. Berlin, Springer, 2009, vol 4, pp 3–63.

2 Cacabelos R: Pharmacogenomics in Alzheimer's disease. Meth Mol Biol 2008;448: 213–357.

3 Cacabelos R, Fernández-Novoa L, Lombardi V, Kubota Y, Takeda M: Molecular genetics of Alzheimer's disease and aging. Meth Find Exper Clin Pharmacol 2005;27(suppl A):1–573.

4 Cacabelos R: Genomic characterization of Alzheimer's disease and genotype-related phenotypic analysis of biological markers in dementia. Pharmacogenomics 2004;5:1049–1105.

5 Cacabelos R: Pharmacogenetic basis for therapeutic optimization in Alzheimer's disease. Mol Diag Ther 2007;11:385–405.

Imaging, Biomarkers, Genetics and Diagnostic Markers

Neuro-degenerative Diseases

Neurodegenerative Dis 2010;7:170–174
DOI: 10.1159/000289231

Published online: March 3, 2010

Common Variant in *GRN* Is a Genetic Risk Factor for Hippocampal Sclerosis in the Elderly

Dennis W. Dickson Matthew Baker Rosa Rademakers

Department of Neuroscience, Mayo Clinic, Jacksonville, Fla., USA

Key Words

Alzheimer's disease · Hippocampal sclerosis · Immunohistochemistry · Progranulin gene

Abstract

Background: Hippocampal sclerosis (HpScl) is common in elderly subjects with dementia, either alone or accompanied by other pathologic processes. It is also found in >70% of frontotemporal lobar degeneration with TDP-43 immunoreactive inclusions (FTLD-TDP). TDP-43 inclusions are detected in >20% of Alzheimer disease (AD) and >70% of HpScl cases. The most common cause of FTLD-TDP is mutation in the progranulin gene *(GRN)*. Recently, a common genetic variant in the 3′ untranslated region (3′UTR) of *GRN* (rs5848; c.*78C>T) located in a microRNA binding site regulated progranulin expression, and the T-allele was increased in FTLD-TDP compared to controls. ***Objective:*** The goal of this study was to determine if the 3′UTR variant in *GRN* was associated with TDP-43 immunoreactivity in AD with and without HpScl. ***Methods:*** 644 cases of pathologically confirmed AD, including 57 with HpScl, were screened for TDP-43 immunoreactivity and were genotyped at the *GRN* 3′UTR single-nucleotide polymorphism rs5848 using previously published methods. ***Results:*** There was a trend ($p = 0.06$) for TDP-43 immunoreactivity, but a very significant ($p = 0.005$) association of HpScl with the variant, with 72% of AD with HpScl carrying a T-allele, compared to 51% of AD without HpScl carrying a T-allele. ***Conclusion:*** The results suggest that a genetic variant in *GRN* leading to decreased levels of progranulin may be a risk factor for HpScl in AD, while its role in TDP-43 immunoreactivity in AD remains less certain.

Introduction

Hippocampal sclerosis (HpScl) is defined by selective neuronal loss and gliosis in CA1 and subiculum sectors of the hippocampus (fig. 1) [1]. HpScl is common in elderly subjects with dementia, either alone or accompanied by other pathologic processes [2]. It is most often associated with pathologic features of frontotemporal lobar degeneration (FTLD) [3, 4] and can be detected in more than 75% of FTLD cases [5]. One of the first studies to draw attention to HpScl in the elderly noted it in more than 20% of demented patients over 80 years of age [1]. The clinical syndrome can be mistaken for amnestic mild cognitive impairment [6, 7], a condition thought to represent prodromal Alzheimer's disease (AD) [8], and in some cases it is the only structural abnormality to explain dementia [9]. It is sometimes associated with tauopathy [10] that resembles argyrophilic grain disease, a medial temporal tauopathy that increases in frequency with age [11] and can also present with amnestic mild cognitive impairment [12]. Focal neuronal loss and gliosis in the

Dennis W. Dickson, MD
Department of Neuroscience, Mayo Clinic
4500 San Pablo Road
Jacksonville, FL 32224 (USA)
Tel. +1 904 953 7137, Fax +1 904 953 7117, E-Mail dickson.dennis@mayo.edu

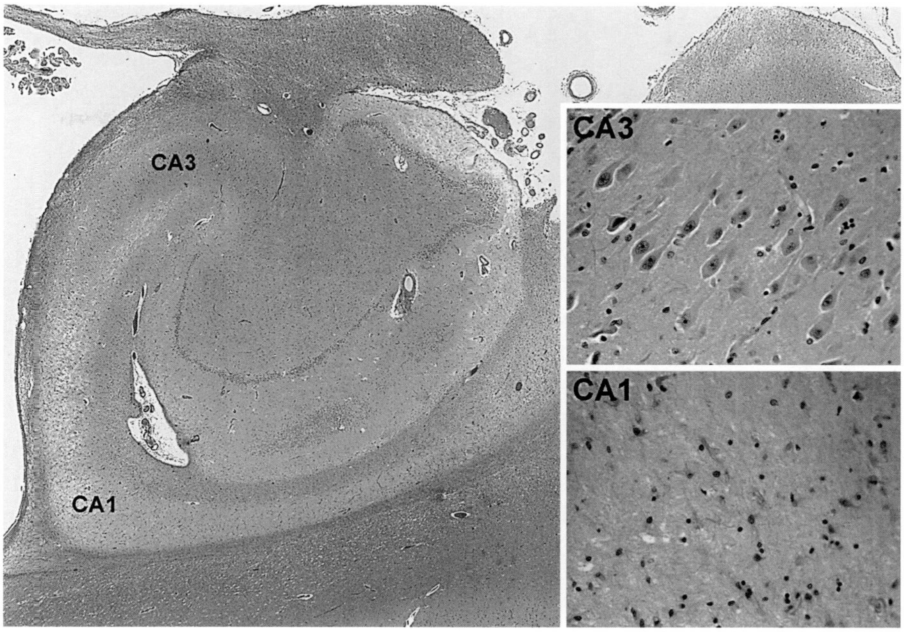

Color version available online

Fig. 1. HpScl is characterized by selective neuronal loss in CA1 with relative preservation of neurons in CA3.

hippocampus can be seen in other degenerative disorders, such as Lewy body disease, but the distribution is different, being most severe in CA2/3 [13, 14].

Immunochemistry using a panel of monoclonal antibodies raised to FTLD brain homogenates led to the discovery of TDP-43 as the major constituent of neuronal inclusions in the most common form of FTLD [15] which is now referred to as FTLD-TDP [16]. TDP-43, for transactivation response protein of 43-kDA molecular weight, is an RNA-binding protein involved in transcriptional regulation that has more recently been implicated in other RNA-dependent cellular functions, such as storage, transport and degradation of mRNA [17]. While initially considered to be a specific marker for FTLD-TDP, this has been called into question as TDP-43 immunoreactivity has been found in 30–50% of AD cases [18, 19] and most cases of HpScl [2, 18, 20].

The most common genetic basis of FTLD-TDP is mutation in the gene for progranulin *(GRN)* [21–23], and the pathology in all cases associated with pathogenic mutations in *GRN* is FTLD-TDP [24, 25]. At present, there are over 125 variants reported in *GRN*, but only 66 that are definitely pathogenic (http://www.molgen.ua.ac.be/FTDMutations). One of the variants is a single-nucleotide polymorphism (rs5848) in the 3′ untranslated region (3′UTR) of *GRN* [26]. Previous studies showed that the T-allele of rs5848 in the 3′UTR of *GRN* was associated with FTLD-TDP [26].

Given that most cases of HpScl are associated with TDP-43 pathology, that many cases of FTLD-TDP have HpScl, and that *GRN* rs5848 is associated with FTLD-TDP, we hypothesized that *GRN* rs5848 would also be associated with HpScl found in AD. As a corollary, if TDP-43 pathology in AD is related to a similar disease process as that seen in FTLD-TDP, the GRN rs5848 T-allele might also associate with AD cases that have TDP-43 immunoreactivity. We set out to test these hypotheses by determining the rs5848 genotype in a series of 644 AD cases that were screened for TDP-43 pathology with immunohistochemistry. A subset of cases had HpScl, which would permit assessment of association of GRN rs5848 with HpScl, as well.

Methods

We obtained frozen brain tissue for DNA extraction and fixed tissue for immunohistochemistry of 644 cases of pathologically confirmed AD. All cases were from the brain bank at Mayo Clinic, Jacksonville and had been evaluated by previously described methods [27]. GRN rs5848 was determined as previously described [26] and TDP-43 immunohistochemistry was also performed as previously described [18]. There were 275 men and 369 women, and the average age at death was 80 ± 9 years; HpScl was detected in 57 cases (9%). Statistical analysis was carried out with SigmaStat for Windows, version 3.0.1a (Systat Software, Richmond, Calif., USA). A significance level was set at 0.05.

Results

TDP-43 immunoreactivity was detected in 219 (34%) of the 644 AD cases. It was present in 44 of 57 (77%) AD cases with HpScl compared to 175 of 587 (30%) AD cases without HpScl (χ^2 49.9, $p < 0.001$). Most often, TDP-43 immunoreactivity was detected in neurons in the limbic distribution, with a smaller subset showing more diffuse distribution, similar to results reported previously [18]. TDP-43 immunoreactivity was not significantly associated with concomitant vascular pathology (Spearman r = 0.052), which was detected in 196 (30%) of the AD cases, or with Lewy bodies (Spearman r = 0.022), which was detected in 185 (29%) of the AD cases.

Presence of TDP-43 immunoreactivity in AD correlated with older age (Spearman r = 0.26, $p < 0.001$), female sex (χ^2 p = 0.04) and presence of HpScl (χ^2 $p < 0.001$). A multiple logistic regression analysis showed that age and presence of HpScl were significant predictors of TDP-43 immunoreactivity (age: OR 1.1, 95% confidence interval 1.04–1.10; HpScl: OR 7.0, 95% confidence interval 3.6–13.6). There was a trend for TDP-43 to be associated with *GRN* rs5848 T-allele (χ^2 p = 0.06), but when included in a multiple regression analysis with age and HpScl, it was not statistically significant (p = 0.093).

The T-allele of *GRN* rs5848 was significantly associated with HpScl in both genotype and allele frequency analyses (table 1). Of the 57 cases of AD and HpScl, 72% carried a T-allele, while only 51% of AD cases without HpScl had a T-allele. The difference in the frequency of the *GRN* rs5848 T-allele in HpScl was greater than chance (p = 0.005). The results suggest that a genetic variant in *GRN* may be a risk factor for HpScl in the elderly.

Table 1. GRN 3′UTR in AD with and without HpScl

	HpScl	No HpScl	p value (χ^2)
Genotype			0.020
rs5848 CC	16	286	
rs5848 CT	33 (58%)	253 (43%)	
rs5848 TT	8 (14%)	48 (8%)	
Allele			0.005
rs5848 C	65	825	
rs5848 T	49 (43%)	349 (31%)	

Discussion

Progranulin is encoded by a single gene on chromosome 17q21 *(GRN)*, and is a 593-amino acid, cysteine-rich protein with an estimated molecular weight of 68.5 kDa that runs at 90 kDa on standard Western blots due to heavy glycosylation [28]. It contains seven granulin-like domains, which consist of highly conserved tandem repeats of a rare 12 cysteinyl motif [29]. Proteolytic cleavage of the precursor protein by extracellular proteases, such as elastase, gives rise to smaller peptide fragments termed granulins [30]. These fragments range in size from 6 to 25 kDa and have been implicated in a range of biological functions, some with properties similar to proinflammatory cytokines [30]. Progranulin plays a role in embryonic development, neoplasia, inflammation and wound healing [28], but its function in the central nervous system is not yet understood [31]. It is widely expressed in neurons, glia and endothelial cells. All known mutations in *GRN* have the same effect; they lead to 50% decreased expression of progranulin and mediate their effects through this deficiency, a process known as haploinsufficiency. Whether FTLD-TDP is caused by deficiencies in trophic actions of progranulin or cytokine-like properties of granulins, or both, and whether the effects of *GRN* are primarily on neurons, glia or endothelial cells is unknown, but these are areas of active investigation.

An emerging topic in the genetics of neurodegenerative diseases is that rare variants in genes (i.e. mutations) cause rare familial forms of the disease, but common variants in the same genes may contribute to risk for the disease in common nonfamilial forms of the disease. A number of examples can be cited, i.e. mutations in *SNCA* cause rare familial Parkinson disease [32], while common variants in *SNCA* are a risk factor for common nonfamilial Parkinson disease [33]. Variants in *GRN* are thus candidate genetic risk factors for nonfamilial forms of FTLD-TDP. Of more that 125 variants described in *GRN*, only 66 segregate with disease (http://www.molgen.ua.ac.be/FTDMutations). One of these variants is located in the 3′UTR of *GRN* with a sequence consistent with a micro-RNA binding site [26], and it is associated with sporadic FTLD-TDP [26].

Recent research has drawn attention to the role of diverse functions of small RNAs, in particular a specific subclass of small RNAs, microRNAs, which have the ability to regulate gene translation through repression or promoting messenger RNA cleavage [34, 35]. At present, there are 851 known microRNAs in humans (http://microrna.sanger.ac.uk) and many target genes, including *GRN*. The *GRN* sequence has at least one micro-RNA binding site for miR-659, a micro-RNA that is expressed in the brain [26]. In addition to GRN, there are 974 other targets of miR-659 (http://microrna.sanger.ac.uk). The presence of the T-allele at the 3′UTR in *GRN* favors miR-659 binding, which lowers levels of progranulin expression without affecting the level of messenger RNA for progranulin. The levels of progranulin in the brains of individuals homozygous for the T-allele are intermediate between wild type (CC homozygous) and individuals carrying a disease-causing mutation in GRN [26]. Similar studies have yet to be performed in AD with TDP-43 immunoreactive inclusions or with HpScl.

The association of the rs5848 T-allele with FTLD-TDP suggests that lower progranulin levels may be one of the factors associated with risk of disease. Similarly, in this study we showed that the T-allele was overrepresented in AD cases with HpScl, most of which (77%) had TDP-43 immunoreactivity, which suggests that *GRN* may also be a risk factor for HpScl. The findings further indicate that HpScl in AD is not merely a reflection of severe neuronal loss due to AD, but rather neuronal loss due to a different mechanism, and perhaps analogous to the mechanism of neuronal loss in FTLD-TDP [36]. While there was a trend for the T-allele to be overrepresented in AD cases with TDP-43 immunoreactive inclusions, in a multivariate analysis this association was lost when HpScl cases were excluded. In addition to HpScl, advanced age was a risk factor for TDP-43 immunoreactivity in AD. The explanation for the age association is not clear at this time.

Selective neuronal loss in the same distribution as that seen in HpScl is also a feature of hypoxic-ischemic injury to the hippocampus. It was of interest that while there was no association of TDP-43 immunoreactivity with vascular pathology, there was a weak association of HpScl with vascular pathology (Spearman r = 0.091, p = 0.021). This may indicate that a subset of HpScl in AD may be related to hypoxic ischemic injury [2]. In this series of AD cases, 196 had concomitant vascular pathology with HpScl in 25 cases, 21 of which had TDP-43 immunoreactivity. The 4 cases without TDP-43 immunoreactivity are likely to be those in which hypoxic-ischemic factors may have contributed to hippocampal neuronal loss.

Acknowledgements

This study was supported by NIH grants P50-NS40256, P01-AG03949, P50-AG16574 and P50-AG25711.

References

1 Dickson DW, Davies P, Bevona C, et al: Hippocampal sclerosis: a common pathological feature of dementia in very old (> or = 80 years of age) humans. Acta Neuropathol 1994;88:212–221.
2 Zarow C, Sitzer TE, Chui HC: Understanding hippocampal sclerosis in the elderly: epidemiology, characterization, and diagnostic issues. Curr Neurol Neurosci Rep 2008;8:363–370.
3 Hatanpaa KJ, Blass DM, Pletnikova O, et al: Most cases of dementia with hippocampal sclerosis may represent frontotemporal dementia. Neurology 2004;63:538–542.
4 Blass DM, Hatanpaa KJ, Brandt J, et al: Dementia in hippocampal sclerosis resembles frontotemporal dementia more than Alzheimer disease. Neurology 2004;63:492–497.
5 Josephs KA, Dickson DW: Hippocampal sclerosis in tau-negative frontotemporal lobar degeneration. Neurobiol Aging 2007;28:1718–1722.
6 Petersen RC, Parisi JE, Dickson DW, et al: Neuropathologic features of amnestic mild cognitive impairment. Arch Neurol 2006;63:665–672.
7 Sepe-Monti M, De Carolis A, Bomboi G, Castri P, Giubilei F: MRI evidence of bilateral hippocampal sclerosis in amnestic mild cognitive impairment. Eur J Neurol 2006;13:1031–1032.
8 Kantarci K, Petersen RC, Przybelski SA, et al: Hippocampal volumes, proton magnetic resonance spectroscopy metabolites, and cerebrovascular disease in mild cognitive impairment subtypes. Arch Neurol 2008;65:1621–1628.
9 Ala TA, Beh GO, Frey WH 2nd: Pure hippocampal sclerosis: a rare cause of dementia mimicking Alzheimer's disease. Neurology 2000;54:843–848.
10 Beach TG, Sue L, Scott S, et al: Hippocampal sclerosis dementia with tauopathy. Brain Pathol 2003;13:263–278.
11 Togo T, Sahara N, Yen SH, et al: Argyrophilic grain disease is a sporadic 4-repeat tauopathy. J Neuropathol Exp Neurol 2002;61:547–556.
12 Jicha GA, Petersen RC, Knopman DS, et al: Argyrophilic grain disease in demented subjects presenting initially with amnestic mild cognitive impairment. J Neuropathol Exp Neurol 2006;65:602–609.
13 Obi T, Nishioka K, Ross OA, et al: Clinicopathologic study of a SNCA gene duplication patient with Parkinson disease and dementia. Neurology 2008;70:238–241.
14 Farrer M, Kachergus J, Forno L, et al: Comparison of kindreds with parkinsonism and alpha-synuclein genomic multiplications. Ann Neurol 2004;55:174–179.
15 Neumann M, Sampathu DM, Kwong LK, et al: Ubiquitinated TDP-43 in frontotemporal lobar degeneration and amyotrophic lateral sclerosis. Science 2006;314:130–133.
16 Mackenzie IR, Neumann M, Bigio EH, et al: Nomenclature for neuropathologic subtypes of frontotemporal lobar degeneration: consensus recommendations. Acta Neuropathol 2009;117:15–18.
17 Wang IF, Wu LS, Shen CK: TDP-43: an emerging new player in neurodegenerative diseases. Trends Mol Med 2008;14:479–485.
18 Amador-Ortiz C, Lin WL, Ahmed Z, et al: TDP-43 immunoreactivity in hippocampal sclerosis and Alzheimer's disease. Ann Neurol 2007;61:435–445.
19 Hasegawa M, Arai T, Nonaka T, et al: Phosphorylated TDP-43 in frontotemporal lobar degeneration and amyotrophic lateral sclerosis. Ann Neurol 2008;64:60–70.

20 Probst A, Taylor KI, Tolnay M: Hippocampal sclerosis dementia: a reappraisal. Acta Neuropathol 2007;114:335–345.
21 Baker M, Mackenzie IR, Pickering-Brown SM, et al: Mutations in progranulin cause tau-negative frontotemporal dementia linked to chromosome 17. Nature 2006;442: 916–919.
22 Cruts M, Gijselinck I, van der Zee J, et al: Null mutations in progranulin cause ubiquitin-positive frontotemporal dementia linked to chromosome 17q21. Nature 2006;442: 920–924.
23 Gass J, Cannon A, Mackenzie IR, et al: Mutations in progranulin are a major cause of ubiquitin-positive frontotemporal lobar degeneration. Hum Mol Genet 2006;15:2988–3001.
24 Josephs KA, Ahmed Z, Katsuse O, et al: Neuropathologic features of frontotemporal lobar degeneration with ubiquitin-positive inclusions with progranulin gene (PGRN) mutations. J Neuropathol Exp Neurol 2007; 66:142–151.
25 Mackenzie IR, Baker M, Pickering-Brown S, et al: The neuropathology of frontotemporal lobar degeneration caused by mutations in the progranulin gene. Brain 2006;129:3081–3090.
26 Rademakers R, Eriksen JL, Baker M, et al: Common variation in the miR-659 binding-site of GRN is a major risk factor for TDP43-positive frontotemporal dementia. Hum Mol Genet 2008;17:3631–3642.
27 Luis CA, Barker WW, Gajaraj K, et al: Sensitivity and specificity of three clinical criteria for dementia with Lewy bodies in an autopsy-verified sample. Int J Geriatr Psychiatry 1999;14:526–533.
28 He Z, Bateman A: Progranulin (granulin-epithelin precursor, PC-cell-derived growth factor, acrogranin) mediates tissue repair and tumorigenesis. J Mol Med 2003;81:600–612.
29 Bhandari V, Palfree RG, Bateman A: Isolation and sequence of the granulin precursor cDNA from human bone marrow reveals tandem cysteine-rich granulin domains. Proc Natl Acad Sci USA 1992;89:1715–1719.
30 Bateman A, Belcourt D, Bennett H, Lazure C, Solomon S: Granulins, a novel class of peptide from leukocytes. Biochem Biophys Res Commun 1990;173:1161–1168.
31 Ahmed Z, Mackenzie IR, Hutton ML, Dickson DW: Progranulin in frontotemporal lobar degeneration and neuroinflammation. J Neuroinflammation 2007;4:7.
32 Polymeropoulos MH, Lavedan C, Leroy E, et al: Mutation in the alpha-synuclein gene identified in families with Parkinson's disease. Science 1997;276:2045–2047.
33 Maraganore DM, de Andrade M, Elbaz A, et al: Collaborative analysis of alpha-synuclein gene promoter variability and Parkinson disease. JAMA 2006;296:661–670.
34 He L, Hannon GJ: MicroRNAs: small RNAs with a big role in gene regulation. Nat Rev Genet 2004;5:522–531.
35 Carthew RW, Sontheimer EJ: Origins and mechanisms of miRNAs and siRNAs. Cell 2009;136:642–655.
36 Dickson DW: TDP-43 immunoreactivity in neurodegenerative disorders: disease versus mechanism specificity. Acta Neuropathol 2008;115:147–149.

Imaging, Biomarkers, Genetics and Diagnostic Markers

Neuro-degenerative Diseases

Neurodegenerative Dis 2010;7:175–179
DOI: 10.1159/000289232

Published online: March 3, 2010

Leucine-Rich Repeat Kinase 2 Gene-Associated Disease: Redefining Genotype-Phenotype Correlation

Christian Wider[a] Dennis W. Dickson[b] Zbigniew K. Wszolek[a]

Departments of [a]Neurology, and [b]Neuropathology, Mayo Clinic, Jacksonville, Fla., USA

Key Words
Leucine-rich repeat kinase 2 gene · Parkinson's disease · Lewy body disease · Progressive supranuclear gaze palsy · Nigral degeneration

Abstract
Background: Leucine-rich repeat kinase 2 *(LRRK2)* has emerged as the most prevalent genetic cause of Parkinson's disease (PD) among Caucasians. Patients carrying an *LRRK2* mutation display significant variability of clinical and pathologic phenotypes across and within affected families. ***Methods:*** Herein, we review available clinical and pathologic data on patients with an *LRRK2* mutation who have come to autopsy. ***Results:*** Thirty-eight patients have been reported who presented clinically with PD; parkinsonism with resistance to levodopa, supranuclear gaze palsy, or autonomic dysfunction; or tremor and dementia. Pathology showed typical PD-type Lewy body disease (LBD) in most patients, whereas in others there was 'pure' nigral degeneration (one with TDP-43-positive inclusions), diffuse LBD, or tau-, α-synuclein- or ubiquitin-positive pathology reminiscent of progressive supranuclear gaze palsy, multisystem atrophy, and frontotemporal dementia with ubiquitin-positive inclusions. ***Conclusions:*** Such clinical and pathologic variability suggests Lrrk2 acts upstream from other proteins implicated in neurodegeneration. Specific mutations may be associated with alternative progressive supranuclear gaze palsy-like or 'pure' nigral degeneration phenotypes. A different effect on Lrrk2 kinase activity may play a role in such heterogeneity.

Introduction

Major breakthroughs in the genetics of Parkinson's disease (PD) have dramatically altered our understanding of the mechanisms leading to neurodegeneration [1]. As the number of genes and loci implicated in PD increased over the past decade, it has become clear that genetic factors play a significant role in risk for both sporadic and familial PD. However, such discoveries have also highlighted the clinical and pathologic variability associated with genetically determined PD. Mutations in the leucine-rich repeat kinase 2 *(LRRK2)* gene have emerged as the major genetic determinants of PD in Caucasian populations [2]. Yet carriers of a given *LRRK2* mutation even from the same family can differ in both their clinical and pathologic presentations [3]. Herein we discuss the implications of recent genetic discoveries for genotype-phenotype correlations in *LRRK2*-associated disease.

KARGER

Fax +41 61 306 12 34
E-Mail karger@karger.ch
www.karger.com

Accessible online at:
www.karger.com/ndd

Zbigniew K. Wszolek, MD
Neurology, Cannaday 2E
Mayo Clinic, 4500 San Pablo Road
Jacksonville, FL 32224 (USA)
Tel. +1 904 953 7229, Fax +1 904 953 0757, E-Mail wszolek.zbigniew@mayo.edu

Table 1. Characteristics of *LRRK2*-associated conditions with reported pathology

First author and year	Name of family	Patients	Lrrk2 (p.) mutation	Age at onset, years	Clinical features	Pathology[1]
Wszolek, 1997, 2004; Zimprich, 2004	D	4	R1441C	48–78	P[2] (3), P+S (1)	BLBD (1), DLBD (1), NFT (1), ND-Ub-TDP-43 (1)
	A	2	Y1699C	51–56	P (1), P+A (1)	ND-Ub[3]
Khan, 2005	Lincolnshire	1	Y1699C	50	P	LBD (few cortical LB)
Gilks, 2005	–	3	G2019S	41–70	P	LBD[4]
Rajput, 2006	SK	1	G2019S	78	P[5]	NFT
Ross, 2006	–	8	G2019S	41–79	P (3), P+Au (2), P+Au+D (1), DLB+Au (1), DLB (1)	BLBD (4), TLBD (3)[6], DLBD (1)
Giasson, 2006	–	3	G2019S	47–76	P (2)[7], P+D (1)	LBD (2)[8], ND[9]
Dachsel, 2007	–	1	G2019S	NR	D, T	FTLD-U pathology
Gaig, 2007	–	1	G2019S	61	P	ND
Gaig, 2008	–	1	G2019S	51	P	LBD (few cortical LB)
Chen-Plotkin, 2008	–	3	G2019S	47–76	P	LBD (diagnosis: PD)
Santpere, 2009	–	1	G2019S	NR	P	LB in SN
	–	1	R1441G	NR	P	ND
Hasegawa, 2009	Sagamihara	8	I2020T	40–74	P	ND (6), ND-GCI (1), BLBD (1)

Figures in parentheses indicate number of cases. A = Amyotrophy with fasciculations; Au = autonomic dysfunction; D = dementia; LB = Lewy bodies; ND = nigral degeneration; ND-GCI = nigral degeneration with α-synuclein-positive glial cytoplasmic inclusions (i.e. multisystem atrophy pathology); ND-Ub = nigral degeneration with ubiquitin-positive cytoplasmic and nuclear inclusions; NFT = neurofibrillary tangles, pathology reminiscent of progressive supranuclear gaze palsy; NR = not reported; P = levodopa-responsive parkinsonism similar to that of idiopathic Parkinson's disease; S = supranuclear gaze palsy; SN = substantia nigra; T = tremor; TLBD = transitional Lewy body disease.

[1] All patients had SN neuronal loss and gliosis. [2] One patient died before levodopa became available. [3] One patient with concurrent AD pathology, and 1 with mild motor neuron loss in lumbar spinal cord. [4] Two with LB in limbic cortex, 1 with mild AD pathology. [5] Poor response to levodopa. [6] One with concurrent AD pathology. [7] One did not tolerate levodopa. [8] One with concurrent AD pathology, and LB and Lewy neurites in the neocortex, and 1 with sparse LB, senile plaques and NFT in neocortex. [9] Rare NFT and senile plaques in neocortex.

***LRRK2*-Associated PD**

The most prevalent mutation in *LRRK2* (p.G2019S) accounts for 1–2% of sporadic PD and about 5% of familial PD in populations of European descent. Figures rise to 10–40% among North-African Arabs and Ashkenazi Jews, whereas Lrrk2 p.G2019S is almost absent in Asian populations. Over forty *LRRK2* variants have been identified in PD patients, but only six of them (p.R1441C, p.R1441G, p.R1441H, p.Y1699C, p.G2019S, and p.I2020T) have been established as definitely pathogenic [4]. The penetrance is reduced and age dependent, with ~75% of mutation carriers displaying clinical PD by age 80 [1, 5]. Two common variants in *LRRK2* (p.G2385R and p.R1628P) were found to increase risk for sporadic PD in Asian populations [6, 7].

Clinically, the majority of PD patients carrying a mutation in *LRRK2* display classic levodopa-responsive late-onset parkinsonism similar to that of idiopathic PD, although a more benign course has been suggested [5]. However, there are notable exceptions. In two of the families that led to the discovery of *LRRK2*, some patients presented with atypical features such as amyotrophy and fasciculations, autonomic dysfunction, supranuclear gaze palsy, dystonia or dementia [8, 9]. Additionally, patients with the Lrrk2 p.G2019S and p.R1441H mutations have been reported with variable phenotypes including corticobasal syndrome [10], progressive supranuclear gaze palsy (PSP) [11], dementia with tremor [12] and levodopa-resistant parkinsonism [13].

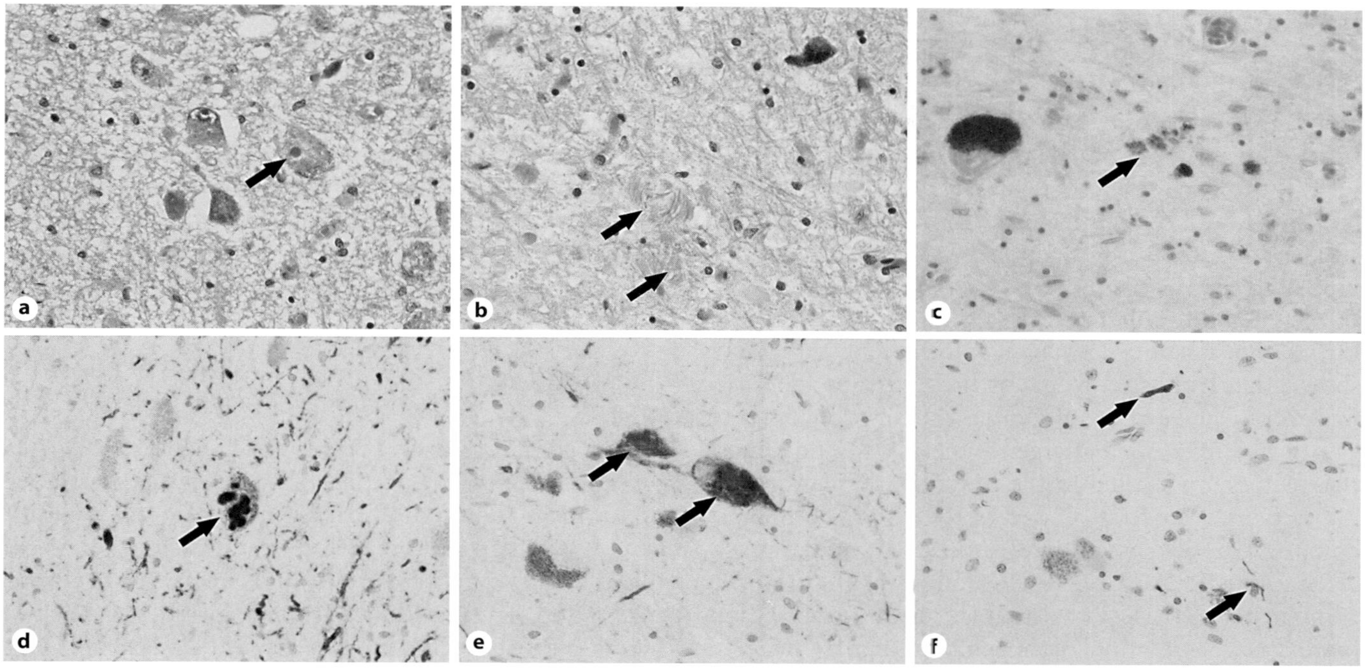

Color version available online

Fig. 1. Histology and immunohistochemistry of 4 PD patients from family D carrying the Lrrk2 p.R1441C mutation. **a, d** DLBD. **b, e** Tauopathy. **c, f** 'Pure' nigral degeneration. **a** Lewy body in periaqueductal gray (arrow; HE). **b** Extracellular neurofibrillary tangles (arrows; HE) in substantia nigra. **c** Nonspecific neuronal loss with neuromelanin in macrophages (arrow; HE). **d** Lewy bodies in periaqueductal gray (arrow; α-synuclein). **e** Neurofibrillary tangles in substantia nigra (arrows; phospho-tau). **f** Neurites in substantia nigra (arrows; TDP-43).

Neuropathology of *LRRK2* Mutation Carriers

Only 38 autopsies of diseased individuals carrying a proven pathogenic *LRRK2* mutation have been reported so far (table 1; fig. 1) [2, 3, 10, 12–21]. Most patients had the p.G2019S mutation (22/38), but some carried the p.I2020T (8/38), p.R1441C (4/38), p.Y1699C (3/38), or p.R1441G (1/38) mutation. Twenty-eight patients had typical levodopa-responsive parkinsonism, whereas others had parkinsonism with levodopa resistance (1/38), supranuclear gaze palsy (1/38), muscular atrophy (1/38), dementia (3/38), or autonomic dysfunction (4/38); one patient had only dementia and tremor.

All patients displayed neuronal loss and gliosis in the substantia nigra. In 20 patients, pathology was deemed compatible with that of idiopathic PD (brainstem or transitional Lewy body disease – LBD, with or without moderate numbers of cortical LB), with concurrent Alzheimer's disease (AD) pathology in 3 of them (fig. 1). Interestingly, the second most common pathology was 'pure' nigral degeneration with no LB, displayed by 12 patients carrying the p.I2020T mutation (6/12) or the p.Y1699C (2/12), p.G2019S (2/12), p.R1441C (1/12), or p.R1441G (1/12) mutation (fig. 1). In the p.R1441C carrier previously reported to have 'pure' nigral degeneration [2], we found that the ubiquitin-positive cytoplasmic inclusions in the nigra were positive for transactive response DNA-binding protein 43 (TDP-43), a feature that has not been emphasized in previous studies (fig. 1). In other patients, predominant pathological features included diffuse LBD (DLBD) (2/38), tau-positive neurofibrillary tangles reminiscent of PSP pathology (2/38), α-synuclein-positive glial cytoplasmic inclusions compatible with multisystem atrophy (MSA) (1/38), and ubiquitin-positive pathology suggestive of frontotemporal dementia (FTLD-U; 1/38). The most striking intrafamilial variability was observed in family D with the Lrrk2 p.R1441C mutation, with brainstem LBD (BLDB), DLBD, PSP-like pathology, and nigral degeneration with ubiquitin-/TDP-43-positive cytoplasmic inclusions (fig. 1) [2, 3]. Most patients from the Sagamihara family with the Lrrk2 p.I2020T mutation had 'pure' nigral degeneration (n = 6); however, one patient had MSA pathology and another one BLBD [16].

From Gene to Disease

LRRK2 is a 144-kb gene with 51 exons that encodes a 2,527 amino-acid multidomain protein. The physiologic function of Lrrk2 remains largely unknown, but experimental evidence suggests it may play a role in neuritic outgrowth and branching [22]. Immunohistochemistry studies in mice and humans have shown that Lrrk2 is mostly a cytoplasmic protein that is widely expressed in the brain and in other organs [17, 23]. While full-length Lrrk2 is not a major component of LB, recent studies have shown that truncated forms of Lrrk2 can be identified within LB, suggesting a potential role in protein aggregate formation [21]. Pathogenic mutations and genetic risk factors are located in the functionally relevant and highly conserved Roc, COR, MAPKKK and WD40 Lrrk2 domains. In vitro assays have shown that mutations located in the Roc and MAPKKK domains enhance Lrrk2 autophosphorylation, consistent with an autosomal dominant 'gain-of-function' pathogenic mechanism with increased kinase activity [24]. However, not all experimental data fit this model, which does not provide an explanation for mutations located in the COR and WD40 domains [22, 25].

Understanding the mechanisms that lead to neurodegeneration in *LRRK2* mutation carriers poses several challenging questions. The widespread expression of the Lrrk2 protein contrasts with the prominent vulnerability of select neuronal populations such as the nigrostriatal system, suggesting interactions with other molecules displaying regional specificity. Moreover, the significant clinical and pathologic phenotypic variability found in *LRRK2* mutation carriers supports the notion that Lrrk2 acts upstream of other proteins implicated in neuronal death, and that additional genetic, environmental and stochastic factors determine the type of pathology that develops in a given individual – α-synuclein, tau, or ubiquitin/TDP-43 positive [2, 19, 22]. The p.R1441 residue may be associated with tau pathology as one patient with the Lrrk2 p.R1441C mutation had supranuclear gaze palsy and PSP-like pathology (fig. 1), and one p.R1441H carrier evolved into clinical PSP [2, 11]. Furthermore, the lack of specific protein aggregation in some *LRRK2* mutation carriers indicates that other pathways exist, which may include accumulation of proteins such as TDP-43 which was identified in one of our patients. Of note, half of the patients with 'pure' nigral degeneration harbor the Lrrk2 p.I2020T mutation, which, in contrast to p.G2019S, was shown to reduce Lrrk2 kinase activity [25]. This may suggest that increased Lrrk2 kinase activity triggers α-synuclein aggregation and LB formation, whereas reduced kinase activity induces nigral degeneration through other pathways. Alternatively, some of the clinical and pathological phenotypes observed may represent incidental co-occurrence of other diseases unrelated to specific *LRRK2* mutations. Such hypothesis may be valid for individuals with pathology reminiscent of MSA, PSP, AD or FTLD-U; however, it would not account for those patients with 'pure' nigral degeneration.

Conclusions

Although recent advances in the genetics of PD have provided mechanistic hypotheses for neurodegenerative pathways, a thorough understanding of disease pathogenesis will require further studies addressing the critical issues of selective vulnerability and genotype-phenotype correlation. The clinical and pathological data reviewed herein suggest specific mutations may be associated with alternative PSP-like or 'pure' nigral degeneration phenotypes. A different effect on Lrrk2 kinase activity may play a role in such heterogeneity.

Acknowledgements

Mayo Clinic Jacksonville is a Morris K. Udall Parkinson's Disease Research Center of Excellence (NINDS P50 No. NS40256; D.W.D., Z.K.W.). Z.K.W. is also partially funded by P01 AG017216, R01 NS057567, R01 AG015866, Pacific Alzheimer Research Foundation grant C06-01, and CIHR 121849. C.W. is supported by the Swiss National Science Foundation (PASMP3-123268/1).

References

1 Farrer MJ: Genetics of Parkinson disease: paradigm shifts and future prospects. Nat Rev Genet 2006;7:306–318.

2 Zimprich A, Biskup S, Leitner P, Lichtner P, Farrer M, Lincoln S, Kachergus J, Hulihan M, Uitti RJ, Calne DB, Stoessl AJ, Pfeiffer RF, Patenge N, Carbajal IC, Vieregge P, Asmus F, Muller-Myhsok B, Dickson DW, Meitinger T, Strom TM, Wszolek ZK, Gasser T: Mutations in LRRK2 cause autosomal-dominant parkinsonism with pleomorphic pathology. Neuron 2004;44:601–607.

3 Wszolek ZK, Pfeiffer RF, Tsuboi Y, Uitti RJ, McComb RD, Stoessl AJ, Strongosky AJ, Zimprich A, Muller-Myhsok B, Farrer MJ, Gasser T, Calne DB, Dickson DW: Autosomal dominant parkinsonism associated with variable synuclein and tau pathology. Neurology 2004;62:1619–1622.

4 Ross OA, Toft M, Haugarvoll K: Corticobasal syndrome and primary progressive aphasia as manifestations of lrrk2 gene mutations. Neurology 2008;71:303; author reply 303–304.
5 Healy DG, Falchi M, O'Sullivan SS, Bonifati V, Durr A, Bressman S, Brice A, Aasly J, Zabetian CP, Goldwurm S, Ferreira JJ, Tolosa E, Kay DM, Klein C, Williams DR, Marras C, Lang AE, Wszolek ZK, Berciano J, Schapira AH, Lynch T, Bhatia KP, Gasser T, Lees AJ, Wood NW: Phenotype, genotype, and worldwide genetic penetrance of LRRK2-associated Parkinson's disease: a case-control study. Lancet Neurol 2008;7:583–590.
6 Di Fonzo A, Wu-Chou YH, Lu CS, van Doeselaar M, Simons EJ, Rohe CF, Chang HC, Chen RS, Weng YH, Vanacore N, Breedveld GJ, Oostra BA, Bonifati V: A common missense variant in the LRRK2 gene, Gly2385Arg, associated with Parkinson's disease risk in Taiwan. Neurogenetics 2006;7:133–138.
7 Ross OA, Wu YR, Lee MC, Funayama M, Chen ML, Soto AI, Mata IF, Lee-Chen GJ, Chen CM, Tang M, Zhao Y, Hattori N, Farrer MJ, Tan EK, Wu RM: Analysis of Lrrk2 R1628P as a risk factor for Parkinson's disease. Ann Neurol 2008;64:88–92.
8 Wszolek ZK, Pfeiffer B, Fulgham JR, Parisi JE, Thompson BM, Uitti RJ, Calne DB, Pfeiffer RF: Western Nebraska family (family D) with autosomal dominant parkinsonism. Neurology 1995;45:502–505.
9 Wszolek ZK, Vieregge P, Uitti RJ, Gasser T, Yasuhara O, McGeer P, Berry K, Calne DB, Vingerhoets FJ, Klein C, Pfeiffer RF: German-Canadian family (family A) with parkinsonism, amyotrophy, and dementia – longitudinal observations. Parkinsonism Relat Disord 1997;3:125–139.
10 Chen-Plotkin AS, Yuan W, Anderson C, McCarty Wood E, Hurtig HI, Clark CM, Miller BL, Lee VM, Trojanowski JQ, Grossman M, Van Deerlin VM: Corticobasal syndrome and primary progressive aphasia as manifestations of LRRK2 gene mutations. Neurology 2008;70:521–527.
11 Spanaki C, Latsoudis H, Plaitakis A: LRRK2 mutations on Crete: R1441H associated with PD evolving to PSP. Neurology 2006;67:1518–1519.
12 Dachsel JC, Ross OA, Mata IF, Kachergus J, Toft M, Cannon A, Baker M, Adamson J, Hutton M, Dickson DW, Farrer MJ: Lrrk2 G2019S substitution in frontotemporal lobar degeneration with ubiquitin-immunoreactive neuronal inclusions. Acta Neuropathol 2007;113:601–606.
13 Rajput A, Dickson DW, Robinson CA, Ross OA, Dachsel JC, Lincoln SJ, Cobb SA, Rajput ML, Farrer MJ: Parkinsonism, Lrrk2 G2019S, and tau neuropathology. Neurology 2006;67:1506–1508.
14 Gaig C, Ezquerra M, Marti MJ, Valldeoriola F, Munoz E, Llado A, Rey MJ, Cardozo A, Molinuevo JL, Tolosa E: Screening for the LRRK2 G2019S and codon-1441 mutations in a pathological series of parkinsonian syndromes and frontotemporal lobar degeneration. J Neurol Sci 2008;270:94–98.
15 Gaig C, Marti MJ, Ezquerra M, Rey MJ, Cardozo A, Tolosa E: G2019S LRRK2 mutation causing Parkinson's disease without Lewy bodies. J Neurol Neurosurg Psychiatry 2007;78:626–628.
16 Hasegawa K, Stoessl AJ, Yokoyama T, Kowa H, Wszolek ZK, Yagishita S: Familial parkinsonism: study of original Sagamihara PARK8 (I2020T) kindred with variable clinicopathologic outcomes. Parkinsonism Relat Disord 2009;15:300–306.
17 Giasson BI, Covy JP, Bonini NM, Hurtig HI, Farrer MJ, Trojanowski JQ, Van Deerlin VM: Biochemical and pathological characterization of Lrrk2. Ann Neurol 2006;59:315–322.
18 Gilks WP, Abou-Sleiman PM, Gandhi S, Jain S, Singleton A, Lees AJ, Shaw K, Bhatia KP, Bonifati V, Quinn NP, Lynch J, Healy DG, Holton JL, Revesz T, Wood NW: A common LRRK2 mutation in idiopathic Parkinson's disease. Lancet 2005;365:415–416.
19 Ross OA, Toft M, Whittle AJ, Johnson JL, Papapetropoulos S, Mash DC, Litvan I, Gordon MF, Wszolek ZK, Farrer MJ, Dickson DW: Lrrk2 and Lewy body disease. Ann Neurol 2006;59:388–393.
20 Khan NL, Jain S, Lynch JM, Pavese N, Abou-Sleiman P, Holton JL, Healy DG, Gilks WP, Sweeney MG, Ganguly M, Gibbons V, Gandhi S, Vaughan J, Eunson LH, Katzenschlager R, Gayton J, Lennox G, Revesz T, Nicholl D, Bhatia KP, Quinn N, Brooks D, Lees AJ, Davis MB, Piccini P, Singleton AB, Wood NW: Mutations in the gene LRRK2 encoding dardarin (PARK8) cause familial Parkinson's disease: clinical, pathological, olfactory and functional imaging and genetic data. Brain 2005;128:2786–2796.
21 Santpere G, Ferrer I: LRRK2 and neurodegeneration. Acta Neuropathol 2009;117:227–246.
22 Devine MJ, Lewis PA: Emerging pathways in genetic Parkinson's disease: tangles, Lewy bodies and LRRK2 FEBS J 2008;275:5748–5757.
23 Melrose HL, Kent CB, Taylor JP, Dachsel JC, Hinkle KM, Lincoln SJ, Mok SS, Culvenor JG, Masters CL, Tyndall GM, Bass DI, Ahmed Z, Andorfer CA, Ross OA, Wszolek ZK, Delldonne A, Dickson DW, Farrer MJ: A comparative analysis of leucine-rich repeat kinase 2 (Lrrk2) expression in mouse brain and Lewy body disease. Neuroscience 2007;147:1047–1058.
24 West AB, Moore DJ, Choi C, Andrabi SA, Li X, Dikeman D, Biskup S, Zhang Z, Lim KL, Dawson VL, Dawson TM: Parkinson's disease-associated mutations in LRRK2 link enhanced GTP-binding and kinase activities to neuronal toxicity. Hum Mol Genet 2007;16:223–232.
25 Jaleel M, Nichols RJ, Deak M, Campbell DG, Gillardon F, Knebel A, Alessi DR: LRRK2 phosphorylates moesin at threonine-558: characterization of how Parkinson's disease mutants affect kinase activity. Biochem J 2007;405:307–317.

Treatment and Prevention

Neuro-degenerative Diseases

Neurodegenerative Dis 2010;7:180–182
DOI: 10.1159/000295659

Published online: March 12, 2010

Lipid-Lowering Treatment Is Related to Decreased Risk of Dementia: A Population-Based Study (FINRISK)

A. Solomon[a] R. Sippola[b] H. Soininen[a] B. Wolozin[c] J. Tuomilehto[b] T. Laatikainen[b] M. Kivipelto[a, d]

[a]Department of Neurology, University of Kuopio, Kuopio, and [b]National Institute of Health and Welfare, Helsinki, Finland; [c]Department of Pharmacology, Boston University School of Medicine, Boston, Mass., USA; [d]Aging Research Center, Karolinska Institutet, Stockholm, Sweden

Key Words

Lipid-lowering drugs · FINRISK study · Dementia prevention

Abstract

Background: Several lines of evidence have linked cholesterol to dementia. ***Objective:*** To investigate lipid-lowering drug use and dementia development in a Finnish population. ***Methods:*** FINRISK is a large population-based survey of cardiovascular risk factors carried out since 1972 every 5 years using independent, random and representative population samples from different parts of Finland. Several cohorts were part of the WHO-MONICA study. Data from cohorts 1972–2002 were linked to the Hospital Discharge Registry and Drug Reimbursement Registry (1995–2007) to ascertain dementia diagnoses and lipid-lowering treatment. Selection criteria for the study were: (1) alive and without dementia in 1995; (2) age ≥60 years (in 1995 for earlier cohorts and in 1997 or 2002 for later cohorts; (3) treatment prescribed at least 1 year before dementia diagnosis. ***Results:*** 17,597 persons were included in the study. Lipid-lowering treatment was related to decreased dementia risk. In Cox proportional hazards model, hazard ratio (95% CI) was 0.42 (0.37–0.49; controlled for age, sex, education, survey region, survey year, baseline cholesterol, body mass index and systolic blood pressure). ***Conclusion:*** Preliminary results from the FINRISK study indicate that lipid-lowering drugs may have a beneficial effect in dementia prevention. Further data linkage is ongoing in order to investigate the roles of different types of lipid-lowering drugs.

Introduction

Current evidence indicates an association between cardiovascular risk factors (such as dyslipidemia) and dementia [1]. Several studies have investigated the role of lipid-lowering drugs in preventing dementia/cognitive impairment, showing either positive effects or no effects [2].

The present study aims to evaluate the relation between lipid-lowering treatment and dementia development in a Finnish population using data from the National FINRISK study.

Subjects and Methods

The National FINRISK study is a large population survey on risk factors of chronic, noncommunicable diseases. The survey is carried out since 1972 every 5 years using independent, random

KARGER

Fax +41 61 306 12 34
E-Mail karger@karger.ch
www.karger.com

1660–2854/10/0073–0180$26.00/0

Accessible online at:
www.karger.com/ndd

Alina Solomon
Department of Neurology
University of Kuopio, PO Box 1627
FI–70211 Kuopio (Finland)
Tel. +46 8 690 5822, Fax +46 8 690 5954, E-Mail alina.solomon@uku.fi

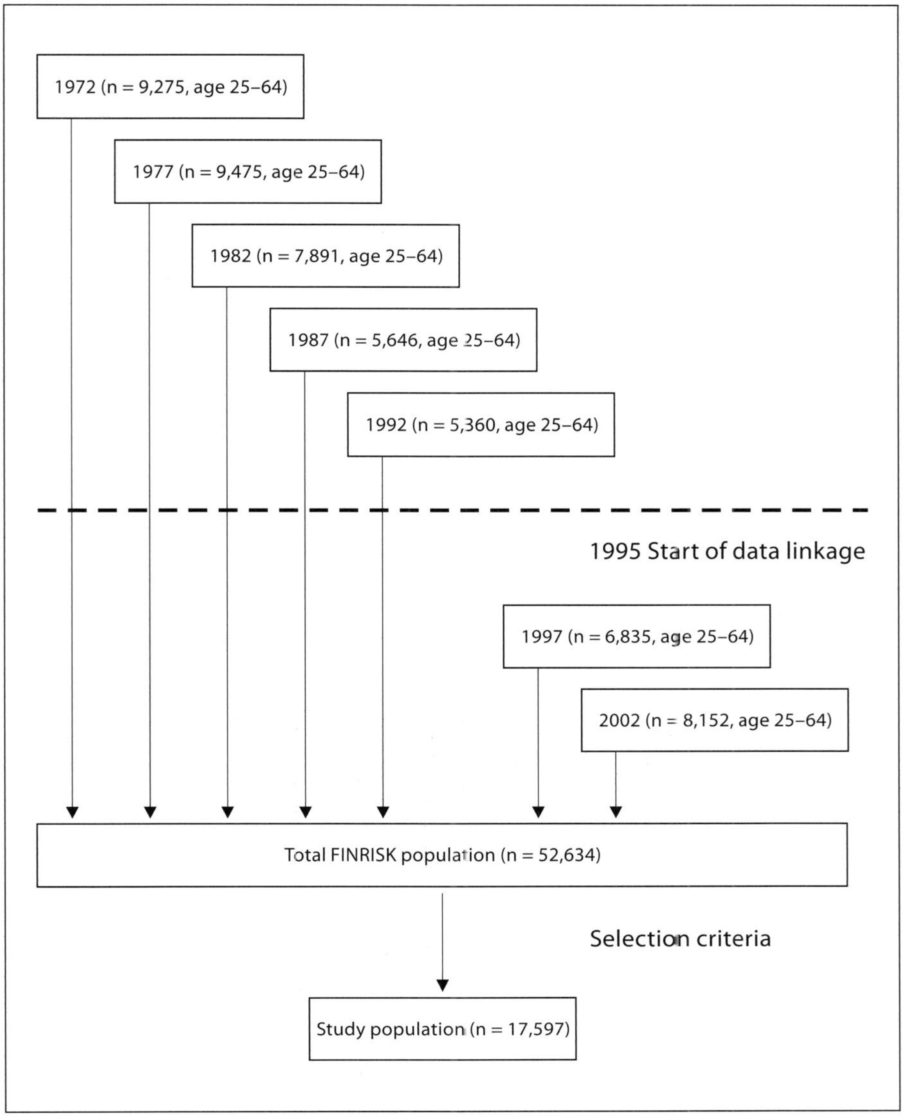

Fig. 1. Formation of the study population.

and representative samples from different parts of Finland, drawn from the national population register. In the first two surveys (1972, 1977), separate independent random samples of 6.6% of the middle-aged population were drawn in both areas. In 1982, 1987, 1992, 1997 and 2002, the samples were stratified by sex and 10-year age categories according to the WHO MONICA protocol [3]. The survey's methods followed the WHO MONICA protocol and were comparable with the methods used in 1972 and 1977 [4]. The participation rates varied between 71 and 95% [4].

Height, weight and blood pressure were measured by nurses specially trained for the survey procedures. Height was measured to the nearest 0.5 cm. Weight was measured in light clothing. Body mass index (BMI) was calculated as weight in kilograms divided by height in meters squared. Blood pressure was measured twice from the right arm of the participant, using a standard mercury sphygmomanometer. The fifth phase of the Korotkoff's sound was recorded as the diastolic BP [4] Total cholesterol was determined by using the Lieberman-Burchard method in 1972 and 1977, and an enzymatic method (CHOD-PAP, Boehringer Mannheim, Mannheim, Germany) since 1982. As the enzymatic method gave 2.4% lower values than the Lieberman-Burchard method, 1972 and 1977 values are corrected by this percentage. All samples were analyzed in the same central laboratory.

Data on dementia diagnoses (year of first diagnosis) and lipid-lowering drug usage (ATC code C10, year of first prescription) were obtained through linkage to the Hospital Discharge Register and Drug Reimbursement Register (KELA) from 1995 to 2007. The Register of Causes of Death was used for mortality data (year of death). The formation of the study population is shown in figure 1. From the total FINRISK population (52,634 subjects), 17,597 persons were selected for the present study. Selection criteria were: (1) age ≥60 years at entry in study (in 1995 for earlier co-

Table 1. General characteristics of the study population

	No dementia (n = 16,036)	Dementia (n = 1,561)	p value
Age at linkage start, years	67.1 (5.6)	72.2 (5.5)	<0.001
Education, years	7.8 (3.3)	6.5 (3.1)	<0.001
Women, %	56.4%	65.1%	<0.001
Baseline total cholesterol, mM	6.6 (1.3)	7.0 (1.3)	<0.001
Baseline BMI	27.3 (4.2)	27.5 (4.2)	0.015
Baseline systolic blood pressure, mm Hg	148.7 (21.4)	151.5 (22.3)	<0.001
Lipid-lowering treatment	6,288 (39.2%)	299 (19.2%)	<0.001

Values are means (standard deviations) unless otherwise specified.

horts, and 1997 and 2002 for later cohorts); (2) alive and without dementia at entry in study; (3) first lipid-lowering drug prescription at least 1 year before dementia diagnosis.

The study was approved by the local ethics committee at the National Institute for Health and Welfare, Helsinki.

Statistical analyses were done using SAS 8.0 and SPSS 16.0. t tests and χ^2 tests were used for evaluating differences between groups. The duration of follow-up was calculated between start of the study (1995 for earlier cohorts, 1997 or 2002 for later cohorts) and death, diagnosis of dementia, or end of the study period, whichever came first. Cox proportional hazards were used for investigating the relation between lipid-lowering treatment and incidence of dementia. All analyses were controlled for survey region, survey year, age, sex, years of formal education, total cholesterol, BMI and systolic blood pressure. Estimated hazard ratios (HRs) and their 95% confidence intervals (CIs) from the fully adjusted models are presented.

Results

General characteristics of the study population are presented in table 1. 1,561 persons developed dementia during the follow-up. As expected, they were older and had a lower education level compared to subjects without dementia. There were significantly more women in the dementia group. Baseline total cholesterol, BMI and systolic blood pressure were higher among subjects who developed dementia. A total of 6,587 subjects had been prescribed lipid-lowering drugs.

A Cox proportional hazards model showed that lipid-lowering treatment was related to decreased dementia risk: HR (95% CI) was 0.42 (0.37–0.49; controlled for survey region, survey year, age, sex, education, baseline total cholesterol, BMI and systolic blood pressure).

Discussion

Preliminary analyses from the FINRISK study indicate that lipid-lowering treatment may have beneficial effects in dementia prevention. However, since treatment was not randomly assigned (as in clinical trials), confounding by indication needs to be considered. Physicians are less likely to prescribe lipid-lowering drugs to people with early signs of dementia; a lag period of at least 1 year before dementia diagnosis was included to minimize this confounding. Further data linkage is ongoing in order to investigate whether different types of lipid-lowering agents (nonstatin or statins; more lipophilic versus more hydrophilic statins, with varying ability to cross the blood-brain barrier) have different effects. The role of other cardiovascular-related medication needs to be considered as well.

Acknowledgments

The authors wish to acknowledge Academy of Finland (grant 120676), EU FP7 project LipiDiDiet 211696, EVO grant 5772720 (Kuopio University Hospital), Marie-Curie EST Program, MEST-CT-176 2005-019217, and Vetenskapsrådet (grant 2007-3577), Stiftelsen Ragnhild och Einar Lundströms mine, and Stohnes Stiftelse, Sweden.

References

1 Fillit H, Nash DT, Rundek T, Zuckerman A: Cardiovascular risk factors and dementia. Am J Geriatr Pharmacother 2008;6:100–118.
2 Solomon A, Kivipelto M: Cholesterol-modifying strategies for Alzheimer's disease. Expert Rev Neurother 2009;9:695–709.
3 WHO MONICA Project Principal Investigators: The World Health Organization MONICA Project (monitoring trends and determinants in cardiovascular disease): a major international collaboration. J Clin Epidemiol 1988;41:105–114.
4 Barengo NC, Kastarinen M, Antikainen R, Nissinen A, Tuomilehto J: The effects of awareness, treatment and control of hypertension on cardiovascular and all-cause mortality in a community-based population. J Hum Hypertens 2009, Epub ahead of print.

Neuro-degenerative Diseases

Neurodegenerative Dis 2010;7:183–186
DOI: 10.1159/000295660

Published online: March 12, 2010

Cholesterol and Cognitive Performance in Normal Controls and the Influence of Elective Statin Use after Conversion to Mild Cognitive Impairment: Results in a Clinical Trial Cohort

D. Larry Sparks[a, b] Richard J. Kryscio[c, d] Donald J. Connor[b]
Marwan N. Sabbagh[b] Lisa M. Sparks[a] Yushun Lin[c] Carolyn Liebsack[b]

[a]Roberts Laboratory for Neurodegenerative Disease Research and [b]Cleo Roberts Clinical Research Center, Sun Health Research Institute, Sun City, Ariz., and Departments of [c]Statistics and [d]Biostatistics, University of Kentucky, Lexington, Ky., USA

Key Words
Alzheimer's disease · Mild cognitive impairment · Cholesterol · Lipid-lowering agents

Abstract

Background: We reported a significant 67% reduction in the hazard risk of incident Alzheimer's disease (AD) with elective statin use in the AD Anti-inflammatory Prevention Trial (ADAPT), without a reduction in risk of incident mild cognitive impairment (MCI). ***Objective:*** To assess if cholesterol levels are associated with cognitive performance and determine if statin use alters cognitive performance after onset of MCI. ***Design:*** Fractionated cholesterol levels, neurological and cognitive status were evaluated annually. Comparisons of non-LLA (lipid-lowering agent) users or statin-LLA users were performed blind to the ADAPT medication randomization. Pearson's correlations were validated using a time-dependent linear mixed model. ***Results:*** The MMSE performance significantly declined over time in non-LLA users, and, after adjusting for this, a significant positive correlation between MMSE and HDL was identified ($p = 0.0002$). A negative correlation between total and LDL cholesterol, and immediate and delayed recall of the Rivermead paragraph was significant (total cholesterol, $p < 0.003$; LDL, $p < 0.02$). Pilot data suggest a positive signal on delayed recall of both the Hopkins word list and Rivermead paragraph with deterioration in the non-LLA users and improvement in the statin users after conversion to MCI. ***Conclusion:*** Cholesterol levels may be associated with differential performance on the MMSE and measures of learning or memory. The trend for improved delayed recall in statin users with MCI compared to non-LLA users with MCI may have contributed to the reduced hazards risk of incident AD without reducing the risk of MCI.

Introduction

Most clinical data suggest that statin treatment may reduce the risk of Alzheimer's disease (AD) later in life. The last three large cohort studies of over 10,000 total subjects [1–3] found significantly reduced risk of incident AD with elective statin use. Data from the Rotterdam study, the largest cohort investigation to date [3], indicate

KARGER

Fax +41 61 306 12 34
E-Mail karger@karger.ch
www.karger.com

Accessible online at:
www.karger.com/ndd

D. Larry Sparks
10515 W. Santa Fe Drive
Sun City, AZ 85351 (USA)
Tel. +1 623 876 5463, Fax +1 623 815 7696
E-Mail Larry.Sparks@BannerHealth.com

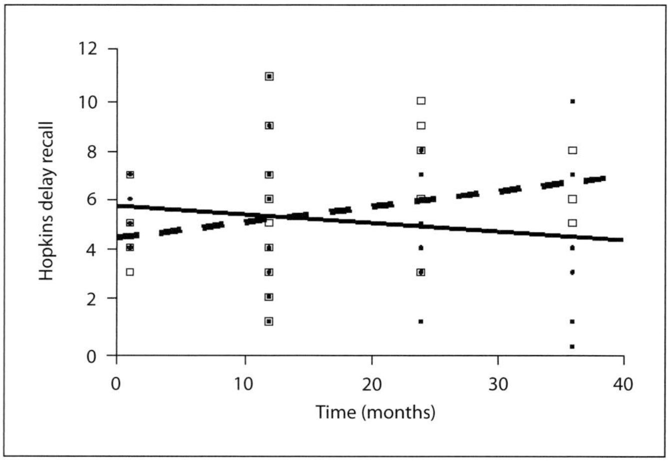

Fig. 1. Plot of estimated performance on delayed recall of the Hopkins word list among individuals with MCI taking statins (dashed line) and those not taking an LLA (solid line) versus time (0–30 months). p value for slope of the statin line is 0.083; p value for slope of the non-LLA line is 0.24; p value for difference in slope is 0.039.

a reduction in the risk of incident AD with elective statin use regardless of an individual's ApoE genotype or statin BBB permeability.

Our study of the effect of elective statin use on the risk of AD comes from the findings in individuals enrolled in the Alzheimer's Disease Anti-inflammatory Prevention Trial (ADAPT) who were allowed the elective use of statins and other lipid-lowering agents (LLAs) [2]. Cognitive performance was not influenced by statin use in cognitively normal controls [2]. We also reported that elective statin use was associated with a significant reduction in the risk of AD associated with ongoing statin use, but there was no reduction in the risk of mild cognitive impairment (MCI) [2]. The objective of the current study was to determine if cholesterol levels were associated with differences in cognitive performance among the 1,309 cognitively normal ADAPT participants not using an LLA during the trial, and to determine if cognitive performance was altered by statin use after conversion to MCI.

Methods

ADAPT was a randomized, double-blind, placebo-controlled, primary prevention trial testing whether NSAIDs prevent or delay incident AD. Specifics regarding study design and eligibility criteria are available elsewhere [4]. Persons regularly using NSAIDs were excluded, but LLA use was permitted and recorded at each scheduled visit.

Eligible participants were randomly assigned to receive NSAIDs or matching placebos irrespective of LLA use. The effect of statin use was analyzed without regard to or knowledge of the primary treatment assignment.

Procedures and outcome assessments are detailed elsewhere [2]. Briefly, the eligibility of prospective participants was established using specified health criteria and scores on an Eligibility Battery, which included the MMSE [5]. Eligible individuals returned for a baseline visit testing their cognitive and functional abilities using a Cognitive Assessment Battery [4], which included delayed recall on the Hopkins Verbal Learning Test and immediate and delayed recall of the Rivermead paragraph. Participants with abnormal cognition received diagnoses of AD using NINCDS/ADRDA criteria, or MCI using published methods [6].

Total cholesterol (TC), LDL, and HDL were correlated with each of the cognitive variables (MMSE, Hopkins word list, Rivermead paragraph) at each visit by calculating Pearson's correlation coefficients and determining if each correlation is statistically significant. We also employed an alternative analysis which relies on a linear mixed model (LMM) in which each clinical variable is regressed on time on study and one of the cholesterol values to determine if that cholesterol measurement is consistently correlated with the end point after adjusting for the decline in the scores over time. The LMM addresses inflation of the type I error rate and accounts for repeated measures made over time.

Analysis of the effect of statins was restricted to the 31 participants who converted to MCI and had at least one observation on their cognition after the date of this diagnosis. Cognitive scores analyzed were limited to all scores after diagnosis as well as the last visit before conversion. Each clinical variable was then regressed on time, statin use (yes or no) and the interaction between stain use and time. Particular interest centered around the interaction, since this would indicate whether decline varied significantly with statin use.

Results

We report the effect of cholesterol levels on cognitive performance in non-LLA using controls and elective statin use compared to non-LLA in MCI, blind to primary anti-inflammatory or placebo use in ADAPT. Based

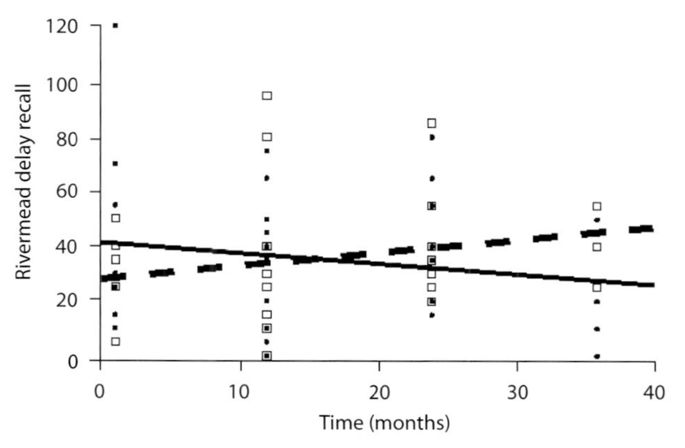

Fig. 2. Plot of estimated performance on delayed recall of the Rivermead paragraph among individuals with MCI taking statins (dashed line) and those not taking an LLA (solid line) versus time (0–30 months). p value for slope of the statin line is 0.23; p value for slope of the non-LLA line is 0.23; p value for difference in slope is 0.096.

on this reclassification, we considered two groups of ADAPT participants in the current study: 1,309 non-LLA users and 759 statin LLA users. Demographic data are reported elsewhere [2]. Of the 50 individuals (33 non-LLA and 17 statin users) converting to MCI, 16 non-LLA users returned for a clinical follow-up visit; 4 were longitudinally assessed, and 15 of the statin-using individuals returned for a follow-up clinical visit; 5 were longitudinally assessed.

MMSE scores declined significantly over time in the non-LLA population. There was a significant positive Pearson's correlation between HDL-cholesterol and MMSE, and after adjusting for time-dependent decrease in MMSE the significant positive correlation between MMSE and HDL remained after LMM analysis ($p = 0.0002$). The negative correlation between TC and LDL cholesterol, and immediate and delayed recall of the Rivermead paragraph remained significant using the LMM analysis (TC, $p < 0.003$, and LDL, $p < 0.02$).

Although there was no significant difference between the non-LLA and statin-LLA users prior to or after conversion to MCI in performance scores on any of the four cognitive measures, the pilot data suggest there is a positive signal on both delayed recall of the Hopkins word list (fig. 1) and the Rivermead paragraph (fig. 2), and the MMSE (not shown) with deterioration in the non-statin users and improvement in the statin users after conversion to MCI. The difference in slope between statin use and non-LLA use groups achieved significance for the Hopkins word list ($p = 0.039$), trended toward significance for the Rivermead paragraph ($p = 0.096$), and was not significant for the MMSE ($p = 0.19$).

Discussion

A modest but significant decrease in global function (MMSE) was identified using a time-dependent assessment (LMM) which was not apparent for measures of learning or memory (Rivermead immediate and delayed recall, and Hopkins delayed recall). Our data tend to confirm previous reports of a positive relationship between HDL cholesterol and cognitive performance, and disclosed a significant deterioration in learning and memory (Rivermead) with increased total and LDL cholesterol.

Consistent with the two very large prospective studies published in 2002 suggesting statins produced no positive effect on cognition in younger individuals at risk for heart disease [7, 8], we found no differences in the mean MMSE performance [2], or recall of the Hopkins word list and Rivermead paragraph between statin users and non-LLA users prior to conversion to MCI. After onset of MCI, elective statin use produced a positive signal on clinical measures of cognition (fig. 1, 2). The trend for improvement on delayed recall of the Hopkins word list and the Rivermead paragraph in statin users with MCI compared to non-LLA users with MCI may have contributed to the reduced hazard risk of incident AD without reducing the risk of incident MCI previously reported [2].

Acknowledgments

We acknowledge the work of the ADAPT Research Group making this Ancillary study possible. The Institute for the Study on Aging provided funding (Ancillary ADAPT study), and the ongoing ADAPT study is funded by the National Institute on Aging, U01 AG15477.

References

1 Cramer C, Haan MN, Galea S, Langa KM, Kalbfleisch JD: Use of statin and incidence of dementia and cognitive impairment without dementia in a cohort study. Neurology 2008;71:344–350.

2 Sparks DL, Kryscio RJ, Sabbagh MN, et al: Reduced risk of incident AD with elective statin use in a clinical trial cohort. Curr Alzheimer Res 2008;5:416–421.

3 Haag MDM, Hofman A, Koudstaal PJ, Stricker BHC, Breteler MMB: Statins are associated with a reduced risk of Alzheimer disease regardless of lipophilicity. The Rotterdam Study. J Neurol Neurosurg Psychiatry 2009;80:13–17.

4 ADAPT Research Group: Cardiovascular and cerebrovascular events in the randomized, controlled Alzheimer's Disease Anti-inflammatory Prevention Trial (ADAPT) PLoS Clin Trials 2006;1:e33.

5 ADAPT Research Group: No immediate reduction in Alzheimer's disease incidence with naproxen or celecoxib: results from ADAPT. Neurology 2007;68:1800–1808.

6 Tschanz J, Welsh-Bohmer KA, Lyketsos CG, et al: Conversion to dementia from mild cognitive disorder. Neurology 2006;67:229–234.

7 Shepherd J: Pravastatin in elderly individuals at risk of vascular disease (PROSPER): a randomized controlled trial. Lancet 2002;360:1623–1630.

8 Heart Protection Study Group: MRC/BHF Heart Protection Study of cholesterol lowering with simvastatin in 20,536 high-risk individuals: a randomized placebo-controlled trial. Lancet 2002;360:7–22.

Treatment and Prevention

Neuro-degenerative Diseases

Neurodegenerative Dis 2010;7:187–189
DOI: 10.1159/000295661

Published online: March 12, 2010

Effect of Heparin on APP Metabolism and Aβ Production in Cortical Neurons

David Klaver[a, c] Amos C. Hung[a] Robert Gasperini[a] Lisa Foa[a, b]
Marie-Isabel Aguilar[c] David H. Small[a, c]

[a]Menzies Research Institute, and [b]School of Medicine, University of Tasmania, Hobart, Tas.,
[c]Department of Biochemistry and Molecular Biology, Monash University, Clayton, Vic., Australia

Key Words
Secretase · Amyloid · Glycosaminoglycan · Heparin · Autocatalysis

Abstract
Background: The β-site APP cleaving enzyme 1 (BACE1) is a major target for drug design in Alzheimer's disease. BACE1 binds strongly to heparin and other glycosaminoglycans, and there is evidence that the enzyme may interact with proteoglycans in vivo. Several studies suggest that heparin or heparan sulfate analogues may have value as therapeutic agents for the treatment of AD. ***Objective:*** To determine whether heparin can inhibit Aβ production in cortical neurons by inhibiting BACE1. ***Methods:*** Cortical neurons from APP (SW) Tg2576 mice were incubated with heparin and the amount of APP processing and Aβ production were measured by enzyme-linked immunosorbent assay and Western blotting. ***Results:*** Treatment of cortical neurons with heparin inhibited Aβ secretion. However, this effect was not mediated via inhibition of BACE1. ***Conclusions:*** Heparin or other glycosaminoglycans may have value for the treatment of Alzheimer's disease. However, the data do not support the view that a heparin-induced decrease in Aβ secretion is due to inhibition of BACE1.

Introduction

The β-site APP cleaving enzyme 1 (BACE1) catalyses the first step in the production of Aβ and is regarded as a key target for drug development [1]. Because the enzyme has a large open active site, it is not ideal for drug development because compounds that fit into the active site tend to be bulky and therefore do not readily cross the blood-brain barrier [2].

Scholefield et al. [3, 4] first reported that BACE1 can bind to heparin and that it can be co-immunoprecipitated with heparan sulfate (HS) proteoglycans. This finding is potentially important because low-molecular-weight heparins may cross the blood-brain barrier [5], and one report suggests that peripheral administration of a low-molecular-weight heparin fraction (enoxaparin) may lower the amyloid load in transgenic mice [6].

The effects of heparin on BACE1 are complex [7]. High concentrations of heparin (100 μg/ml) inhibit the enzyme, whereas lower concentrations (1 μg/ml) stimulate its activity. Heparin (1 μg/ml) also stimulates autocatalytic cleavage of proBACE1 [7], which leads to inactivation

D.K. and A.C.H. contributed equally to the preparation of the manuscript.

KARGER
Fax +41 61 306 12 34
E-Mail karger@karger.ch
www.karger.com

1660–2854/10/0073–0187$26.00/0

Accessible online at:
www.karger.com/ndd

Prof. David H. Small, PhD
Menzies Research Institute, University of Tasmania
Private Bag 24
Hobart, Tas. 7001 (Australia)
Tel. +61 3 6226 7348, Fax +61 3 6226 2679, E-Mail d.h.small@menzies.utas.edu.au

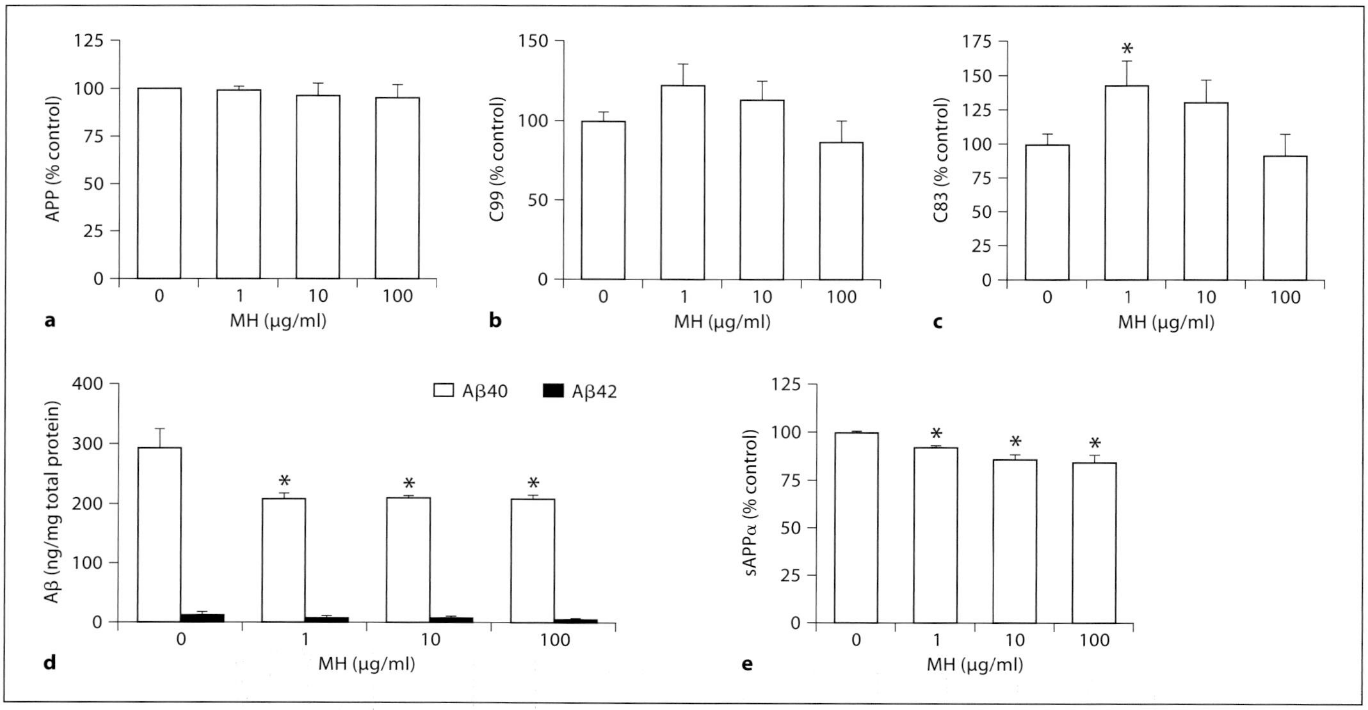

Fig. 1. Effect of MH on levels of APP and its proteolytic fragments in isolated cortical neurons derived from APP (SW) Tg2576 mice. Cells were treated for 24 h with MH. Levels of APP (**a**), C99 (**b**) and C83 (**c**) were then measured in cell lysates by Western blotting, whereas levels of Aβ peptides (**d**) and sAPPα (**e**) in the culture medium were measured by ELISA and Western blotting, respectively. **a–c**, **e** Means ± SEM of four observations. **d** Means ± SEM of eight observations. Asterisks show values that are significantly different from control values (no MH; $p < 0.05$).

of the enzyme with prolonged incubation times. Analysis of the products of cleavage by tandem mass spectrometry revealed that one of the heparin-stimulated autocatalytic cleavage sites was at phenylalanine-99, close to one of the active site aspartate residues (aspartate-93) which is critical for enzyme activity. It is possible that cleavage at this position (or at another position close to the active site) may account for the loss of enzyme activity.

As BACE1 may bind to endogenous proteoglycans, heparin could potentially interfere with Aβ production by inhibiting BACE1 trafficking. Indeed, exogenously added heparin inhibits β-secretase processing in N1e neuroblastoma cells [3], although the significance of this result is unclear, as Leveugle et al. [8] reported that heparin could stimulate β-secretase processing of APP in SH-SY5Y neuroblastoma cells.

To determine whether glycosaminoglycans can influence BACE1 activity in cortical neurons, we have examined the effect of heparin on APP processing in primary cortical neurons derived from Tg2576 transgenic mice which express human sequence APP [9]. This culture system allows for the easy detection of APP and Aβ-containing APP fragments using human sequence-specific antibodies.

Methods

Cortical neurons were prepared from the brains of newborn APP (SW) Tg2576 mice [9]. Cerebral cortices were dissected and incubated in Ca^{2+}- and Mg^{2+}-free HBSS containing 0.25% papain and 0.06% DNase I in the presence of 1.8 g/l glucose for 15 min at 37°C, followed by two washes with neurobasal medium (Invitrogen Australia, Mount Waverley, Vic., Australia). Individual cells were then obtained by gentle mechanical dissociation and plated onto poly-D-lysine-coated 12-well culture plates, and maintained in neurobasal medium containing 2% B27 supplement (Invitrogen), 1 mM glutamine, and 1% penicillin/streptomycin in an atmosphere of 5% CO_2-95% air at 37°C. After 3 days in vitro (DIV), half of the culture medium was replaced with fresh medium. All experiments were performed on 6 DIV cultures. Neurons were then incubated with various concentrations of mucosal heparin (MH). After incubation for 24 h, the medium was removed and assayed for Aβ peptides by enzyme-linked immunosorbent assay (ELISA) and for sAPPα by Western blotting.

The amount of Aβ40 or Aβ42 in cell culture supernatants was determined by specific Aβ ELISAs as described previously [10] with some modification. For the Aβ40-specific ELISA, 6E10 monoclonal antibody (Covance, San Diego, Calif., USA; 1:500) was coated onto 96-well plates overnight. Each well was then blocked in 5% (w/v) bovine serum albumin for 1 h before loading the cell culture fractions which were further incubated for 2 h. Aβ40 or Aβ42 was subsequently detected by incubation with an Aβ40- or Aβ42-specific polyclonal antibody (Invitrogen; 1 μg/ml) for another 2 h, followed by 1 h incubation with the HRP-conjugated anti-rabbit secondary antibody (1:2,000). The bound antibody was detected by the colorimetric development in the presence of TMB, and the reaction stopped with 1 N HCl. Absorbance was monitored at 450 nm. Recombinant Aβ40 or Aβ42 peptides were used to generate a standard curve and included in every assay performed.

For Western blotting, cells were lysed in lysis buffer (150 mM NaCl, 50 mM Tris, 0.5% w/v Na deoxycholate, 1% v/v Nonidet P-40) and then cell lysates or media were applied to SDS-polyacrylamide gels. To determine levels of full-length APP, C99 and C83, cell lysates were loaded (10 μg protein/lane) onto 16.5% Tris-tricine polyacrylamide gels, and subjected to Western blotting using an antibody (1:4,000 dilution) directed against the C-terminus of the APP protein (Sigma-Aldrich Pty. Ltd., Sydney, N.S.W., Australia). Blots were then stripped and reprobed with a monoclonal antibody directed against β-actin (clone AC-15; Sigma-Aldrich Pty. Ltd.) to control for loading. To determine the level of sAPPα, cell culture media were analyzed on 8% Tris-glycine polyacrylamide gels and subjected to Western blotting using the monoclonal anti-Aβ antibody 6E10 (1:1,000 dilution). Immunoreactive proteins were detected using an HRP-conjugated secondary antibody (1:5,000 dilution) and with an ECL Plus kit (GE Healthcare, Sydney, N.S.W., Australia). Image density was quantified by image-capture analysis using ImageJ software (RSB; NIH, http://rsbweb.nih.gov/ij/index.htm).

Results and Discussion

To determine whether exogenously derived glycosaminoglycans can influence Aβ production and β-secretase processing of APP in cortical neurons, the effect of MH on APP, sAPPα, Aβ40, Aβ42, C99 and C83 was examined (fig. 1). The results showed that MH (1 μg/ml) produced a significant decrease in the level of Aβ40 secretion. The level of Aβ42 secretion was not significantly decreased by treatment, although only low levels of Aβ42 were detectable in the culture medium.

The effect of MH on Aβ was not due to an effect on BACE1 activity as there was no decrease in the level of C99 production. The level of full-length APP was not decreased by MH either. There was a small, but significant increase in the level of C83 at a concentration of 1 μg/ml MH. While the mean level of C99 was also higher at this concentration, the difference from control levels was not statistically significant.

The results support the view that while heparin can inhibit Aβ production and/or secretion, this effect is not due to inhibition of β-secretase processing by BACE1. It was interesting to note that a small inhibition of sAPPα secretion also occurred in the presence of MH, raising the possibility that heparin may inhibit secretion in general. Thus, the effect of MH on Aβ could have been caused by inhibition of secretion of the peptide. However, such a mechanism needs to be tested in further experiments.

References

1 Cole SL, Vassar R: The role of amyloid precursor protein processing by BACE1, the β-secretase, in Alzheimer disease pathophysiology. J Biol Chem 2008;283:29621–29625.
2 Silvestri R: Boom in the development of non-peptidic β-secretase (BACE1) inhibitors for the treatment of Alzheimer's disease. Med Res Rev 2009;29:295–338.
3 Scholefield Z, Yates EA, Wayne G, Amour A, McDowell W, Turnbull JE: Heparan sulfate regulates amyloid precursor protein processing by BACE1, the Alzheimer's β-secretase. J Cell Biol 2003;163:97–107.
4 Patey SJ, Edwards EA, Yates EA, Turnbull JE: Heparin derivatives as inhibitors of BACE-1, the Alzheimer's β-secretase, with reduced activity against factor Xa and other proteases. J Med Chem 2006;49:6129–6132.
5 Leveugle B, Ding W, Laurence F, Dehouck MP, Scanameo A, Cecchelli R, Fillit H: Heparin oligosaccharides that pass the blood-brain barrier inhibit β-amyloid precursor protein secretion and heparin binding to β-amyloid peptide. J Neurochem 1998;70:736–744.
6 Bergamaschini L, Rossi E, Storini C, Pizzimenti S, Distaso M, Perego C, De Luigi A, Vergani C, De Simoni MG: Peripheral treatment with enoxaparin, a low molecular weight heparin, reduces plaques and β-amyloid accumulation in a mouse model of Alzheimer's disease. J Neurosci 2004;24: 4181–4186.
7 Beckman M, Holsinger RM, Small DH: Heparin activates β-secretase (BACE1) of Alzheimer's disease and increases autocatalysis of the enzyme. Biochemistry 2006;45:6703–6714.
8 Leveugle B, Ding W, Durkin JT, Mistretta S, Eisle J, Matic M, Siman R, Greenberg BD, Fillit HM: Heparin promotes β-secretase cleavage of the Alzheimer's amyloid precursor protein. Neurochem Int 1997;30:543–548.
9 Hsiao K, Chapman P, Nilsen S, Eckman C, Harigaya Y, Younkin S, Yang F, Cole G: Correlative memory deficits, Abeta elevation, and amyloid plaques in transgenic mice. Science 1996;274:99–102.
10 Savage MJ, Trusko SP, Howland DS, Pinsker LR, Mistretta S, Reaume AG, Greenberg BD, Siman R, Scott RW: Turnover of amyloid β-protein in mouse brain and acute reduction of its level by phorbol ester. J Neurosci 1998; 18:1743–1752.

Treatment and Prevention

Neuro-degenerative Diseases

Neurodegenerative Dis 2010;7:190–192
DOI: 10.1159/000295662

Published online: March 12, 2010

Retinoids as a Perspective in Treatment of Alzheimer's Disease

Falk Fahrenholz Frank Tippmann Kristina Endres

Institute of Biochemistry, Johannes Gutenberg-University, Mainz, Germany

Key Words
Alzheimer's disease · Disintegrin metalloproteinase ADAM10 · Promoter activity · Retinoids

Abstract
Background: In the past, we demonstrated that the disintegrin metalloproteinase ADAM10 has α-secretase activity in vitro and in cultured cells. We also found out that moderate overexpression of this proteinase inhibits Aβ peptide production and prevents the formation of amyloid plaques in an Alzheimer's disease (AD) mouse model. Moreover, it corrects early hippocampal defects like LTP impairment and increases cortical synaptogenesis. ***Objective:*** Upregulation of ADAM10 might be an alternative approach concerning AD therapy. Our current research therefore focuses on substances and/or pathways which regulate ADAM10 gene expression. ***Methods:*** Analyses of ADAM10 promoter activity were performed in human and murine neuroblastoma cell lines and important findings were validated in an AD mouse model. ***Results:*** The outcome of our investigations indicates that a heterodimeric retinoid receptor mediates the activation of the ADAM10 promoter by all-*trans*-retinoic acid. This then results in enhanced ADAM10 expression, pronounced APPs-α secretion and diminished proteolytic processing products of the amyloidogenic pathway (APPs-β, Aβ). ***Conclusion:*** Nontoxic synthetic retinoids – like acitretin – offer a valuable therapeutic approach in treatment of AD by moderately enhancing ADAM10 gene expression.

Processing of the amyloid precursor protein (APP) occurs via two distinct pathways: in the initial step β-secretase in the amyloidogenic pathway and α-secretase in the nonamyloidogenic pathway compete for their substrate. Cleavage of APP by the α-secretase in the middle of the Aβ sequence prevents the formation of synaptotoxic Aβ peptides [1]. Additionally, many results provide evidence that the alternatively released soluble fragment (APPs-α) has neuroprotective, neurotrophic and memory-enhancing properties [2, 3].

Several reports traced nutritional factors as a possible clue to Alzheimer's disease treatment. These include caloric restriction and cholesterol reduction [4, 5] or ω3 fatty acids [6, 7]. In addition, there is ample genetic, biochemical and dietary evidence for the bioreactive metabolite of vitamin A – all-*trans*-retinoic acid (atRA) – having a role in Alzheimer's disease [8, 9]. Vitamin A (retinol) is incorporated by food and transported via chylomicrons to the liver. Retinol bound to the retinol-binding protein and to transthyretin then can be delivered across the blood brain barrier into neurons. Here, a two-step oxidation takes place and retinoic acid subsequently can be released within cells to translocate to the nucleus and bind to its receptors: the dimeric receptors consist of retinoic X receptors (RXRs) only or of RXRs in

KARGER

Fax +41 61 306 12 34
E-Mail karger@karger.ch
www.karger.com

1660–2854/10/0073–0190$26.00/0

Accessible online at:
www.karger.com/ndd

Dr. Kristina Endres
Department of Psychiatry and Psychotherapy, Clinical Research Group
Johannes Gutenberg-Universität, Untere Zahlbacher Str. 8
DE–55131 Mainz (Germany)
Tel. +49 6131 172 133, E-Mail endres_k@psychiatrie.klinik.uni-mainz.de

Co-corresponding author:
Prof. Falk Fahrenholz
E-mail fahrenho@uni-mainz.de

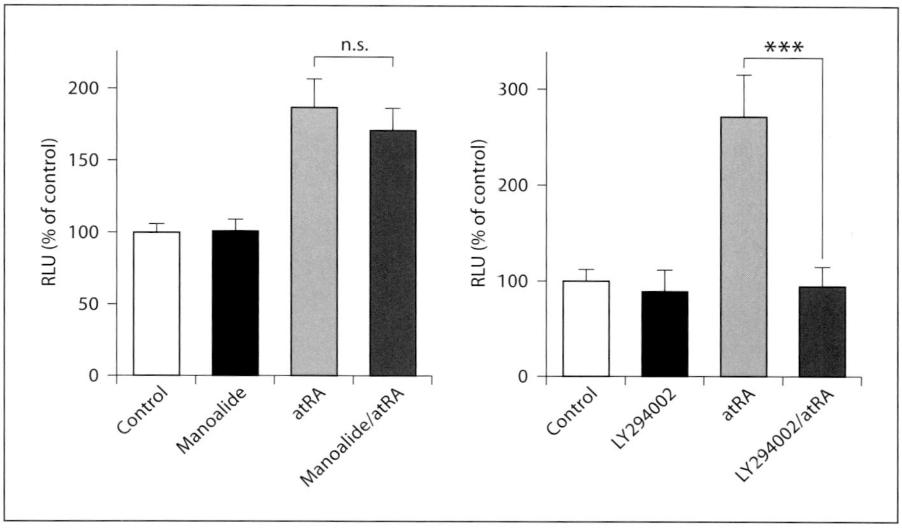

Fig. 1. Effect of PLA2 and PI3K inhibitors on atRA-stimulated promoter activity of human ADAM10. Human neuroblastoma cells (SH-SY5Y) were transiently transfected with an hADAM10-luciferase-reporter construct as previously described [12] and subsequently treated with atRA (2 µM) with or without manoalide (2 µM) or LY294002 (10 µM) for 48 h. Promoter activity was measured in cell lysates and normalized to protein content (relative light units, RLU). Values from solvent-treated cells (control) were set to 100%. Data represent means ± SD (left n = 6, right n ≥ 9; n.s., $p > 0.05$; *** $p < 0.001$).

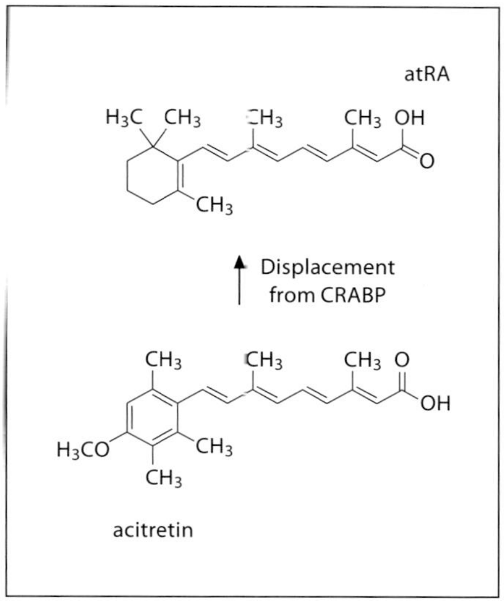

Fig. 2. Structure of the naturally occurring atRA and the synthetic retinoid acitretin. Acitretin displaces atRA from the cellular retinoic acid-binding protein (CRABP) and increases atRA availability for nuclear receptor binding.

combination with a wide variety of receptors like retinoic acid receptor (RAR), vitamin D receptor or PPARγ.

We discovered that human, mouse and rat ADAM10 genes contain two potential RXR binding sites in the conserved region of their promoter [10]. To investigate the physiological context in which ADAM10 might be regulated by vitamin A metabolites, we treated several human cell lines, representing different tissues, with atRA: while cells of hepatic or kidney origin showed no significant response to the treatment, ADAM10 mRNA of neuroblastoma as well as monocyte precursors displayed enhanced ADAM10 transcription [11, 12]. This suggested that we might be able to upregulate ADAM10 in the brain without a general upregulation in peripheral tissue. Using specific ligands for RXR dimerization partners, we were able to identify RAR/RXR heterodimers as regulators of ADAM10 expression. By coexpression studies, two of the RAR isotypes – RAR-α and RAR-β – were identified to take part in the stimulation of the ADAM10 promoter. Interestingly, these subtypes are highly expressed in the hippocampus and discussed to play a role in synaptic plasticity.

Direct binding of a protein complex has been shown on one of the two potential retinoid receptor binding sites on the ADAM10 promoter [10], suggesting a direct mechanism of action for atRA on the ADAM10 promoter. However, atRA can also influence cellular mechanisms in addition to directly binding to its nuclear receptors: it has been revealed that phospholipase 2 (PLA2) [13], and also phosphatidylinositol-3-kinase (PI3K) [14], signaling is modified by the vitamin A derivative. Therefore, we tested this possibility using the inhibitor manoalide for PLA2 and LY294002 for PI3K (fig. 1). Manoalide changed neither the ADAM10 basal promoter activity nor the atRA-stimulated activity, although PLA2 has been described to be involved in muscarinic receptor-driven APPs-α release [15]. For LY294002, we observed a significant reduction in retinoid-driven promoter activity. This is in accordance with findings from Holback et al. [16] who demonstrated a strong decrease in atRA-induced ADAM10 protein level by this compound.

As vitamin A and retinoic acid bear too many side effects to be of value in therapeutic concerns, we tested synthetic retinoids used in clinical application in dermatology and oncology for their potential to act on ADAM10 expression. Acitretin, which has replaced its ethyl ester etretinate for long-term oral treatment of psoriasis due to a more favorable pharmacokinetic profile [17], was identified as a potent activator of ADAM10 gene expression (fig. 2). When applied to human as well as murine neuroblastoma cells, acitretin enhanced ADAM10 promoter activity, followed by increased amounts of ADAM10 protein and a shift towards the nonamyloidogenic processing pathway. To demonstrate this effect in vivo, APP/presenilin 1 double-transgenic mice were injected intracerebrally with acitretin. Within 48 h after treatment, we observed an enhanced APPs-α/-β ratio and reduction in Aβ peptides of approximately 50% [12]. Since it was evident in animal studies that acitretin reaches the brain in higher concentrations than several other peripheral tissues [18], it is an interesting compound for further studies and for application in humans.

Acknowledgements

This work was supported by the Federal Ministry of Education and Research within the framework of the National Genome Research Network, Förderkennzeichen FKZ01GS08130.

References

1 Postina R, Schroeder A, Dewachter I, Bohl J, Schmitt U, Kojro E, Prinzen C, Endres K, Hiemke C, Blessing M, Flamez P, Dequenne A, Godaux E, van Leuven F, Fahrenholz F: A disintegrin-metalloproteinase prevents amyloid plaque formation and hippocampal defects in an Alzheimer disease mouse model. J Clin Invest 2004;113:1456–1464.

2 Gralle M, Botelho MG, Wouters FS: Neuroprotective secreted amyloid precursor protein acts by disrupting amyloid precursor protein dimers. J Biol Chem 2009;284:15016–15025.

3 Ring S, Weyer SW, Kilian SB, Waldron E, Pietrzik CU, Filippov MA, Herms J, Buchholz C, Eckman CB, Korte M, Wolfer DP, Muller UC: The secreted beta amyloid precursor protein ectodomain APPs alpha is sufficient to rescue the anatomical, behavioral, and electrophysiological abnormalities of APP-deficient mice. J Neurosci 2007;27:7817–7826.

4 Patel NV, Gordon MN, Connor KE, Good RA, Engelman RW, Mason J, Morgan DG, Morgan TE, Finch CE: Caloric restriction attenuates Abeta-deposition in Alzheimer transgenic models. Neurobiol Aging 2005;26:995–1000.

5 Kojro E, Gimpl G, Lammich S, Marz W, Fahrenholz F: Low cholesterol stimulates the nonamyloidogenic pathway by its effect on the alpha-secretase ADAM 10. Proc Natl Acad Sci USA 2001;98:5815–5820.

6 Sahlin C, Pettersson FE, Nilsson LN, Lannfelt L, Johansson AS: Docosahexaenoic acid stimulates non-amyloidogenic APP processing resulting in reduced Abeta levels in cellular models of Alzheimer's disease. Eur J Neurosci 2007;26:882–889.

7 Hooijmans CR, Van der Zee CE, Dederen PJ, Brouwer KM, Reijmer YD, van Groen T, Broersen LM, Lutjohann D, Heerschap A, Kiliaan AJ: DHA and cholesterol containing diets influence Alzheimer-like pathology, cognition and cerebral vasculature in APPswe/PS1dE9 mice. Neurobiol Dis 2009;33:482–498.

8 Goodman AB, Pardee AB: Evidence for defective retinoid transport and function in late onset Alzheimer's disease. Proc Natl Acad Sci USA 2003;100:2901–2905.

9 Goodman AB: Retinoid receptors, transporters, and metabolizers as therapeutic targets in late onset Alzheimer disease. J Cell Physiol 2006;209:598–603.

10 Prinzen C, Muller U, Endres K, Fahrenholz F, Postina R: Genomic structure and functional characterization of the human ADAM10 promoter. FASEB J 2005;19:1522–1524.

11 Endres K, Postina R, Schroeder A, Mueller U, Fahrenholz F: Shedding of the amyloid precursor protein-like protein APLP2 by disintegrin-metalloproteinases. FEBS J 2005;272:5808–5820.

12 Tippmann F, Hundt J, Schneider A, Endres K, Fahrenholz F: Up-regulation of the alpha-secretase ADAM10 by retinoic acid receptors and acitretin. FASEB J 2009;23:1643–1654.

13 Abe A, Poucher HK, Hiraoka M, Shayman JA: Induction of lysosomal phospholipase A2 through the retinoid X receptor in THP-1 cells. J Lipid Res 2004;45:667–673.

14 Masia S, Alvarez S, de Lera AR, Barettino D: Rapid, nongenomic actions of retinoic acid on phosphatidylinositol-3-kinase signaling pathway mediated by the retinoic acid receptor. Mol Endocrinol 2007;21:2391–2402.

15 Cho HW, Kim JH, Choi S, Kim HJ: Phospholipase A2 is involved in muscarinic receptor-mediated sAPPalpha release independently of cyclooxygenase or lypoxygenase activity in SH-SY5Y cells. Neurosci Lett 2006;397:214–218.

16 Holback S, Adlerz L, Gatsinzi T, Jacobsen KT, Iverfeldt K: PI3-K- and PKC-dependent up-regulation of APP processing enzymes by retinoic acid. Biochem Biophys Res Commun 2008;365:298–303.

17 Pang ML, Murase JE, Koo J: An updated review of acitretin – a systemic retinoid for the treatment of psoriasis. Expert Opin Drug Metab Toxicol 2008;4:953–964.

18 Eisenhardt EU, Bickel MH: Kinetics of tissue distribution and elimination of retinoid drugs in the rat. I. Acitretin. Drug Metab Dispos 1994;22:26–30.

Treatment and Prevention

Neuro-degenerative Diseases

Neurodegenerative Dis 2010;7:193–202
DOI: 10.1159/000295663

Published online: March 12, 2010

Treatment of Alzheimer's Disease with a Cholinesterase Inhibitor Combined with Antioxidants

Umberto Cornelli

Loyola University Chicago School of Medicine, Maywood, Ill., USA

Key Words

Alzheimer's disease · d-ROMs test · Glutathione · Homocysteine · Sickle erythrocytes

Abstract

A formula (formula F) was prepared to counteract oxidative stress (OS) in the brain. The formula contained the most common antioxidants and was intended to: (a) protect proteins, lipids, DNA and proteoglycans from oxidation (carnosine, coenzyme Q_{10}, vitamin E, vitamin C, β-carotene, selenium, L-cysteine and ginkgo biloba); (b) reduce homocysteine (HCy) blood levels (vitamins B_6, B_9 and B_{12}), and (c) sustain the pentose phosphate cycle in circulating cells (vitamins B_1, B_2 and B_3). Formula F contained low doses of each antioxidant component and was administered in a two-phase ampoule. A cohort of 52 patients (21 males and 31 females) affected with moderate probable AD (according to NINCDS-ARDA and NINCS-AIREN criteria) already being treated with donepezil (5 mg/day for at least two months) was randomly divided into two groups, and followed for 6 months. A double-blind design was used in which 26 cases were treated once a day with formula F plus donepezil, and the other 26 with placebo plus donepezil. The level of OS was measured on the basis of a d-ROMs test (which measures plasma hydroperoxides), plasma HCy and glutathione, and percentage of sickle erythrocytes. The two patient groups were comparable for all variables (age, sex, concomitant diseases, ApoE ε4, MMSE II score, OS, antioxidant reserve and sickle erythrocytes). Forty-eight subjects completed the trial. Significant decreases in OS and HCy were only observed when there was an increase in glutathione (in erythrocytes) and a decrease in sickle erythrocytes in patients treated with formula F. The MMSE II score remained almost the same in the group treated with donepezil and placebo, whereas some significant improvements were found in the group treated with donepezil plus formula F.

Introduction

The brain has certain characteristics that make it very sensitive to oxidative stress (OS). Although it accounts for 2% of body weight, the brain consumes 20% of the total O_2 inhaled. It also has the highest concentration of docosahexaenoic acid, an unsaturated fatty acid that is extremely sensitive to oxidation. The iron concentration in some areas of the brain, such as the red nucleus and basal ganglia, lays the ground for substantial oxidation. This is also supported by the reactive oxygen species (ROS) generated by dopamine auto-oxidation.

KARGER

Fax +41 61 306 12 34
E-Mail karger@karger.ch
www.karger.com

1660–2854/10/0073–0193$26.00/0

Accessible online at:
www.karger.com/ndd

Umberto Cornelli, MD, PhD
Loyola University Chicago School of Medicine
Maywood, IL 60153 (USA)
Tel. +39 02 7012 1867, Fax +39 02 714 904
E-Mail umbertocornelli@cornelliconsulting.it

Another peculiarity of the brain is its lack of a lymphatic system, which means that tissue drainage has to take place through the blood vessels because CSF circulation is too low (25 ml/h) to support this task.

All these characteristics make the brain very sensitive to OS, which may be one of the causes of many degenerative diseases [1–3], especially Alzheimer's disease (AD). It is not enough, however, to administer one or two antioxidants at high doses to improve the antioxidant network in the brain. It is necessary to consider many aspects of oxidation. At least six elements take part in the OS process in AD: vessels/blood brain barrier (BBB), mitochondria, homocysteine (HCy), amyloid, erythrocytes and proteoglycans (PGs).

The brain vessels do not support blood flow to tissue efficiently in AD. The brain's attempt to compensate with vasodilatation is clear from the increase in nitric oxide production. This can be seen from the dramatic increase in dimethylargininase, which is one of the key enzymes in nitric oxide production [4–7]. However, the concomitant presence of superoxide ($O_2\cdot$), owing to local inflammatory processes, generates peroxynitrate ($ONOO^-$) and hydroxyl radicals ($OH\cdot$), which may cause vasoconstriction [8, 9] when produced in large quantities. The brain vasculature (about 600 km of vessels) ends up at the BBB, which consists of many components (endothelial cells, pericytes, neuron feet, astrocytes, etc.) connected in a highly coordinated structure. It is so coordinated that it has to be considered a true neurovascular unit [10, 11]. Because of its nature, lesion of one component directly affects all the others. Consequently, the BBB is one of the first structures damaged in AD.

The second structures on the list are mitochondria. BBB endothelial cells are characterized by tight junctions that require large quantities of energy to keep the barrier effective. Consequently many mitochondria are found in the cells to provide the necessary ATP. Another source of this high energy production is the presence of ROS, which can only be sufficiently quenched by a very efficient antioxidant system [12]. There are at least seven different systems that produce ROS in mitochondria, and any alterations to the respiratory chain cytochromes end up in two parallel phenomena: a decrease in ATP and an increase in ROS production [13–15]. ATP may be imported from the cytoplasm to compensate for the shortage in energy production. If this is not possible, the cell undergoes apoptosis.

At least three mitochondrial systems relating to energy production have been shown to be deficient in AD: pyruvate dehydrogenase, α-ketoglutarate dehydrogenase, and cytochrome oxidase [16, 17]. Mitochondrial abnormalities related to OS have been described in neurons, lymphocytes [18], endothelial cells [11] and fibroblasts [19] of subjects affected with AD. This condition may be one of the main causes of the loss in efficiency of endothelial cell function and consequently of BBB activity [20, 21].

The third element is HCy. An increase in HCy plasma levels has been correlated with alterations in the EEG of patients with AD [22] and is a known cause of endothelial damage [23, 24]. HCy is produced during metabolism in strict connection with methionine, cellular methylation, DNA and glutathione (GSH) synthesis. A few details of the HCy metabolic pathway are needed to point out the key steps in reducing its plasma levels (fig. 1).

HCy turnover is very complex and related to many different activities. Supplementation with vitamins B_6, B_9 and B_{12} or even B_6 alone has been found to reduce HCy levels [25–27]. Some clinical trials have shown that cardiovascular mortality is not affected by the use of the vitamin B group despite the decrease in HCy levels [28, 29]. However, the doses administered to patients were extremely high: 40 mg of vitamin B_6 and 0.4 mg of vitamin B_{12}, i.e. 20 and 200 times the RDA, respectively. These amounts may cause damaging effects in the long-term.

The fourth important factor is amyloid formation from amyloid precursor protein [30, 31]. Peptides Aβ 1–40/42 have both antioxidant and pro-oxidant activity, but they are definitely pro-oxidant [32, 33] and, when produced in large amounts, cause vasoconstriction in cerebral vessels [34]. The pro-oxidant activity damages proteins by forming advanced glycated end products and protein cross-linking. Carnosine may be used to protect against this specific brain oxidation [35, 36]. The first aggregate forms of Aβ peptides are soluble dimers and trimers [37, 38] which are neurotoxic. The oligomers and fibrillar forms, on the other hand, seem to lack both oxidant activity and neurotoxicity. As a consequence, brain cell proteins have to be protected from the damage caused mainly by the initial aggregation of Aβ peptides (2–4 peptides).

This is the task of erythrocytes, which are the fifth important element in brain protection. The main activity of erythrocytes is hemoglobin O_2 transport. This task is done very efficiently since each erythrocyte contains about 300 million hemoglobin molecules. All the hemoglobin is protected from oxidation basically by the NAD(P)H obtained through the pentose phosphate cycle.

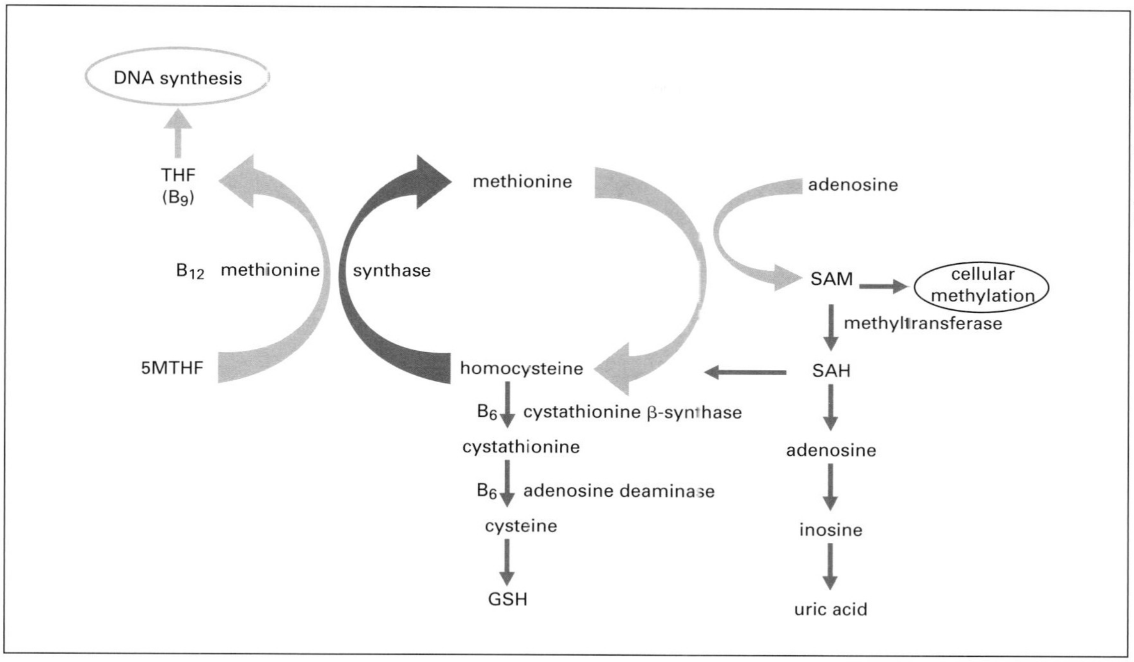

Fig. 1. Metabolic pathway of HCy. HCy is methylated by 5-methyltetrahydrofolate (5MTHF) in the presence of vitamin B_{12} to form tetrahydrofolate (THF), the active form of vitamin B_9. If there is a shortage of 5MTHF, DNA/RNA synthesis is impaired. Methionine is needed to produce S-adenosyl methionine (SAM), which is the main cellular methyl donor. HCy is also produced by S-adenosyl HCy (SAH). The cysteine which is derived from HCy in the presence of vitamin B_6 is needed to form GSH. Adapted from Pogribna et al. [78].

In this cycle (fig. 2), glucose is activated to glucose 6 phosphate (G6P) by ATP and becomes ribulose 5 phosphate (R5P), with the presence of vitamin B_1 as a cofactor. This allows the production of four ATP molecules.

GSH is produced from NAD(P)H and is used to protect the hemoglobin from oxidation and to conjugate toxic products, which are exported from erythrocytes by active pumps [39, 40].

Vitamins B_3 and B_2 are needed as cofactors to produce NADP and activate this process. Since large quantities of GSH are needed when erythrocytes undergo OS, they can produce tripeptides from single amino acids (L-cysteine, glycine and glutamine) and also need selenium (Se) to produce the 'anti-stress' enzyme glutathione peroxidase (GPx 1). GPx 1 contains a particular GSH formed with Se-L-cysteine instead of L-cysteine as a prosthetic part.

Erythrocytes bind amyloid dimers or trimers [41, 42] that generate pore-like structures on the erythrocyte membrane and can alter the cell membrane and volume. They exhibit ionophore-like properties [43] and undergo OS, resulting in an increase in erythrocyte size and the assumption of an elongated shape (sickle erythrocytes). In these OS conditions, erythrocytes may deposit their amyloid burden on endothelial cells [44]. In patients suffering from AD, sickle erythrocytes increase in number until reaching around 20%, whereas in comparable control cases it is far less than 10% [41].

The sixth important element in the development of AD is proteoglycans (PGs). PGs are found both on cells and in the extracellular matrix. They consist of a few glycosaminoglycans (GAGs) linked to a core protein, and between 100,000 and 1 million of them are found on every cell. The core proteins differ according to the type of PG, but they are usually large proteins (>500 kDa). However, both core proteins and GAGs may have highly variable dimensions.

GAGs are usually highly sulphated and consist of heparan sulphate, dermatan sulphate, chondroitin sulphate or keratan sulphate. All these molecules consist of chains of disaccharides, either glucose or galactose derivatives [45–47], and the chains are made up of polymers of several saccharides (usually >50). PGs are chemically well defined and have different names, such as perlecan, glyp-

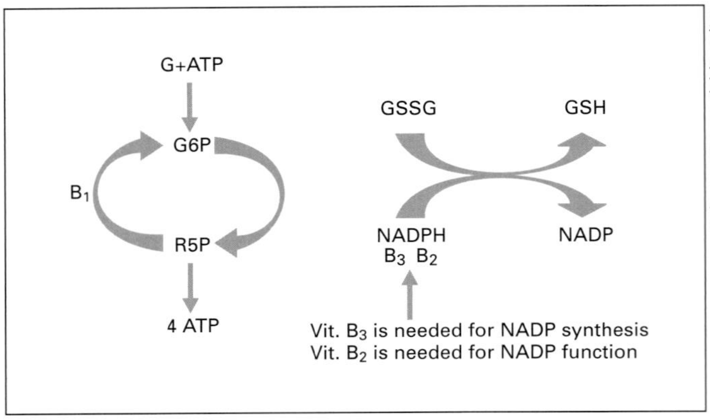

Fig. 2. Pentose phosphate cycle and vitamins B_1, B_2 and B_3. Part of the R5P is also used for trioses, which generate four molecules of ATP, and part returns to G6P. During the passage from G6P to R5P, a reducing unit (NADPH) is generated, which donates hydrogen in order to transform oxidized glutathione (GSSG) into GSH.

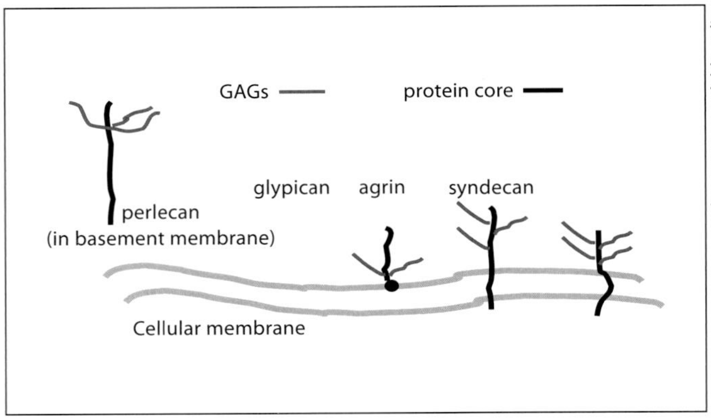

Fig. 3. PGs are a sort of signal indicating the receptor. The GAG is specific for the ligand that interacts with the receptor. The GAGs found on PGs are negatively charged owing to the presence of many sulphate groups on the saccharides, and may drive different ligands by charge repulsion or charge attraction. Fibroblast growth factors for instance only bind to their receptor after dimerization triggered by the heparan sulphate of the PG.

ican, syndecan, agrin, etc. They differ from the core protein and according to the type and number of GAGs. The location of PGs is also characteristic; perlecan is only found in the basement membrane of the BBB and glomeruli, whereas agrin and syndecan are very often found in BBB endothelial cells. Figure 3 shows some PGs and their respective locations on the cellular membrane.

Oxidized PGs [48, 49] have to be internalized for substitution. Owing to the high negative charge of their GAGs, they can attract all compounds with positive charges, such as Aβ peptides. This charge binding can trigger amyloid formation inside endothelial cells (vascular amyloid) or within neurons and astrocytes (cerebral amyloid).

The formation of neurofibrillary tangles (NFTs) is also related to the PGs internalized for substitution, as shown in figures 4 and 5. The internal aggregation of hyperphosphorylated tau protein with PG interferes with microtubule repair (fig. 4). This aggregation is self-maintaining up to the formation of a NFT (fig. 5) and any attempt to repair microtubules ends up with a sort of 'abortion'.

Basically, the process starts with the aggregation of hyperphosphorylated tau protein triggered by the internalized PGs that have to be substituted for repair.

In conclusion, damaged PGs are involved both in the formation of amyloid and NFTs. These are the most important markers of neuronal damage in Alzheimer's disease, seen in the form of neuritic and/or senile plaques.

Brain Antioxidant: Formula F

Considering all aspects of OS in the brain (BBB, mitochondria, HCy, amyloid, erythrocytes and PGs), a specific antioxidant formula (table 1) was created to improve the antioxidant network in subjects suffering from AD.

The components were combined according to the following concepts: carnosine to protect proteins from amyloid oxidation, which produces advanced glycated end products and cross-linking; vitamins B_1, B_2 and B_3 to support the pentose phosphate cycle in erythrocytes and brain cells; vitamins B_6, B_9, B_{12} to reduce HCy plasma levels; Se and L-cysteine to increase GSH production [50–52]; coenzyme Q_{10} to improve mitochondrial function [53]; vitamin E, β-carotene and vitamin C to protect cell membranes from oxidation; ginkgo biloba to support the vasodilatation of micro- and macrovessels and for its antioxidant activity [54–56].

We tested formula F in patients in a controlled, clinical study. The aim of the double-blind clinical trial was to treat patients suffering from mild AD in combination with donepezil for a period of 6 months, and to evaluate changes in plasma OS.

Materials and Methods

A cohort of 52 patients suffering from probable AD was randomly divided into two groups and followed for a period of 6

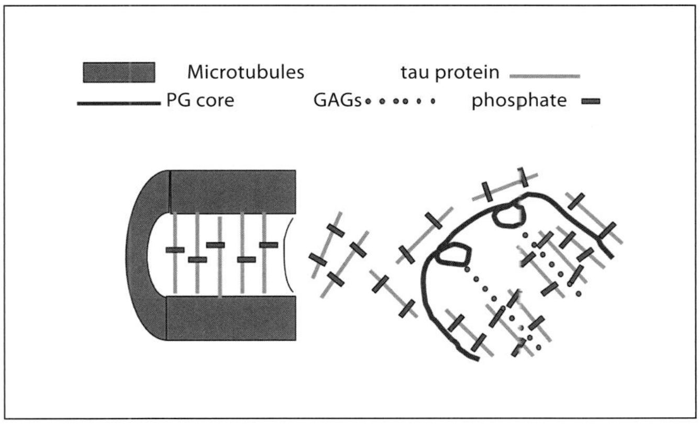

Fig. 4. Components of an NFT: hyperphosphorylated tau protein, PGs and amyloid. Tau protein becomes hyperphosphorylated to repair microtubules and its aggregation is triggered by PGs, which also impair microtubule repair.

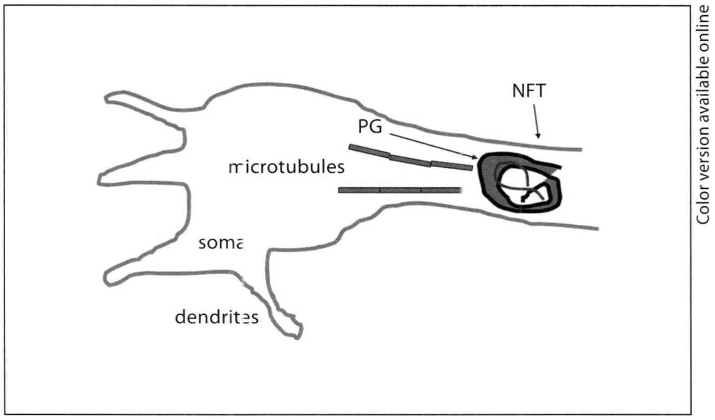

Fig. 5. Formation of NFTs in neurons. Microtubules transport substances from the soma of a neuron to its periphery (dendrites or synapses) and vice versa, and the initial NFT formation does not allow them to be repaired.

Table 1. Formula to protect brain from aging: formula F (AR_D Cogiton®)

Antioxidant	Dose	RDA
Carnosine	100 mg	–
Thiamine (B_1)	1.4 mg	100
Riboflavin (B_2)	1.6 mg	100
Nicotinamide (B_3)	18 mg	100
Pyridoxine (B_6)	2 mg	100
Folic acid (B_9)	200 μg	100
Cyanocobalamin (B_{12})	1 μg	100
Vitamin C	30 mg	50
Vitamin E	20 mg	200
Coenzyme Q_{10}	10 mg	–
β-Carotene	800 RE	100
Selenium	27.5 μg	25
L-cysteine	10 mg	–
Ginkgo biloba	25 mg	–

months according to a double-blind design. A group of 26 subjects was treated with formula F ampoules, and a similar group of 26 cases with placebo ampoules. Treating AD patients with placebo only (without any specific AD treatment) was not allowed by the ethics committee. Consequently, the experiment was performed on patients already being treated with donepezil. All the subjects were referred to a UVA centre (Unit for Alzheimer' Disease Evaluation and Assistance) and the protocol was approved by the center's ethics committee.

Admission Criteria

Cases were diagnosed according to NINCDS-ADRDA [57] and NINDS-AIREN [58]. Patients with an MMSE II score >21 with diagnosis of probable AD were admitted, provided they had been treated with donepezil at 5 mg/day for at least 2 months and had been receiving stable treatment (for at least 3 months) for any other concomitant chronic diseases. The type of ApoE ε alleles was not considered as an inclusion/exclusion criterion but was simply measured as a routine variable.

Exclusion Criteria

Patients not assisted by a caregiver, with malignancies or receiving chemotherapy were not admitted. Patients with an MMSE II score <21, alcohol abuse or severe depression were excluded. Patients being treated with donepezil for less than 2 months or with dosages of donepezil of >5 mg/day were also excluded.

A patient register was kept in order to record the number of subjects who referred to the centre during the enrolment period and the reason for their exclusion. Enrolment was completed in less than 2 weeks. One hundred and twenty patients were considered and 52 cases complied with the admission criteria.

Most of the exclusions were related to the severity of the disease (MMSE II score <21), the short period of donepezil treatment (<2 months) or because patients were undergoing treatment with drugs other than donepezil. It was decided to exclude subjects being treated with drugs other than donepezil because their interactions with the antioxidants may be different and this might lead to misinterpretation of results.

Treatments

All patients were undergoing treatment with 5 mg of donepezil. One group was treated with antioxidant formula F at a dose of one ampoule/day in the morning immediately before breakfast, and the other group was treated with placebo (excipients plus 500 mg of fructose and flavoring) at one ampoule/day. The placebo ampoule was identical to the formula F ampoule.

All treatments were administered for a period of 6 months. A 3-month supply of either formula F or placebo was given to each patient (9 boxes of 10 ampoules each). Compliance with the antioxidant treatment was measured by counting the remaining am-

Table 2. Characteristics of patients treated with formula F and placebo

Variables	Formula F	Placebo	p[1]
Sex			NS
Males	9	10	
Females	14	15	
Age	75 ± 4.2	74 ± 4.9	NS
Hypertension	6	5	NS
NIDD	6	5	NS
MI	5	6	NS
Hyperlipidemia	6	6	NS
ApoE ε4[2]	4	5	NS

NIDD = Non-insulin-dependent diabetes; MI = previous myocardial infarction (at least 3 years before). Some patients were also affected with other chronic diseases (urological/gynecological), but their frequencies were too low to be evaluated statistically.

[1] χ^2 test with Yates correction or t test for independent data; NS = $p > 0.05$.

[2] At least one ε4 allele.

poules returned by the subject during the checks. Compliance was also checked for donepezil on the basis of a tablet count (four boxes of 28 tablets were given to each patient). No other treatments were checked for compliance.

After the first 3-month period, patients were asked to refer to the centre again for an intermediate check and treatment supply.

Principal and Secondary Parameters

The main parameter considered was oxidative status measured using the d-ROMs test [59, 60] on plasma. HCy, plasma GSH levels, and the percentage of sickle erythrocytes were considered as secondary parameters. The overall clinical condition measured with MMSE II score was also considered as a secondary parameter.

Laboratory Assessment and Rating Scales

At each check (baseline, 3 months and 6 months), blood samples were collected in heparinized and nonheparinized tubes in the morning (between 8 and 10 a.m.) after overnight fasting. Three different aliquots of 5 ml each (two for plasma and one for serum) were taken from the brachial vein. They were immediately centrifuged and kept at –80°C until the measurements were taken. One further aliquot of 2 ml was also taken (without heparin) for sickle erythrocyte analysis at baseline and after 6 months only.

The d-ROMs test, erythrocyte GSH [61] and plasma HCy [62] were measured as described elsewhere. The d-ROMs test was performed at each check, whereas all the other tests were done at baseline and after 6 months only.

To measure the percentage of sickle erythrocytes, an erythrocyte pellet was isolated by centrifugation (1,000 *g* for 15 min at 4°C) immediately after the collection of a 2-ml sample in 2 ml citrate-phosphate-dextrose solution with adenine. The top of the tube was discarded and the process was repeated three times using CDPA for resuspension. Immediately after preparation, the percentage of sickle erythrocytes was calculated manually (on 400 erythrocytes) using Nomarski optics [41].

An MMSE II was performed at baseline and after 3 and 6 months, no more than 1 day before or after blood sampling. A change of at least 1 point in the MMSE II score compared with the baseline value was considered clinically relevant both in terms of improvement (≥+1) and worsening (≤–1).

Sleeping was also measured using a three-point scale (no change, better or worse).

Sample Size and Statistical Analysis

The sample size was based on the expected decrease in plasma hydroperoxides measured using the d-ROMs test, which is a test for measuring OS. Preliminary experiments on patients suffering from AD in non-blind conditions (2 months of treatment) gave some indication of the expected d-ROMs test values. An average decrease of at least 70–80 ± 10 (SD) CARR.U. was expected in the treated group (corresponding to a decrease of about 20% compared with the baseline value), whereas the placebo group was expected to show no more than a 20 ± 10 CARR.U. decrease (corresponding to a decrease of about 5% of the baseline value).

For a value of $\alpha = 0.05$ and $1\text{-}\beta = 0.9$, groups of 20 subjects are sufficient to obtain a power of at least >0.9. Assuming a maximum dropout of 30%, a total number of 26 patients were added to each group. Average values ± SD were calculated for all variables. The t tests for independent and interdependent data were used in order to measure the differences between baseline values and final values and between treatments, respectively.

Correlation coefficients were calculated between all the variables, and the exact χ^2 (Fisher) was used to measure the improvement/worsening in MMSE II score.

Results

Two subjects in the group treated with formula F underwent major orthopedic surgery a few weeks after starting the trial and were excluded from the evaluation.

One patient treated with formula F and one with placebo did not come to the first check (after 3 months) and were excluded from the analysis. Consequently, 48 of the initial 52 cases concluded the trial: 23 cases with formula F and 25 with placebo.

The general characteristics of the patients are shown in table 2.

The antioxidant treatment was very well tolerated, and no relevant side effects that could be interpreted as due to the antioxidant treatment were reported by any group member. Compliance was excellent since the remaining dose count was in line with expected values. None of the concomitant chronic diseases (hypertension, diabetes type II, hyperlipidemia, etc.) was affected by the treatments.

The main results are shown in tables 3 and 4. The baseline data and data after 6 months of treatment are shown for the variables assessed in the laboratory (table 3).

A significant reduction in OS was only found in subjects treated with the antioxidant. As regards the OS values recorded after 3 months of treatment, only the d-ROMs test data were available for all patients. In a few cases, other variables were also available (data not shown).

The measurements relating to the MMSE II score recorded at baseline, 3 and 6 months are shown in table 4.

The average improvement in MMSE II score was not very substantial in either group. However, considering each case singularly, an improvement in MMSE II score (≥+1) was found in 12 patients in the formula F group and in only 4 cases treated with placebo. This difference is statistically significant according to the Fisher test ($p < 0.05$).

A fall (≤–1) in MMSE II score was also observed in one case treated with the antioxidant and 2 cases treated with placebo. These numbers are too small to draw conclusions.

The correlation coefficients between the differences in the values recorded at baseline and after 6 months were calculated for the group treated with antioxidant supplementation (table 5). The same calculation was not possible for the placebo group because there were not enough cases of improvement for this type of analysis.

Significant correlation was found between the MMSE II differential (6 months – baseline) and the decrease in sickle erythrocytes. The increase in GSH was also strongly correlated with the improvement in MMSE II score. The decrease in d-ROMs test values was correlated with both the decrease in sickle erythrocytes and increase in GSH. The latter two variables also showed significant internal correlation ($p < 0.01$).

All the variables were tested for correlation and against each other at baseline, using the combined data from both groups. None of the variables were significantly correlated.

Discussion

Since all the patients were being treated with donepezil, the results obtained from this experiment have to be considered as the combined effect of a cholinesterase inhibitor with antioxidant supplementation.

One initial limitation of this trial stems from the type of patients included, since the diagnosis of AD was concomitant with other chronic diseases which may all also

Table 3. Laboratory assessment of patients suffering from AD

Variables	Period	Formula F	Placebo
d-ROMs test, CARR.U.	baseline	380 ± 44.6	365 ± 37.8
	6 months	295 ± 26.3[1,2]	356 ± 40.2
HCy, μmol/l	baseline	27 ± 5.4	29 ± 5.9
	6 months	20 ± 2.9[1,2]	27 ± 2.3
GSH, μmol/ml	baseline	2.6 ± 0.72	2.9 ± 0.84
	6 months	3.2 ± 0.82[1]	3.0 ± 0.79
Sickle erythrocytes, %[3]	baseline	18 ± 4.4	20 ± 4.2
	6 months	12 ± 3.8[1,2]	17 ± 3.7[1]

Values shown are mean ± SD.
[1] t test $p < 0.05$ for dependent data (before vs. 6 months).
[2] t test $p < 0.05$ for independent data (formula F vs. placebo at 6 months).
[3] Measurement in the group treated with formula F was only performed in 20 subjects.

Table 4. MMSE II score in the two patient groups (mean ± SD)

Treatment	Period	MMSE II	Cases improved/ worsened
Donepezil + formula F	baseline	23.2 ± 1.14	
	3 months	24.0 ± 1.57	4/0
	6 months	24.3 ± 1.43	11*/1
Donepezil + placebo	baseline	23.9 ± 1.04	
	3 months	23.6 ± 1.11	0
	6 months	24.2 ± 1.28	4/2

* $p < 0.05$, exact χ^2 test (Fisher), formula F vs. placebo.

Table 5. Correlation coefficients for all variables in the group treated with antioxidant formula

Variables	MMSE II	d-ROMs test	HCy	Sickle erythrocytes	GSH
MMSE II	1				
d-ROMs test	0.388	1			
HCy	0.242	–0.194	1		
Sickle erythrocytes[1]	0.816**	0.489*	0.179	1	
GSH	0.881**	0.499*	0.307	0.621**	1

* $p < 0.05$; ** $p < 0.01$.
[1] Measurement was done in only 20 cases.

cause OS. The improvement shown by the antioxidants administered in formula F may not be specifically related to AD, but to the other diseases as well. Furthermore, the sample size was sufficient for the d-ROMs test (the principal variable), but was not big enough to detect any significant change in the MMSE II score with sufficient power. In this case, the number of patients needed would be much greater. Sickle erythrocytes were studied in relation to amyloid only [41, 42], but theoretically their increase could be detected in many other diseases. Therefore, to draw correct clinical conclusions, more studies will have to be conducted in this area.

Despite all these limitations, formula F treatment was shown to substantially reduce OS and to improve the clinical results obtained with donepezil. Consequently, all the differences in the results of the two groups may be attributed to the antioxidant treatment.

The data showing a decrease in the number of sickle erythrocytes are particularly interesting. These data show that oxygen transport to the brain is greater owing to the presence of more deformable erythrocytes, thus with positive consequences on microcirculation. This effect could be very positive in the case of high levels of amyloid in the vasculature, as usually occurs even before AD symptoms become evident.

The antioxidant treatment was found to improve the antioxidant network substantially as shown by the increase in plasma GSH. This is mainly a measure of the antioxidant capability of circulating cells and especially erythrocytes, which make up the majority. This effect acts in parallel with the decrease in sickle erythrocytes.

These two tests were found to be highly correlated with the improvement in MMSE II score. Plasma GSH is merely a biochemical measurement, whereas the number of sickle erythrocytes is more related to function. The correlation between these two parameters indicates that the increase in circulating antioxidant may improve erythrocyte membrane function. Consequently, the whole brain may benefit from higher O_2 availability and this may have a favorable impact on cognitive function.

HCy was not found to be related to clinical outcome measured in terms of MMSE II score. This lack of correlation between HCy and clinical improvement was also found by other authors for cardiovascular diseases [28, 29]. One explanation might be that HCy is only one of many epiphenomena of a more complex equilibrium with other inflammatory markers [63], and that its decrease is due to a more general reduction in OS and not specifically to microvessel endothelial cell stress. This may explain why some authors found that its reduction was concomitant with a decrease in the risk of stroke [64], and that short-term treatment is effective on carotid intima-media thickness, whereas long-term treatment is not [65]. However, regardless of its origin, HCy can be a cytotoxic oxidant [66] and its decrease helps quench OS. All known HCy metabolic pathways were considered in the current formulation, especially its transformation into GSH through efficient NAD(P)H turnover. This was done by administering a more complete vitamin B group and not just vitamins B_6, B_9, and B_{12} alone.

This is the first time that a combination of antioxidants at doses within the RDA has been found to be active in decreasing OS in patients with AD. Excessive doses of vitamin E and vitamin C are usually administered [67, 68], which may behave as pro-oxidants [69]. Supplementation with vitamin B_6 and vitamin B_{12} at high doses [70] with or without vitamin B_9 [71] was also found to be ineffective in the treatment of cognitive decline. Combinations of different types of antioxidant at lower doses (within the RDA) should be tested with the aim of improving the whole antioxidant network.

The variability in the intake of antioxidants with diet makes comparing clinical data derived from different countries very complex. Patients should use antioxidants according to their needs as determined by measuring OS. The amount of oxidized vitamin E, for instance, was recently found to be directly related to the severity of cognitive impairment [72].

Despite the need for further larger studies, the idea of simultaneously tackling brain oxidation in many different compartments seems to be promising.

Donepezil has been found to be active in the treatment of cognitive impairment [73, 74], but association with vitamin E at high doses has not been seen to improve its activity [75]. In contrast, the larger spectrum of antioxidants at doses close to the RDA used in this trial was found to be helpful. Treatment with these types and doses of antioxidants could be even more useful in preventing/delaying the onset of the disease in those patients who have risk factors without any overt AD symptoms.

Age is the most important risk factor. The risk of AD doubles for every 5 years of age increase, and millions of people in every developed country are at risk of this disease, which is becoming a real economic problem for all societies. There is no alternative to aging. Aging instead can be faced with some preventive measures. In other words, when a subject is 60 years old and has some risk factors, he should be carefully monitored for the additional risk of OS and particular importance should be placed on its measurement.

Further studies with a larger population and involving other types of AD therapy are needed to clarify the role of antioxidants in the treatment of AD. Furthermore, more specific tests for brain oxidation [76, 77] should become available for routine studies in the field to understand the real clinical value of reducing brain oxidation.

References

1 Ding Q, Dimayuga E, Keller JN: Oxidative damage, protein synthesis, and protein degradation in Alzheimer's disease. Curr Alzheimer Res 2007;4:73–79.
2 Dröge W, Schipper MH: Oxidative stress and aberrant signaling in aging and cognitive decline. Aging Cell 2007;6:361–370.
3 Christen Y: Oxidative stress and Alzheimer disease. Am J Clin Nutr 2000;71:621S–629S.
4 Smith MA, Vasak K, Knipp M, et al: Dimethylargininase, a nitric oxide regulatory protein, in Alzheimer's disease. Free Radic Biol Med 1998;25:898–902.
5 Luth HJ, Munch G, Gartner U, et al: Expression of endothelial and inducible NOS-isoforms is increased in Alzheimer's disease, in APP23 transgenic mice and after experimental brain lesions in rats: evidence for an induction by amyloid pathology. Brain Res 2001;913:57–67.
6 Heneka MT, Wiesinger H, Dumitrescu-Ozimek L, et al: Neuronal and glial coexpression of arginosuccinate synthetase and inducible nitric oxide synthase in Alzheimer disease. J Neuropathol Exp Neurol 2001;60:906–916.
7 Lee SC, Zhao ML, Hirano A, Dickson DW: Inducible nitric oxide synthase immunoreactivity in the Alzheimer disease hippocampus: association with Hirano bodies, neurofibrillary tangles, and senile plaques. J Neuropathol Exp Neurol 199;58:1163–1169.
8 Soneja A, Drews M, Malinski T: Role of nitric oxide, nitroxidative and oxidative stress in wound healing. Pharmac Report 2005;57:108–119.
9 Malinski T: Nitric oxide and nitroxidative stress in Alzheimer's disease. J Alzheimers Dis 2007;11:207–218.
10 Hawkins BT, Davis T: The blood-brain barrier/neurovascular unit in health and disease. Pharmacol Rev 2005;57:173–185.
11 Stewart PA, Hayakawa K, Akers MA, Vinters HV: A morphometric study of the blood-brain barrier in Alzheimer's disease. Lab Invest 1992;67:734–742.
12 Andreyev AY, Kushnareva YE, Starkov AA: Mitochondrial metabolism of reactive species. Biochemistry (Moscow) 2005;70:200–214.
13 Wang J, Xiong S, Xie C, et al: Increased oxidative damage in nuclear and mitochondrial DNA in Alzheimer's disease. J Neurochem 2005;93:933–962.
14 Lin MT, Beal MF: Mitochondrial dysfunction and oxidative stress in neurodegenerative diseases. Nature 2006;433:787–795.
15 Sas K, Robotka H, Toldi J, Vécsei L: Mitochondria, metabolic disturbances, oxidative stress and kynurenine system, with focus on neurodegenerative disorders. J Neurol Sci 2007;257:221–239.
16 Marlatt M, Lee H, Perry G, et al: Sources and mechanism of cytoplasmatic oxidative damage in Alzheimer's disease. Acta Neurobiol Exp 2004;64:81–87.
17 Hirai K, Aliev G, Nunomura A, et al: Mitochondrial abnormalities in Alzheimers disease. J Neurosci 2001;21:3017–3023.
18 Mecocci P, Polidori MC, Cherubini A, et al: Lymphocyte oxidative DNA damage and plasma antioxidants in Alzheimer disease. Arch Neurol 2002;59:794–798.
19 Blass JP, Gibson GE: The role of oxidative abnormalities in the pathophysiology of Alzheimer's disease. Rev Neurol (Paris) 1991;147:513–525.
20 Zhu X, Smith MA, Honda K, et al: Vascular oxidative stress in Alzheimers disease. J Neurol Sci 2007;257:240–246.
21 Hachinski V, Munoz DG: Cerebrovascular pathology in Alzheimer's disease: cause, effect or epiphenomenon? Ann NY Acad Sci 1997;826:1–6.
22 Babiloni C, Bosco P, Ghidoni R, et al: Homocysteine and electroencephalographic rhythms in Alzheimer disease: a multicentric study. Neuroscience 2007;143:942–954.
23 Seshadri S, Beiser A, Selhub J, et al: Plasma HCy as risk factor for dementia and Alzheimer's disease. NEJM 2002;346:476–483.
24 Ravaglia G, Forti P, Maioli F, et al: HCy and folate as risk factors for dementia and Alzheimer disease. Am J Clin Nutr 2005;82:636–643.
25 Bleie Ø, Refsum H, Ueland PM, et al: Changes in basal and postmethionine load concentration of total HCy and cystationine after B vitamin intervention. Am J Clin Nutr 2004;80:641–648.
26 Lee BJ, Huang MC, Chung LJ, et al: Folic acid and vitamin B_{12} are more effective than vitamin B_6 in lowering fasting plasma homocysteine concentration in patients with coronary artery disease. Eur J Clin Nutr 2004;58:481–487.
27 NcKinley MC, McNulty H, McPartlin J, et al: Low-dose vitamin B_6 effectively lowers fasting HCy in healthy elderly person who are folate and riboflavin replete. Am J Clin Nutr 2001;73:759–764.
28 Bønaa KH, Njølstad NJ, Ueland PM, et al: Homocysteine lowering and cardiovascular events after acute myocardial infarction. NEJM 2006;354:1578–1588.
29 Ebbing M, Bleie Ø, Ueland PM, et al: Mortality cardiovascular events in patients treated with HCy-lowering B vitamin after coronary angiography: a randomized clinical trial. JAMA 2008;300:795–804.
30 Selkoe DJ: Normal and abnormal biology of the β-amyloid precursor protein. Annu Rev Neurosci 1994;17:439–517.
31 Näslund J, Haroutonian V, Mohs R, et al: Correlation between elevated levels of amyloid β-peptide in the brain and cognitive decline. JAMA 2000;283:1571–1577.
32 Butterfield DA: Amyloid beta-peptide (1–42)-induced oxidative stress and neurotoxicity: implication for neurodegeneration in Alzheimer's disease brain. A review. Free Radic Res 2002;36:1307–1313.
33 Kontush A: Amyloid-beta: an antioxidant that becomes a pro-oxidant and critically contributes to Alzheimer's disease. Free Radic Biol Med 2001;31:1120–1131.
34 Suo Z, Su G, Kundtz A, et al: A beta vasoactivity in vivo. Ann NY Acad Sci 2000;903:156–163.
35 Guiotto A, Calderan A, Ruzza P, Borin G: Carnosine and carnosine-related antioxidants: a review. Curr Med Chem 2005;12:2293–2315.
36 Hipkiss AR: Could carnosine or related structures suppress Alzheimer's disease? J Alzheimers Dis 2007;11:229–240.
37 Cleary JP, Walsh DM, Hofmeister JJ, et al: Natural oligomers of the amyloid-beta protein specifically disrupt cognitive function. Nat Neurosci 2005 8:79–84.
38 Walsh DM, Selkoe DJ: Oligomers on the brain: the emerging role of soluble protein aggregates in neurodegeneration. Protein Pept Lett 2004;11:213–228.

39 Alhamdani MSS: Impairment of glutathione biosynthetic pathway in uremia and dialysis. Nephrol Dial Transplant 2005;20:124–128.
40 Reid M, Badaloo A, Forrester T, Jahoor F: In vivo rates of erythrocytes glutathione synthesis in adults with sickle cell disease. Am J Physiol Endocrinol Metab 2006;291:E73–E79.
41 Mohanty JG, Eckley DM, Williamson JD, et al: Do red blood cell-β-amyloid interaction alter oxygen delivery in Alzheimer's disease? Adv Exp Med Biol 2008;614:29–35.
42 Singer SJ, Dewji NN: Evidence that Perutz's double-β-stranded subunit structure for β-amyloid also applies to their channel-forming structures in membranes. PNAS 2006; 103:1546–1550.
43 Engström I, Ronquist G, Petterson L, Waldenström A: Alzheimer amyloid beta-peptides exhibit ionophore-like properties in human erythrocytes. Eur J Clin Invest 1995;25:471–476.
44 Ravi LB, Mohanty JG, Chrest FJ, et al: Influence of beta-amyloid fibrils on the interactions between red blood cells and endothelial cells. Neurol Res 2004;26:579–585.
45 Cornelli U: Glycosaminoglycans as potential future treatment of Alzheimer's disease; in Richter RW, Richter BZ (eds): Alzheimer's Disease. A Physician Guide to Practical Management. Totowa, Humana Press, 2004.
46 Van Vactor D, Wall DP, Johnson KG: Heparan sulphate proteoglycans and the emergence of neuronal connectivity. Curr Opin Neurobiol 2006;16:50–51.
47 Galtrey CM, Fawcett JW: The role of condroitin sulphate proteoglycans in regeneration and plasticity in the central nervous system. Brain Res Rev 2007;54:1–18.
48 Metcalfe DD, Thompson HL, Klebanoff SJ, Henderson WR: Oxidative degradation of rat mast-cell proteoglycan. Biochem J 1990; 272:51–57.
49 Roberts CR, Roughley PJ, Mort JS: Degradation of human proteoglycan aggregates induced by hydrogen peroxide. Biochem J 1989;259:805–811.
50 Wessjohann LA, Schneider A, Abbas M, Brandt W: Selenium in chemistry and biochemistry in comparison to sulfur. Biol Chem 2007;388:997–1006.
51 Wu G, Fang YZ, Yang S, et al: Glutathione metabolism and its implications for health. J Nutr 2004;134:489–492.
52 Franco R, Schoneveld OJ, Pappa A, Panayioditis MI: The central role of glutathione in the pathophysiology of human diseases. Arch Physiol Biochem 2007;113:234–258.
53 Littarru GP, Tiano L: Bioenergetic and antioxidant properties of coenzyme Q10: recent developments. Mol Biotechnol 2007;37:31–37.
54 Koltermann A, Harkorn A, Koch E, et al: Ginkgo biloba extract Egb 761 increases endothelial nitric oxide production in vitro and vivo. Cell Mol Life Sci 2007;64:1715–1722.
55 Napryeyenko O, Borzenko I, GINDEM-NP Study Group: Ginkgo biloba special extract in dementia with neuropsychiatric features. A randomized placebo-controlled double-blind clinical trial. Arzneimittelforschung 2007;57:4–11.
56 Mazza M, Capuano A, Bria P, Mazza S: Ginkgo biloba and donepezil: a comparison in the treatment of Alzheimer's dementia in a randomized placebo-controlled double-blind study. Eur J Neurol 2006;13:981–985.
57 McKhann G, Drachman D, Folstein M, et al: Clinical diagnosis of Alzheimer's disease: report of the NINCDS-ADRDA Work Group under auspices of Department of Health and Human Services Task Force on Alzheimer's Disease. Neurology 1984;34:939–944.
58 Romàn GC, Tatemichi TK, Erkinjuntti T, et al: Vascular dementia: diagnostic criteria for research studies: report of the NINDS-AIREN International Workshop. Neurology 1993;43:250–260.
59 Cesarone MR, Belcaro G, Carratelli M, et al: A simple test to monitor oxidative stress. Int Angiol 1999;18:127–130.
60 Cornelli U, Terranova R, Luca S, et al: Bioavailability and antioxidant activity of some food supplements in men and women using the D-Roms test as a marker of oxidative stress. J Nutr 2001;131:3208–3211.
61 Reid M, Badaloo A, Forrester T, Jahoor F: In vivo rates of erythrocyte glutathione synthesis in adults with sickle cell disease. Am J Physiol Endocrinol Metab 2006;291:E73–E79.
62 Bleie Ø, Refsum H, Ueland PM, et al: Changes in basal and postmethionine load concentration of total homocysteine and cystationine after B vitamin intervention. Am J Clin Nutr 2004;80:641–648.
63 McDermott MM, Liu K, Ferrucci L, et al: Circulating markers and functional impairment in peripheral arterial disease. J Am Geriatr Soc 2008,56:1504–1510.
64 Wang X, Qin X, Demitras H, et al: Efficacy of folic acid supplementation in stroke prevention: a meta analysis. Lancet 2007;369: 1876–1882.
65 Potter K, Hankey GJ, Green DJ, et al: The effect of long term homocysteine-lowering on carotid intima-media thickness and flow-mediated vasodilation in stroke patients: a randomized controlled trial and meta-analysis. BMC Cardiovasc Disord 2008;8:24.
66 Stanger O, Herrmann W, Pietrzik K, et al: DACH-LIGA Homocystein (German, Austrian and Swiss Homocysteine Society): consensus paper on the rational clinical use of homocysteine, folic acid and B-vitamins in cardiovascular and thrombotic disease: guidelines and recommendation. Clin Chem Lab Med 2003;41:1392–1403.
67 Yaffe K, Clemons TE, McBee WL, et al: Impact of antioxidants, zinc, and copper, on cognition in the elderly: a randomized clinical trial. Neurology 2004;63:1705–1707.
68 Gray SL, Anderson ML, Crane PK, et al: Antioxidant vitamin supplement use and risk of dementia or Alzheimer's disease in older adults. J Am Geriatr Soc 2008;56:291–295.
69 Miller ER 3rd, Pastor-Barriuso R, Dalal D, et al: Meta-analysis: high dosages vitamin E supplementation may increase all-cause mortality. Ann Intern Med 2005;142:37–46.
70 Aisen PS, Schneider LS, Sano M, et al: High-dose B vitamin supplementation and cognitive decline in Alzheimer disease: a randomized controlled trial. JAMA 2008;300: 1774–1783.
71 Malouf M, Grimley EJ, Areosa SA: Folic acid with or without vitamin B_{12} for cognition and dementia. Cochrane Database Syst Rev 2003;CD004514.
72 Ravaglia G, et al: Plasma tocopherol and risk of cognitive impairment in an elderly Italian cohort. Am J Clin Nutr 2008;87:1306–1313.
73 Ringman JM: Donepezil improves cognitive function and reduces decline in activities of daily living in people with severe Alzheimer's disease. Evid Based Ment Health 2006; 9:104–117.
74 Setzer B: Donepezil an update. Expert Opin Pharmacother 2007:8:1011–1023.
75 Petersen RC, Thomas RG, Grundman M, et al: Vitamin E and donepezil for the treatment of mild cognitive impairment. NEJM 2005;352:2379–2388.
76 Montine TJ, Montine KF, McMahan W, et al: F2-isoprostanes in Alzheimer and other neurodegenerative diseases. Antiox Redox Signal 2005;7:269–275.
77 Montine TJ, Quinn J, Kaie J, Morrow JD: F(2)-isoprostanes as biomarkers of late-onset Alzheimer's disease. J Mol Neurosci 2007; 33:114–119.
78 Pogribna M, Melnik S, Pogribni I, Chango P, et al: HCy metabolism with Down syndrome: in vitro stimulation. Am J Hum Genet 2001; 69:88–95.

Neuro-degenerative Diseases

Neurodegenerative Dis 2010;7:203–205
DOI: 10.1159/000295664

Published online: March 12, 2010

Filamentous Phages Reduce α-Synuclein Oligomerization in the Membrane Fraction of SH-SY5Y Cells

Hemi Dimant Beka Solomon

Department of Molecular Microbiology and Biotechnology, George S. Wise Faculty of Life Sciences, Tel-Aviv University, Tel-Aviv, Israel

Key Words
Membrane α-synuclein · Filamentous phages · Disaggregation · SH-SY5Y cells

Abstract
Background: α-Synuclein (AS) is an abundant neuronal protein predominantly localized in presynaptic terminals in the central nervous system. AS aggregation is a molecular hallmark of several neurodegenerative diseases, including Parkinson's disease, and is thought to play a significant role in the etiology of the disease. Recent experimental evidence indicates that AS exists in two forms, a membrane-bound form and a disordered cytosolic form. Much effort is dedicated to prevent and dissolve AS aggregates, specifically AS oligomers and protofibrils, which are thought to be the more toxic form of aggregates. ***Methods:*** The effect of filamentous phages on AS aggregation in SH-SY5Y cells overexpressing wild-type AS was quantified in ELISA designed to detect and quantify AS oligomers. ***Results:*** We found reduced levels of AS oligomers in the membrane fraction in cells treated with filamentous phages compared to non-treated cells. ***Conclusion:*** The reduction in AS oligomers from the plasma membrane in treated cells may suggest further therapeutic application.

Introduction

Fibrillar aggregates of α-synuclein (AS) are the main pathological hallmark of Parkinson's disease (PD). Missense mutations and gene multiplication in the AS gene are linked to familial forms of PD [1–3]. These mutations result in amino acid substitution and acceleration of pathogenic AS aggregation [4]. Transgenic animal models overexpressing AS exhibit selective degeneration of dopaminergic neurons and protein aggregation [5, 6]. These facts and other accumulating data suggest that AS aggregation plays a critical role in the etiology of the disease.

AS is a natively unfolded protein localized at presynaptic terminals. AS readily incorporates into membranes through the N-terminus and thus exists in the cell in two forms: a membrane-bound and a disordered cytosolic form. Accumulating data indicate that the membrane form of AS plays a role in cellular toxicity. Protofibrils can form annular structures embedded on the cell membrane and cause membrane permeability [7]. It was recently demonstrated that AS has a higher aggregation propensity in the presence of lipids and that the membrane aggregates can induce aggregation of the cytosolic form of AS [8].

KARGER

Fax +41 61 306 12 34
E-Mail karger@karger.ch
www.karger.com

1660–2854/10/0073–0203$26.00/0

Accessible online at:
www.karger.com/ndd

Beka Solomon
Department of Molecular Microbiology and Biotechnology
George S. Wise Faculty of Life Sciences, Tel-Aviv University
Ramat Aviv, Tel-Aviv 69978 (Israel)
Tel. +972 3 640 9711, Fax +972 3 640 5871, E-Mail beka@post.tau.ac.il

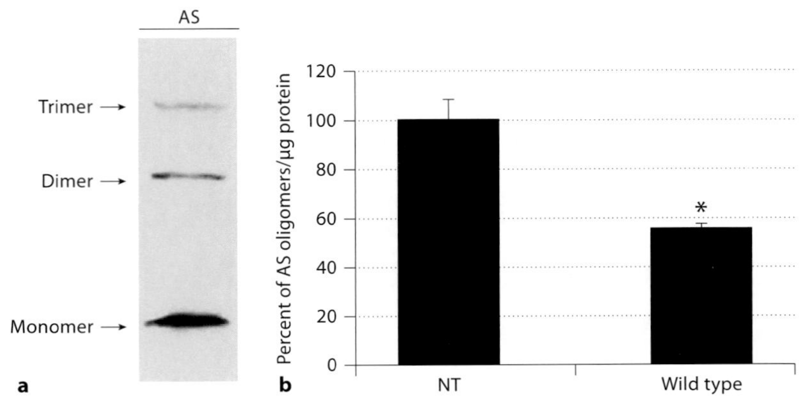

Fig. 1. a Western blot analysis of the membrane fraction of SH-SY5Y cells, demonstrating the presence of various AS oligomers. **b** The amount of AS oligomers from the membrane fraction was quantified in an ELISA specific for AS oligomers. A significant (*) reduction in the amount of AS oligomers was measured in the membrane fraction of SH-SY5Y cells treated with wild-type filamentous phages.

Although the mechanisms of in vivo aggregation and toxicity are not well understood, much focus has been directed towards intervention in the aggregation process of AS.

Here, we present reduction in the level of AS oligomers following treatment with wild-type filamentous phages in SH-SY5Y cells overexpressing wild-type AS.

Results and Discussion

AS is a natively unstructured, highly soluble protein which incorporates easily into membranes and is thus present in the cell, either in the cytoplasm or the membrane. Lewy bodies, the hallmark of PD, are intracellular aggregates composed primarily of AS. The intracellular aggregates of AS were targeted with filamentous phages using the f88 system which present on its major coat protein (pVIII) a cyclic RGD motif. This sequence is known to mediate binding to integrin receptors on the cell surface with subsequent integrin-dependent internalization. Indeed we have demonstrated the binding of RGD phages to integrin and their internalization to SH-SY5Y cells. We separated the soluble fraction of the cells following incubation with RGD phages and evaluated the level of soluble AS oligomers using an ELISA in which only oligomers are detected. A significant reduction in the amount of oligomers was measured in the cells treated with the RGD phages [9].

The membrane fraction of AS in the cell and its relation to disease etiology has recently drawn more interest. Oligomers and protofibrils of AS are associated with the plasma membrane in pathological circumstances of PD leading to neurodegeneration.

In order to examine this effect, SH-SY5Y cells were treated with wild-type phages. These phages do not present the RGD motif on pVIII and thus are not able to internalize in an integrin-dependent manner. Nonetheless, in immunocytochemistry wild-type phages were stained on the membrane of SH-SY5Y cells. Furthermore, in SH-SY5Y cells incubated with wild-type phages, a small percentage of plaque forming units were counted from cellular extracts following an acidic wash, suggesting that a small portion of the phages may internalize into the cells.

We extracted the membrane fraction of the cells using a membrane extraction kit. Indeed, AS was detected in Western blot analysis, verifying the presence of AS in the cell membrane. Not only AS monomers were detected but also AS dimers and trimers were detected in the membrane fraction (fig. 1a), demonstrating the existence of AS oligomers in membrane compartments in our cellular model. We examined the effect of filamentous phages on the oligomerization on membrane AS following incubation with filamentous phages. SH-SY5Y cells were differentiated using retinoic acid and were incubated with wild-type phages. Cells were incubated with 10^{11} phages/ml overnight. The membrane fractions were extracted the following day, and samples of each extraction were measured for the amount of AS oligomers in an ELISA designed to recognize only oligomeric species of AS [10]. A significant reduction in AS oligomers from the membrane fraction was measured in SH-SY5Y cells following incubation with filamentous phages. The effect of wild-type phages on AS aggregation extracted from the membrane fraction suggests that the wild-type phages affect AS on the plasma membrane, possibly via direct interaction with AS through a previously demonstrated region of interaction located at amino acids 73–85 of AS [9]. It is also possible that, due to the long incubation of the cells with phages, a small percentage of the phages are internalized into the cells affecting other membranous compartments in the cell other than the plasma membrane. Binding of the phages to the cells with possible internalization may promote clearance of AS from the plasma membrane through activation of lysosmal degradation [11].

Data presented here demonstrate that wild-type filamentous phages incubated with SH-SY5Y cells reduced the level of AS oligomerization, possibly directly through the plasma membrane, as indicated by the reduction of oligomers in the membrane fraction of the cells. This suggests further therapeutic application in the treatment of PD.

References

1 Polymeropoulos MH, Lavedan C, Leroy E, Ide SE, Dehejia A, Dutra A, Pike B, Root H, Rubenstein J, Boyer R, Stenroos ES, Chandrasekharappa S, Athanassiadou A, Papapetropoulos T, Johnson WG, Lazzarini AM, Duvoisin RC, Di Iorio G, Golbe LI, Nussbaum RL: Mutation in the alpha-synuclein gene identified in families with Parkinson's disease. Science 1997;276:2045–2047.

2 Zarranz JJ, Alegre J, Gomez-Esteban JC, Lezcano E, Ros R, Ampuero I, Vidal L, Hoenicka J, Rodriguez O, Atares B, Llorens V, Gomez Tortosa E, del Ser T, Munoz DG, de Yebenes JG: The new mutation, E46K, of alpha-synuclein causes Parkinson and Lewy body dementia. Ann Neurol 2004;55:164–173.

3 Kruger R, Kuhn W, Muller T, Woitalla D, Graeber M, Kosel S, Przuntek H, Epplen JT, Schols L, Riess O: Ala30Pro mutation in the gene encoding alpha-synuclein in Parkinson's disease. Nat Genet 1998;18:106–108.

4 Conway KA, Harper JD, Lansbury PT: Accelerated in vitro fibril formation by a mutant alpha-synuclein linked to early-onset Parkinson disease. Nat Med 1998;4:1318–1320.

5 Masliah E, Rockenstein E, Veinbergs I, Mallory M, Hashimoto M, Takeda A, Sagara Y, Sisk A, Mucke L: Dopaminergic loss and inclusion body formation in alpha-synuclein mice: implications for neurodegenerative disorders. Science 2000;287:1265–1269.

6 Feany MB, Bender WW: A Drosophila model of Parkinson's disease. Nature 2000;404:394–398.

7 Lashuel HA, Petre BM, Wall J, Simon M, Nowak RJ, Walz T, Lansbury PT Jr: Alpha-synuclein, especially the Parkinson's disease-associated mutants, forms pore-like annular and tubular protofibrils. J Mol Biol 2002;322:1089–1102.

8 Lee H-J, Choi C, Lee S-J: Membrane-bound alpha-synuclein has a high aggregation propensity and the ability to seed the aggregation of the cytosolic form. J Biol Chem 2002;277:671–678.

9 Dimant H, Sharon N, Solomon B: Modulation effect of filamentous phage on alpha-synuclein aggregation. Biochem Biophys Res Commun 2009;383:491–496.

10 El-Agnaf OMA, Salem SA, Paleologou KE, Curran MD, Gibson MJ, Court JA, Schlossmacher MG, Allsop D: Detection of oligomeric forms of alpha-synuclein protein in human plasma as a potential biomarker for Parkinson's disease. FASEB J 2006;20:419–425.

11 Masliah E, Rockenstein E, Adame A, Alford M, Crews L, Hashimoto M, Seubert P, Lee M, Goldstein J, Chilcote T, Games D, Schenk D: Effects of alpha-synuclein immunization in a mouse model of Parkinson's disease. Neuron 2005;46:857–868.

Neuro-degenerative Diseases

Neurodegenerative Dis 2010;7:206–209
DOI: 10.1159/000295665

Published online: March 12, 2010

Effects of Dopamine Agonists on Neuropsychiatric Symptoms of Parkinson's Disease

Irena Rektorová

First Department of Neurology, Masaryk University and St. Anne's Hospital, Brno, Czech Republic

Key Words
Dopamine agonists · Parkinson's disease · Depression · Cognition · Functional imaging

Abstract
The efficacy of dopamine (DA) agonists in the treatment of motor symptoms of Parkinson's disease (PD) has been clearly demonstrated. It has also been documented that DA agonists may have both a positive and a negative impact on neuropsychiatric symptoms in PD patients. This paper will focus on the effects of DA agonists on depressive and cognitive symptoms of PD.

Although L-dopa is still the most effective and most widely used therapy for symptomatic management in Parkinson's disease (PD), dopamine (DA) agonists may have several potential advantages over L-dopa. For example, in contrast to L-dopa, DA agonists are supposed to act directly at the level of the postsynaptic DA receptors, most DA agonists have a longer elimination half-life than L-dopa and some of them can be easily delivered continuously via transdermal patches (e.g. rotigotine) or via subcutaneous pumps (e.g. apomorphine, lisuride). It is possible that an abnormal pulsatile dopaminergic stimulation, as induced by daily oral L-dopa administration, deregulates dopaminergic and nondopaminergic receptors at the level of the basal ganglia, leading to the occurrence of abnormal motor responses, like fluctuations and dyskinesias. In line with this hypothesis, the results of several double-blind studies have shown that DA agonists, when added to L-dopa, significantly reduce the total time spent in the 'off' state, and when started in monotherapy, DA agonists as compared to L-dopa alone prevent and delay the incidence of L-dopa-induced dyskinesias in particular [1].

Despite the emphasis on motor function, several studies have shown that the non-motor symptoms of PD have greater significance than the motor symptoms when assessed in terms of quality of life measures, institutionalization rates, or health economics [2]. Recent work from different groups shows that DA replacement therapy in PD (and high doses of DA agonists in particular) can lead to several neuropsychiatric side effects such as development of hallucinations, psychosis, excessive daytime sleepiness, disorders of impulse control such as patho-

KARGER
Fax +41 61 306 12 34
E-Mail karger@karger.ch
www.karger.com

1660–2854/10/0073–0206$26.00/0

Accessible online at:
www.karger.com/ndd

Irena Rektorová
First Department of Neurology
Masaryk University and St. Anne's Hospital
Pekarska 53, CZ–656 91 Brno (Czech Republic)
Tel. +420 54318 2639, Fax +420 54318 2624, E-Mail irena.rektorova@fnusa.cz

logical gambling, and 'DA dysregulation syndrome' (compulsive use of dopaminergic medication associated with disabling dyskinesias). The following text will briefly touch upon two rather controversial issues: the impact of DA agonists on depressive and cognitive symptoms of PD. It is based on published and unpublished work of the author.

Prevalence rates of depression in PD have been reported to be as high as 40%. Depressive symptoms precede those of motor dysfunction in 12–37% of patients with PD. Although mood and anxiety fluctuations may parallel motor fluctuations, the natural history of depression does not parallel the progression of physical symptoms of PD, suggesting that it is an independent process. Biological factors involved include probably dopaminergic, serotonergic, and noradrenergic deficits. With respect to DA, both the mesolimbic DA ('reward circuits') and frontal-subcortical (basal ganglia-thalamo-cortical circuits) systems seem to be implicated in the pathophysiology of PD depression [3].

With respect to cognitive deficits, it has been documented that particularly executive functions are affected in nondemented patients with PD. This impairment has been related to the dysfunction of the dorsolateral striato-prefrontal loop following the loss of dopaminergic nigral neurons, as well as the mesocortical pathway in which neurons project predominantly from the ventral tegmental area and medial substantia nigra pars compacta to the neocortex [4, 5]. In addition to DA deficits, the cholinergic system has also been implicated in cognitive dysfunction and in PD dementia in particular, and serotonergic, glutamatergic or noradrenergic systems could also be involved [6]. It has been demonstrated that the presence of visual hallucinations and specific cognitive deficits may predict the occurrence of dementia later during the disease progression. Prevalence of dementia in PD is 30%, and its incidence is 4–6 times greater compared to the general age-matched population [7].

Utilizing functional imaging, we studied whether the ^{123}I-FP-CIT uptake in the striatum (i.e. a marker of dopaminergic neuronal density) correlates with depressive symptoms and cognitive performance in patients with PD [8]. Twenty patients with PD without major depression and/or dementia (mean age 61.7 ± 12.7 years) were enrolled. The ratios of striatal to occipital binding for the entire striatum, putamina, and putamen to the caudate (put/caud) index were calculated in the basal ganglia. The association between neuropsychiatric measures and DA transporter availability was calculated; multiple regression analysis was used to assess association with age and disease duration. We found significant correlations between Montgomery and Asberg Depression Rating Scale (MADRS) and Tower of London (TOL) task scores and ^{123}I-FP-CIT uptake in various striatal ROIs. Multiple regression analysis confirmed the significant relationship between TOL performance and put/caud ratio ($p = 0.001$) and age ($p = 0.001$), and between MADRS and left striatal ($p = 0.005$) and putaminal DA transporter availability ($p = 0.003$). Our results are in line with those of recent studies [9–12] and support the notion that depressive symptoms in patients with PD are at least partly related to the dopaminergic hypofunction in the left putamen in particular, whereas the cognitive performance on the TOL task is related to both the dopaminergic deficit in the caudate nucleus and the patient's age.

Following the functional imaging study, we performed several pharmacological studies in order to assess the impact of DA agonists on depressive symptoms and cognitive functions in PD. Our 8-month multicenter prospective randomized study was designed to compare the effects of DA agonists pramipexole (PPX) and pergolide (PRG) as add-ons to L-dopa therapy on depressive symptoms (assessed by the MADRS, and the Self-Rating Depression Scale by Zung) in 41 nondemented advanced PD patients (25 men, 16 women) suffering also from depression [13]. The average total daily doses of both preparations were comparable (2.7 ± 0.5 mg for PPX and 3.0 ± 0.3 mg for PRG). The average value of Zung scores decreased significantly in both groups and paralleled improvement of motor complications as measured by the UPDRS IV. The average value of MADRS scores decreased in both groups (dropped from an average value of 15.11 points at the first visit to 9.28 points at the last visit for PPX and from 11.25 to 10.06 for PRG). While mean entry MADRS values did not differ statistically, there was a statistically significant decrease observed only in the PPX group (at the 5% significance level). The decrease was significantly more pronounced in the PPX group than in the PRG group (at the 5% significance level), and the difference was still observed when the effect of motor symptom changes as measured by UPDRS III was controlled for (analysis of covariance, $p = 0.036$). The number of MADRS responders (defined as the number of patients for whom the decrease in MADRS between the first and last visit was at least 50%) was 8 of 18 (44%) in the PPX group and 3 of 16 (18.7 %) in the PRG group. Our results demonstrated for the first time a possible antidepressant effect of PPX (a D2/D3 DA agonist) in PD patients with depression.

In another study, we evaluated the effects of ropinirole (another D2/D3 DA agonist) on anxiety, depressive symptoms and sleep disturbances in addition to other selected non-motor symptoms of PD [14]. Forty-four PD patients with or without motor complications (MC+ group and MC– group, respectively) were enrolled in this open-label 6-month prospective study. The median ropinirole dose was 10 mg. In addition to improvement in motor symptoms and motor complications, both median Hamilton Anxiety Scale (HAMA) and MADRS scores dropped significantly in the MC+ group (median scores of both HAMA and MADRS changed from 12 to 8 points; $p = 0.002$ and 0.007, respectively); patients in our MC– group had little or no anxiety and depression at the baseline visit. Changes in HAMA and MADRS correlated significantly only with changes of sleep quality, as measured by the Parkinson's Disease Sleep Scale.

Finally, we tested the impact of DA agonists on cognitive performance in the same group of 41 nondemented PD patients in whom the effects of PPX and PRG were studied with regard to depression [15]. The Trail Making Test (TMT), the Stroop Test and four subtests (arithmetic, picture completion, digit symbols and similarities) of the Wechsler Adult Intelligence Scale-Revised (WAIS-R) were performed prior to and 8 months after the administration of either PPX or PRG. We found no statistically significant difference between the two tested drugs or between the first and the last visit in any of the above-listed neuropsychological tests. Both PPX and PRG in combination with L-dopa were safe in terms of their effect on cognitive performance. It is noteworthy that the mean adjusted profile scores and T scores in all tests performed were within normal ranges, except for the tests reflecting motor speed (such as TMT or the Digit symbols subtest of WAIS-R) where none of the patients had hallucinations. The absence of cognitive effects of DA agonists, in contrast to the modulation of motor and mood symptoms, indicates that the pathological mechanisms of cognitive, motor and affective disturbances are different in advanced non-demented PD patients. Interestingly, these results are also in line with results of the EWO study (Epidemiology of Wearing Off Phenomena in PD) [Rektorová et al., unpubl.]: the total daily dose of dopaminergic treatment as expressed by L-dopa-equivalent doses in 208 PD patients had no effect on the Montreal Cognitive Assessment Score ($p = 0.555$; generalized linear regression model adjusted for patients' age and depressive symptoms as measured by MADRS). Conversely, the long-term treatment with continuous subcutaneous apomorphine infusions led to statistically and clinically significant impairment in the Verbal Fluency tasks and Mattis Dementia Rating Scale in PD patients with visual hallucinations and dementia [Kubikova et al., unpubl.].

Taken together, our results are in line with other studies published so far with respect to effects of D2/D3 DA agonists on depressive symptoms of PD [16–18]. The D3 DA receptors are widely expressed in the mesolimbic pathways. Stimulation of these receptors may be responsible for antidepressive effects. DA agonists are probably effective for depressive symptoms in PD, but to date there have been no well-designed randomized double-blind studies in PD depression. The contribution of DA to cognitive impairment is still a matter of debate. Studies which specifically examined the effect of dopaminergic treatment on cognition suggest that the effect depends on many variables, including the specific task demands, the PD population tested (de novo versus chronically treated fluctuating patients; presence or absence of cognitive decline/dementia), genetic and perhaps other factors – with treatment sometimes improving, sometimes having no effect, and sometimes impairing cognition [19–21]. In conclusion, DA agonists are safe for treatment of motor symptoms of PD and they may have both a positive and a negative impact on neuropsychiatric symptoms in PD patients. Therefore, careful observation of patients under treatment is recommended.

Acknowledgement

The study was supported by the Research Project of the Czech Ministry of Education MSM 0021622404.

References

1 Goetz CG, Poewe W, Rascol O, Sampaio C: Evidence-based medical review update: pharmacological and surgical treatments of Parkinson's disease: 2001 to 2004. Mov Disord 2005;20:523–539.

2 Chaudhuri KR, Healy DG, Schapira AHV: Non-motor symptoms of Parkinson's disease: diagnosis and management. Lancet Neurol 2006;5:235–245.

3 Burn DJ: Beyond the iron mask: towards better recognition and treatment of depression associated with Parkinson's disease. Mov Disord 2002;17:445–454.

4 Mega MS, Cummings JL: Frontal-subcortical circuits and neuropsychiatric disorders. J Neuropsychiatry Clin Neurosci 1994;6:358–370.

5 Jellinger KA: The pathology of Parkinson's disease. Adv Neurol 2001;86:55–72.

6 Pillon B, Dubois B, Cusimano G, Bonnet AM, Lhemitte F, Agid Y: Does cognitive impairment in Parkinson's disease result from non-dopaminergic lesions? J Neurol Neurosurg Psychiatry 1989;52:201–206.
7 Emre M, Aarsland D, Brown R, et al: Clinical diagnostic criteria for dementia associated with Parkinson's disease. Mov Disord 2007; 22:1689–1707.
8 Rektorova I, Srovnalova H, Kubikova R, Prasek J: Striatal dopamine transporter imaging correlates with depressive symptoms and tower of London task performance in Parkinson's disease. Mov Disord 2008;23: 1580–1587.
9 Remy P, Samson Y: The role of dopamine in cognition: evidence from functional imaging studies. Curr Opin Neurol 2003;16(suppl 2):S37–S41.
10 Cheesman AL, Barker RA, Lewis SJ, Robbins TW, Owen AM, Brooks DJ: Lateralisation of striatal function: evidence from 18F-dopa PET in Parkinson's disease. J Neurol Neurosurg Psychiatry 2005;76:1204–1210.
11 Weintraub D, Newberg AB, Cary MS, et al: Striatal dopamine transporter imaging correlates with anxiety and depression symptoms in Parkinson's disease. J Nucl Med 2005;46:227–232.
12 Koerts J, Leenders KL, Koning M, Portman AT, van Beilen M: Striatal dopaminergic activity (FDOPA-PET) associated with cognitive items of a depression scale (MADRS) in Parkinson's disease. Eur J Neurosci 2007;25: 3132–3136.
13 Rektorová I, Rektor I, Bares M, et al: Pramipexole and pergolide in the treatment of depression in Parkinson's disease: a national multi-centre prospective randomized study. Eur J Neurol 2003;10:399–406.
14 Rektorova I, Balaz M, Svatova J, et al: Effects of ropinirole on nonmotor symptoms of Parkinson disease: a prospective multicenter study. Clin Neuropharmacol 2008;31:261–266.
15 Rektorová I, Rektor I, Bares M, et al: Cognitive performance in people with Parkinson's disease and mild or moderate depression: effects of dopamine agonists in an add-on to L-dopa therapy. Eur J Neurol 2005;12:9–15.
16 Lemke MR, Brecht HM, Koester J, Kraus PH, Reichmann H: Anhedonia, depression, and motor functioning in Parkinson's disease during treatment with pramipexole. J Neuropsychiatry Clin Neurosci 2005;17:214–220.
17 Barone P, Scarzella L, Marconi R, et al: Pramipexole versus sertraline in the treatment of depression in Parkinson's disease. A national multicenter parallel-group randomized study. J Neurol 2006;253:555–561.
18 Pahwa R, Stacy MA, Factor SA, et al: Ropinirole 24-hour prolonged release: randomized, controlled study in advanced Parkinson's disease. Neurology 2007;68:1108–1115.
19 Kulisevsky J, García-Sánchez C, Berthier ML, et al: Chronic effects of dopaminergic replacement on cognitive function in Parkinson's disease: a two-year follow-up study of previously untreated patients. Mov Disord 2000;15:613–626.
20 Cools R: Dopaminergic modulation of cognitive function-implications for L-DOPA treatment in Parkinson's disease. Neurosci Biobehav Rev 2006;30:1–23.
21 Nieoullon A: Dopamine and the regulation of cognition and attention. Prog Neurobiol 2002;67:53–83.

Neurodegenerative Diseases

Neurodegenerative Dis 2010;7:210–212
DOI: 10.1159/000295666

Published online: March 12, 2010

Future Strategies for Neuroprotection in Parkinson's Disease

Anthony H.V. Schapira

Department of Clinical Neurosciences, Institute of Neurology, University College London, London, UK

Key Words
Parkinson's disease · Mitochondria · Oxidative stress · α-Synuclein · Phosphorylation

Abstract
The development of a drug or combination of drugs to slow or stop the progression of Parkinson's disease is the most important goal in this disease area. An understanding of the complex etiology and pathogenesis of the disorder is essential in this process. However, the current pathways to disease pathogenesis identified from the genetic causes of Parkinson's disease offer optimism in the sense that they appear to converge and interconnect rather than diverge. Problems include the limited applicability of current models and the ability to test drugs at the right dose in clinical trials with suitable end points. Trials conducted so far have provided some indication of a positive effect, although the mechanism underlying this is not yet known.

Introduction

It is generally accepted that the ability to slow, or preferably stop the progress of Parkinson's disease (PD) is a major unmet need. The motor symptoms and other symptoms of PD that are a consequence of dopaminergic cell loss are generally amenable to therapeutic intervention with levodopa, dopamine agonists or monoamine oxidase inhibitors [1]. These drugs are likely to be used in combination with advancing disease and the emergence of levodopa-related motor complications [2, 3]. However, the progressive loss of dopaminergic and other neuronal populations result in symptoms increasingly refractory to treatment. These features dominate the later stages of PD and lead to considerable impairment of quality of life [4].

It is reasonable to presume that effective treatments to slow progression in PD will be the result of a better understanding of the etiology and pathogenesis of the disease [5]. There have been several reviews on the topic of the causation of PD [6–8]. There is increasing evidence that although there may be several different causes of PD, they appear to mediate neuronal cell dysfunction and death through converging pathways, and these pathways are interconnected at strategic points. This is important for the future development of drug interventions and is discussed below.

Pathways to PD

Mitochondria play fundamental roles in energy production, free radical production and apoptosis. Defects of mitochondria have therefore been associated with neuromuscular disorders [9], in free radical-mediated damage that is also present in PD brain [10], in association with apoptosis and complex I inhibitors [11] and in conditions of primary oxidative damage [12]. Mitochondrial dys-

KARGER

Fax +41 61 306 12 34
E-Mail karger@karger.ch
www.karger.com

1660–2854/10/0073–0210$26.00/0

Accessible online at:
www.karger.com/ndd

Prof. A. Schapira
Department of Clinical Neurosciences, Institute of Neurology
University College London, Rowland Hill Street
London, NW3 2PF (UK)
Tel. +44 20 7830 2012, Fax +44 20 7472 6829, E-Mail a.schapira@medsch.ucl.ac.uk

function in the form of complex I deficiency was the first evidence for a bioenergetic defect in PD [13, 14] and was found to have specificity within the brain for the substantia nigra [15], although peripheral tissues do express mitochondrial abnormalities in a proportion of cases [16]. Parkin mutations have been associated with mitochondrial structural and functional defects in patients and animal models, and parkin protein has recently been confirmed to have a mitochondrial localization and to regulate mitochondrial DNA function and mitochondrial morphology [17–19]. Furthermore, parkin is selectively recruited to dysfunctional mitochondria with low membrane potential and mediates the destruction of the organelle by autophagy (mitophagy) [20]. PTEN-induced kinase 1 *(PINK1)* gene mutations induce a reduction of mitochondrial DNA, defective ATP production, impaired mitochondrial calcium handling and increased free radical generation, which in turn result in a fall in mitochondrial membrane potential and an increased susceptibility to apoptosis in neuronal cells and patient-derived fibroblasts [21–24]. Overexpression of parkin protein can rescue *PINK1* mutation effects in *Drosophila*, suggesting participation in related pathways [25].

Another important and related area of pathogenesis is that of protein aggregation. The presence of α-synuclein-rich Lewy bodies indicated an abnormality of protein handling that may reflect a toxic process or potentially a successful response to an increase in the protofibrillar form of the protein. It is notable that the majority of α-synuclein in Lewy bodies is phosphorylated and that this is of relevance to the free radical pathway that also is active in the PD nigra [26]. The issue of post-translational modification of proteins, particularly in the context of phosphorylation is emerging as important given that both *PINK1* and *LRRK2* are kinases. Indeed, the kinase activity of *LRRK2* is already considered a drug target for PD neuroprotection.

Clinical Trials

Monoamine oxidase B inhibitors have shown promise in the laboratory and the clinic. Selegiline was the first to be tested and was successful in delaying the need for levodopa, although the interpretation of the study was confounded by the symptomatic effects of selegiline. Rasagiline has shown benefit in a delayed start design, and the 1-mg dose of this drug has recently been shown to improve motor outcome if given earlier as opposed to 9 months later. The dopamine agonists pramipexole and ropinirole have both shown that compared to levodopa they can slow the loss of dopaminergic neurons as determined by PET or SPECT. However, these studies too have been the subject of debate regarding interpretation. Several other drugs have been tested for neuroprotective properties, but with varying results [for review see 27–29].

In conclusion, insight into the etiology of PD is likely to provide novel targets for drug action in PD neuroprotection, and an important next step is to develop a clear understanding of the means by which such drugs can be tested in the clinic.

References

1 Chaudhuri KR, Schapira AH: Non-motor symptoms of Parkinson's disease: dopaminergic pathophysiology and treatment. Lancet Neurol 2009;8:464–474.
2 Schapira AH, Emre M, Jenner P, Poewe W: Levodopa in the treatment of Parkinson's disease. Eur J Neurol 2009;16:982–989.
3 Schapira AH: Treatment options in the modern management of Parkinson disease. Arch Neurol 2007;64:1083–1088.
4 Chaudhuri KR, Healy DG, Schapira AH: Non-motor symptoms of Parkinson's disease: diagnosis and management. Lancet Neurol 2006;5:235–245.
5 Schapira AH, Agid Y, Barone P, Jenner P, Lemke MR, Poewe W, Rascol O, Reichmann H, Tolosa E: Perspectives on recent advances in the understanding and treatment of Parkinson's disease. Eur J Neurol 2009;16:1090–1099.
6 Schapira AH: Molecular and clinical pathways to neuroprotection of dopaminergic drugs in Parkinson disease. Neurology 2009;72:S44–S50.
7 Schapira AH: Neurobiology and treatment of Parkinson's disease. Trends Pharmacol Sci 2009;30:41–47.
8 Schapira AH: Mitochondria in the aetiology and pathogenesis of Parkinson's disease. Lancet Neurol 2008;7:97–109.
9 Morgan-Hughes JA, Schapira AH, Cooper JM, Clark JB: Molecular defects of NADH-ubiquinone oxidoreductase (complex I) in mitochondrial diseases. J Bioenerg Biomembr 1988;20:365–382.
10 Owen AD, Schapira AH, Jenner P, Marsden CD: Oxidative stress and Parkinson's disease. Ann NY Acad Sci 1996;786:217–223.
11 Seaton TA, Cooper JM, Schapira AH: Cyclosporin inhibition of apoptosis induced by mitochondrial complex I toxins. Brain Res 1998;809:12–17.
12 Thomas PK, Cooper JM, King RH, Workman JM, Schapira AH, Goss-Sampson MA, Muller DP: Myopathy in vitamin E deficient rats: muscle fibre necrosis associated with disturbances of mitochondrial function. J Anat 1993;183:451–461.
13 Schapira AH, Cooper JM, Dexter D, Jenner P, Clark JB, Marsden CD: Mitochondrial complex I deficiency in Parkinson's disease. Lancet 1989;1:1269.
14 Schapira AH, Cooper JM, Dexter D, Clark JB, Jenner P, Marsden CD: Mitochondrial complex I deficiency in Parkinson's disease. J Neurochem 1990;54:823–827.

15 Schapira AH, Mann VM, Cooper JM, Dexter D, Daniel SE, Jenner P, Clark JB, Marsden CD: Anatomic and disease specificity of NADH CoQ1 reductase (complex I) deficiency in Parkinson's disease. J Neurochem 1990;55:2142–2145.
16 Schapira AH: Evidence for mitochondrial dysfunction in Parkinson's disease – a critical appraisal. Mov Disord 1994;9:125–138.
17 Kuroda Y, Mitsui T, Kunishige M, Shono M, Akaike M, Azuma H, Matsumoto T: Parkin enhances mitochondrial biogenesis in proliferating cells. Hum Mol Genet 2006;15: 883–895.
18 Poole AC, Thomas RE, Andrews LA, McBride HM, Whitworth AJ, Pallanck LJ: The PINK1/Parkin pathway regulates mitochondrial morphology. Proc Natl Acad Sci USA 2008;105:1638–1643.
19 Deng H, Dodson MW, Huang H, Guo M: The Parkinson's disease genes pink1 and parkin promote mitochondrial fission and/or inhibit fusion in *Drosophila*. Proc Natl Acad Sci USA 2008;105:14503–14508.
20 Narendra D, Tanaka A, Suen DF, Youle RJ: Parkin is recruited selectively to impaired mitochondria and promotes their autophagy. J Cell Biol 2008;183:795–803.
21 Gegg ME, Cooper JM, Schapira AH, Taanman JW: Silencing of PINK1 expression affects mitochondrial DNA and oxidative phosphorylation in dopaminergic cells. PLoS One 2009;4:e4756.
22 Grunewald A, Gegg ME, Taanman JW, King RH, Kock N, Klein C, Schapira AH: Differential effects of PINK1 nonsense and missense mutations on mitochondrial function and morphology. Exp Neurol 2009;219:266–273.
23 Gandhi S, Wood-Kaczmar A, Yao Z, Plun-Favreau H, Deas E, Klupsch K, Downward J, Latchman DS, Tabrizi SJ, Wood NW, Duchen MR, Abramov AY: PINK1-associated Parkinson's disease is caused by neuronal vulnerability to calcium-induced cell death. Mol Cell 2009;33:627–638.
24 Morais VA, Verstreken P, Roethig A, Smet J, Snellinx A, Vanbrabant M, Haddad D, Frezza C, Mandemakers W, Vogt-Weisenhorn D, Van Coster R, Wurst W, Scorrano L, De Strooper B: Parkinson's disease mutations in PINK1 result in decreased Complex 1 activity and deficient synaptic function. EMBO Mol Med 2009;1:99–111.
25 Park J, Lee SB, Lee S, Kim Y, Song S, Kim S, Bae E, Kim J, Shong M, Kim JM, Chung J: Mitochondrial dysfunction in *Drosophila* PINK1 mutants is complemented by parkin. Nature 2006;441:1157–1161.
26 Chau KY, Ching HL, Schapira AH, Cooper JM: Relationship between alpha synuclein phosphorylation, proteasomal inhibition and cell death: relevance to Parkinson's disease pathogenesis. J Neurochem 2009;110: 1005–1013.
27 Olanow CW, Kieburtz K, Schapira AH: Why have we failed to achieve neuroprotection in Parkinson's disease? Ann Neurol 2008; 64(suppl 2):S101–S110.
28 Olanow CW, Schapira AH, LeWitt PA, Kieburtz K, Sauer D, Olivieri G, Pohlmann H, Hubble J: TCH346 as a neuroprotective drug in Parkinson's disease: a double-blind, randomised, controlled trial. Lancet Neurol 2006;5:1013–1020.
29 Schapira AH, Bezard E, Brotchie J, Calon F, Collingridge GL, Ferger B, Hengerer B, Hirsch E, Jenner P, Le NN, Obeso JA, Schwarzschild MA, Spampinato U, Davidai G: Novel pharmacological targets for the treatment of Parkinson's disease. Nat Rev Drug Discov 2006;5:845–854.

Neuro-degenerative Diseases

Neurodegenerative Dis 2010;7:213–215
DOI: 10.1159/000295667

Published online: March 12, 2010

The Concept of Continuous Dopaminergic Stimulation: What We Should Consider when Starting Parkinson's Disease Treatment

Fabrizio Stocchi

Department of Neurology, Institute of Research and Medical Care IRCCS San Raffaele, Rome, Italy

Key Words
Continuous dopaminergic stimulation · Dopamine agonists · Parkinson's disease · Early Parkinson's disease treatment · Rasagiline · Ropinirole · Rotigotine

Abstract
Treatment of early Parkinson's disease (PD) should pursue objectives like possible disease-modifying effect, more physiological dopaminergic stimulation, and avoidance of motor fluctuations. The recent published ADAGIO trial showed that rasagiline (1 mg/day), used in early PD, has a disease-modifying effect. Dopaminergic drugs administered to provide more continuous dopaminergic stimulation prevent or minimize motor fluctuations in experimental animals. Dopamine (DA) agonists delay motor fluctuations in humans providing a more continuous dopaminergic stimulation. New formulations of DA agonists, such as once a day preparations and patch technology, have been developed to provide a more continuous delivery of drug and consequently a more physiological stimulation. According to patient characteristics, treatment of PD should be started with rasagiline and/or with long-acting DA agonists.

Introduction

When treatment of Parkinson's disease (PD) is introduced, there are some criteria to consider and objectives to pursue: patient characteristics (age, severity of disease, more affected site, cognitive status, job) and balance between symptomatic improvement and possible side effects; presence of non-motor symptoms and quality of life should also be taken into account. Modification of natural disease progression, improvement of symptoms and quality of life, induction of a physiological dopaminergic stimulation, avoidance or delay of complications and dyskinesia, patient compliance, and minimizing side effects are the objectives of good treatment. In this paper, treatment choices that pursue the objectives mentioned above are illustrated.

Disease-Modifying Effect

Modification of the natural course of the disease is a primary goal in the treatment of PD. Many studies with different agents had been conducted over the past 20 years with the aim to demonstrate neuroprotection. Unfortunately, for many different reasons all of them failed. Recently, a study using a novel study design showed a disease-modifying effect of rasagiline in patients with early PD. The study (ADAGIO) was a randomized double-

KARGER

Fax +41 61 306 12 34
E-Mail karger@karger.ch
www.karger.com

1660–2854/10/0073–0213$26.00/0

Accessible online at:
www.karger.com/ndd

Fabrizio Stocchi, MD, PhD
IRCCS San Raffaele
Via della Pisana 235
IT–00163 Rome (Italy)
Tel. +39 06 6605 8456, Fax +39 06 789 158, E-Mail fabrizio.stocchi@sanraffaele.it

blind trial using the delayed start design and a novel analytical approach to prospectively examine the possibility that the compound has disease-modifying effects in PD [1].

The delayed start design has been developed to avoid the possibility of a symptomatic confounding when testing putative disease-modifying therapies. 1,176 untreated patients with PD participated in the study and were randomized to receive rasagiline (1 or 2 mg/day) for 72 weeks (early start) or placebo for 36 weeks followed by rasagiline (1 or 2 mg/day) for 36 weeks (delayed start). The primary analysis included three hierarchical endpoints based on the total Unified Parkinson Disease Rating Scale score comparing the early with delayed start groups: (a) superiority in slope of progression between weeks 12–36; (b) superiority in change from baseline to week 72, and (c) noninferiority of slope during weeks 48–72. Rasagiline (1 mg/day) met all three primary endpoints. The 2 mg/day dose did not meet all endpoints [1]. The results of the ADAGIO trial should be taken into account when the diagnosis of PD is made and rasagiline considered as the drug to start the treatment in the early stage, considering that it also has symptomatic effects [2].

Whenever a drug with stronger symptomatic effect is needed, immediately or during the course of the disease, the drug of choice should ensure a continuous dopaminergic stimulation (CDS) to reduce the risk of motor complications.

Continuous Dopaminergic Stimulation

Substantia nigra pars compacta dopaminergic neurons can fire both tonically and phasically (i.e. bursting), but striatal and synaptic dopamine (DA) are normally maintained at relatively constant levels [3]. DA acts presynaptically to modulate the glutamate-mediated excitability of medium spiny striatal neurons (in both up and down directions) so as to further maintain the stability of the basal ganglia network [4]. Under normal circumstances, DA neurons fire continuously at a rate of about 3–4 cycles per second, independent of movement, and dopaminergic receptors are continuously stimulated.

The situation changes when there is degeneration of substantia nigra pars compacta dopaminergic neurons, as in PD. In the DA-depleted state, striatal DA levels become increasingly dependent on the peripheral availability of levodopa. In this setting, fluctuations in plasma levels of levodopa may be directly translated into fluctuations in striatal levels of DA; intermittent doses of a standard short-acting oral formulation of levodopa do not fully restore the DA-denervated basal ganglia to normal. Repeated oral doses of short-acting levodopa result in marked oscillations in the plasma levodopa concentration, as well as in striatal and synaptic DA levels of PD patients, as illustrated by microdialysis and amperometry in rodents and [^{11}C]raclopride-PET [5]. In this situation, striatal DA receptors are no longer exposed to relatively constant DA levels as they would be in a normal situation, but rather to alternating high and low concentrations of DA. This intermittent or discontinuous activation of DA receptors is known as pulsatile stimulation, and further destabilizes the already unstable DA-denervated basal ganglia. Over time, this pulsatile stimulation is associated with gene and protein changes in striatal neurons, altered firing patterns in basal ganglia output neurons, and the development of motor complications [5, 6].

The deleterious effect of abnormal, nonphysiological pulsatile stimulation of DA receptors has been demonstrated in animal models of PD. In an MPTP-lesioned monkey, treatment with either levodopa or a short-acting DA agonist induces behavioral benefits which are complicated by the rapid onset of severe dyskinesia. In contrast, treatment with a long-acting DA agonist provides comparable benefit, but this is associated with much less or even no dyskinesia. The differences between pulsatile and continuous infusion are particularly well illustrated in experiments in which intermittent doses of a short-acting DA agonist are shown to induce dyskinesia, while continuous infusion of the same drug administered in the same dose provides comparable benefits without dyskinesia [7].

CDS-based therapies have been shown to reduce the risk of developing motor complications when used as initial therapy in untreated PD patients. Several prospective, double-blind trials have compared the time at onset of motor complications in untreated PD patients randomized to initiate therapy with a standard, oral, short-acting formulation of levodopa compared with a long-acting DA agonist [8]. In each of these studies, the time at onset of dyskinesia and/or wearing off was significantly delayed in patients receiving initial treatment with a long-acting DA agonist, even though patients in both groups could receive supplemental therapy with open-label levodopa if required.

DA Agonists as Early Monotherapy

Based on a consistent body of evidence from randomized controlled trials, the DA agonists dihydroergocryptine, pergolide, pramipexole, and ropinirole have all been assessed as effective monotherapy in early PD [8]. For methodological reasons, such evidence was found less strong for bromocriptine, cabergoline and lisuride [9], and recently placebo-controlled trials have also shown efficacy of rotigotine [10] and piribedil [11] in early disease. Importantly, cabergoline, pergolide, pramipexole and ropinirole have also been tested against levodopa in large randomized trials. These trials have all demonstrated a significantly reduced risk of motor complications, in particular dyskinesias, over double-blind follow-up periods of up to 5 years. At the same time, symptomatic effect size, as assessed by the Unified Parkinson Disease Rating Scale, was consistently greater for levodopa.

DA agonists remain the best therapeutic option to provide CDS in the early stage of the disease. New formulations of DA agonists are now available. These formulations (oral prolonged release and patch technology) have made these drugs easier to use, and ensure a more continuous dopaminergic stimulation. Ropinirole PR (prolonged release) has been successfully tested in patients at different stages of their disease. In a non-inferiority study, ropinirole PR was shown, to be as efficacious as ropinirole IR (immediate release) in de novo patients, but the titration was easier and the once-a-day tablet offered a clear advantage for the patients and increased their compliance with the treatment [12].

Rotigotine is a novel non-ergot DA agonist which is administered transdermally using patch technology. The patch ensures a stable plasma level of rotigotine over 24 h. In controlled trials, rotigotine monotherapy proved to be efficacious in the treatment of early parkinsonian patients [10]. Studies with a prolonged release preparation of pramipexole are ongoing.

Conclusion

When treatment of PD is initiated, patient characteristics should be considered and objectives such as disease modifications and avoidance of motor complications pursued. The ADAGIO trial showed that rasagiline (1 mg) administered in the early stage of PD has a disease-modifying action and a symptomatic effect; therefore, it should be considered when starting treatment. When starting treatment with a dopaminergic drug, those able to provide a more physiological dopaminergic stimulation should be taken into account because they may avoid or delay motor complications. In the early stage of the disease, DA agonists have been used in monotherapy and they proved to delay motor complications. The new long-acting formulations of DA agonists are more convenient for patients, and can provide CDS.

References

1 Olanow CW, Rascol O, Hauser R, et al: A double-blind, delayed-start trial of rasagiline in Parkinson's disease. N Engl J Med 2009;361:1268–1278.

2 Stocchi F: Rasagiline: defining the role of a novel therapy in the treatment of Parkinson's disease. Int J Clin Pract 2006;60:215–221.

3 Bamford NS, Robinson S, Palmiter RD, Joyce JA, Moore C, Meshul CK: Dopamine modulates release from corticostriatal terminals. J Neurosci 2004;24:9541–9552.

4 Rodriguez M, Gonzalez J, Sabate M, Obeso J, Pereda E: Firing regulation in dopaminergic cells: effect of the partial degeneration of nigrostriatal system in surviving neurons. Eur J Neurosci 2003;18:53–60.

5 Olanow CW, Obeso JA, Stocchi F: Continuous dopamine-receptor treatment of Parkinson's disease: scientific rationale and clinical implications. Lancet Neurol 2006;5:677–687.

6 Jenner P: Factors influencing the onset and persistence of dyskinesia in MPTP-treated primates. Ann Neurol 2000;47:S90–S99.

7 Bibbiani F, Costantini LC, Patel R, Chase TN: Continuous dopaminergic stimulation reduces risk of motor complications in parkinsonian primates. Exp Neurol 2005;192:73–78.

8 Horstink M, Tolosa E, Bonuccelli U, Deuschl G, Friedman A, Kanovsky P, et al: Review of the therapeutic management of Parkinson's disease. Report of a joint task force of the European Federation of Neurological Societies and the Movement Disorder Society European Section. I. Early (uncomplicated) Parkinson's disease. Eur J Neurol 2006;13:1170–1185.

9 Goetz CG, Poewe W, Rascol O, Sampaio C: Evidence-based medical review update: pharmacological and surgical treatments of Parkinson's disease: 2001 to 2004. Mov Disord 2005;20:523–539.

10 Jankovic J, Watts RL, Martin W, Boroojerdi B: Transdermal rotigotine: double-blind, placebo-controlled trial in Parkinson disease. Arch Neurol 2007;64:676–682.

11 Rascol O, Dubois B, Caldas AC, Senn S, Del Signore S, Lees A: Early piribedil monotherapy of Parkinson's disease: a planned seven-month report of the REGAIN study. Mov Disord 2006;21:2110–2115.

12 Stocchi F, Hersh BP, Scott BL, Nausieda PA, Giorgi L, Ease-PD Monotherapy Study Investigators: Ropinirole 24-hour prolonged release and ropinirole immediate release in early Parkinson's disease: a randomized, double-blind, non-inferiority crossover study. Curr Med Res Opin 2008;24:2883–2895.

Neuro-degenerative Diseases

Author Index Vol. 7, No. 1–3, 2010

Aguilar, M.-I. 187
Albinson, K. 153
Alves da Costa, C. 50
Andel, R. 148
Avila, J. 13

Baker, M. 170
Baláž, M. 160
Barcikowska, M. 143
Belinson, H. 16
Berson, A. 60
Berti, V. 131
Bočková, M. 160
Bonini, S.A. 143
Brouillette, J. 88
Bruno, M.A. 96

Cacabelos, R. 167
Canneva, F. 96
Cavalieri, M. 122
Cenini, G. 143
Chabot, J.-G. 88
Chan, D. 68
Checler, F. 50
Choi, S.H. 46
Comery, T.A. 153
Connor, D.J. 183
Cornelli, U. 193
Cuello, A.C. 96

de la Torre, J.C. 116
de Leon, M.J. 131
De Santi, S. 131
Dennissen, F.J.A. 76
Dickson, D.W. 170, 175
Dimant, H. 203
Doggui, S. 88
Ducatenzeiler, A. 96
Dunys, J. 50

Eckert, A. 10
Eikelenboom, P. 38
Endres, K. 190
Engel, T. 13
Enzinger, C. 122

Fahrenholz, F. 190
Farso, M. 88
Fazekas, F. 122
Ferretti, M.T. 96
Fisher, A. 5
Fishman-Jacob, T. 108
Foa, L. 187
Fuster-Matanzo, A. 13

Gasperini, R. 187
Gómez de Barreda, E. 13
Goñi-Oliver, P. 13
Götz, J. 10
Greenberg, D.S. 60
Grossardt, B.R. 163

Haass, C. 99
Hanin, I. 5
Hernández, F. 13
Homayoon, N. 122
Hoozemans, J.J.M. 38
Hort, J. 148
Hsu, C.H. 68
Hung, A.C. 187

Inbar, D. 16
Ittner, L.M. 10
Iulita, M.F. 96

Jellinger, K.A. 112

Kalvach, P. 6
Kalvach, Z. 6
Ke, Y.D. 10
Kholod, N. 76
Kivipelto, M. 180
Klaver, D. 187
Korczyn, A.D. 127
Kovacech, B. 24
Krüger, U. 103
Kryscio, R.J. 183
Kubek, K. 153

Laatikainen, T. 180
Laczó, J. 148
Leddy, L. 153
Leon, W.C. 96
Leurgans, S. 139
Li, Y. 131
Liebsack, C. 183
Lim, Y.-A. 10
Lin, Y. 183
Lucas, J.J. 13

Magerova, H. 148
Mandel, S.A. 108
Mandelkow, E. 103
Mandelkow, E.-M. 28, 103
Martín-Maestro, P. 13
Melis, T. 96
Memo, M. 143
Michaelson, D.M. 16
Monaghan, M.M. 153
Mosconi, L. 131
Mufson, E.J. 139

Nagatsu, T. 64
Nitsch, R. 5
Nordberg, A. 136
Novak, M. 24

Okochi, M. 42
Osorio, R.S. 131

Pangalos, M.N. 153
Paquet, D. 99
Pardossi-Piquard, R. 50
Pérez, M. 13
Perry, G. 56
Petrovic, K. 122
Pluta-Fuerst, A. 122

Quirion, R. 88

Rademakers, R. 170
Reinhart, P.H. 153
Rektor, I. 160
Rektorová, I. 206
Robakis, N.K. 32
Rocca, W.A. 163
Rosenman, H. 16
Rozemuller, A.J.M. 38

Sabbagh, M.N. 183
Sawada, H. 64
Sawada, M. 64
Schapira, A.H.V. 210
Schmid, B. 99
Schmidt, H. 122
Schmidt, R. 122
Shen, J. 80
Shuster, L.T. 163
Sippola, R. 180
Sisodia, S.S. 46
Skrabana, R. 24
Small, D.H. 187
Smith, M.A. 56
Soininen, H. 180
Solomon, A. 180
Solomon, B. 203
Soreq, H. 60
Sparks, D.L. 183
Sparks, L.M. 183
Steinbusch, H.W.M. 76
Stocchi, F. 213
Styczynska, M. 143
Sugaya, K. 84
Sung, M.-L.A. 153
Suzuki, H. 64
Sydow, A. 28
Szybinska, A. 143

Tagami, S. 42
Takeda, M. 42
Tippmann, F. 190
Toiber, D. 60
Tolar, M. 148
Tuomilehto, J. 180

Uberti, D. 143

van Exel, E. 38
van Gool, W.A. 38
Van Leeuwen, F.W. 76
Varjassyova, A. 148
Veeraraghavalu, K. 46
Veerhuis, R. 38
Vlcek, K. 148
Vyhnalek, M. 148

Wang, X. 56
Wang, Y. 103
Wider, C. 175
Windisch, M. 5
Wolozin, B. 68, 180
Wszolek, Z.K. 175

Youdim, M.B.H. 108

Zaleska, M.M. 153
Zhu, X. 56

KARGER
Fax +41 61 306 12 34
E-Mail karger@karger.ch
www.karger.com

Accessible online at:
www.karger.com/ndd

Neuro-degenerative Diseases

Acetylcholinesterase 60
Acute phase reactants 38
Adult hippocampal neurogenesis 46
Age-related neurodegeneration 80
Aggregation 28
Alzheimer('s) disease 10, 13, 16, 24, 28, 32, 38, 50, 56, 60, 88, 96, 99, 103, 112, 136, 148, 167, 170, 183, 190, 193
– – biomarker(s) 42, 131, 139
Amyloid 60, 187
– cascade 16
– imaging 136
– lesions 131
– β-peptides 50
– precursor protein 32, 76, 84
– precursor-like protein 1 42
Amyloid-β peptide 42 42
β-Amyloid 38
Apolipoprotein E 16, 148, 167
Apoptosis 60
Autocatalysis 187
Autophagy 103
Axonal transport 10, 56
Aβ oligomers and minocycline 96
– peptides 32
Aβ-derived diffusible ligands 56

Basal ganglia 160
Biomarkers 167
Brain imaging 122

Cardiovascular disease 116
Carotid artery stenosis 116
– – ultrasound 116
Caspases 60
CD44 gene 143
Cell culture model 108
– cycle 108
Central nervous system 96
Cerebral hypoperfusion 116
Cerebrospinal fluid 42
Cerebrovascular lesions 112
Cholesterol 183
c-jun NH2-terminal kinase 68
Cognition 206
Cognitive activities 160
– impairment 163
Conformational change 24
Continuous dopaminergic stimulation 213
CSF biomarkers 136
Cytokines 38
Czech psychiatry 6

Dementia 127, 163
– prevention 180
– research 6
– with Lewy bodies 112
Dentate gyrus 13
Deposition of β-amyloid 88
Depression 206
Diagnostic criteria 122
Disaggregation 203
Disintegrin metalloproteinase ADAM10 190
Dopamine agonists 206, 213
Dopaminergic markers 108
d-ROMs test 193
Drug screening 99

Early diagnostic markers 136
– – tools 131
– Parkinson's disease treatment 213
Echocardiography 116
Enriched environment 46
Estrogen 163
Ethanol 64
Event-related desynchronization/synchronization 160

Filamentous phages 203
FINRISK study 180
Frontotemporal dementia 10, 99
Functional imaging 206

Gal4-UAS 99
Glutathione 193
Glycosaminoglycan 187
GSK3 activity 13

Heparin 187
Hippocampal sclerosis 170
Homocysteine 193
Human amyloid precursor protein transgenic mouse 88

Immunohistochemistry 170
Immunoprecipitation 68
Inflammaging 38
Inflammation 96
Innate immunity 38
Intima media thickness 116
Intracellular Aβ 96
Intrinsically disordered tau 24
Isoprostane 139

Kinesin 10

Leucine-rich repeat kinase 2 gene 175
Lewy body disease 112, 175
Lipid-lowering agents 183
– drugs 180
Lymphocyte 143

MAP kinase 68
Membrane α-synuclein 203
Memory 153
Menopause 163
1-Methyl-4-phenyl-1,2,3,6-tetrahydropyridine 64
Microglia 38, 46, 64
Mild cognitive impairment 136, 139, 148, 183
Mitochondria 56, 210
Molecular misreading 76
Morris water maze 88
MPTP 153

Neonatal mice 64
Neprilysin 16
Neural stem cell 84
Neuroinflammation 60
Neuronal loss 32
Neuroprotection 163
Nicastrin 80
Nigral degeneration 175

Olfaction 153
Oligomer 10
Oophorectomy 163
Oxidative stress 139, 210

P3-like potential 160
Paired helical filaments 103
Parkin 80
Parkinson('s) disease 68, 112, 127, 153, 175, 206, 210, 213
Peripheral marker 143
PET neuroimaging 131
Pharmacogenomics 167
Phosphorylation 210
Pittsburgh compound B 136
Positron emission tomography 136
Prague 6
Presenilin 50, 80
Presenilin 1 46
Progranulin gene 170
Progressive supranuclear gaze palsy 175
Promoter activity 190
Protein aggregation 103
– quality control 76
Proteolysis 103

Rasagiline 213
Reelin 84
Retinoids 190
Ropinirole 213
Rotigotine 213

Scaffold proteins 68
Secretase 187
γ-Secretase complex 50
Senile plaques 6
Short hairpin RNA 108
SH-SY5Y cells 203
Sickle erythrocytes 193
SKP1, Cullin, F-box complex 108
Spatial learning 88
– memory 148
Sporadic Parkinson's disease 108
St. Catherine asylum 6
Subthalamic nucleus 160
Surrogate marker 122
Synapse 80
α-Synuclein 210

Tau 10, 13, 28, 99
– kinase I 13
– phosphorylation 16
– protein 103
– transition 24
Tauopathy 28
TgCRND8 mouse 88
Timing hypothesis 163
Transgenic mice 10
– mouse models 28
Transthyretin 88
Truncation 24
Tumor suppressor p53 50
Type 2 diabetes 10

Ubiquitin 76
Ubiquitin-proteasome system 76
Unfolded p53 isoform 143

Vascular dementia 122
– hypothesis of Alzheimer's disease 116
– lesions 127

Water maze task 148

Zebrafish 99

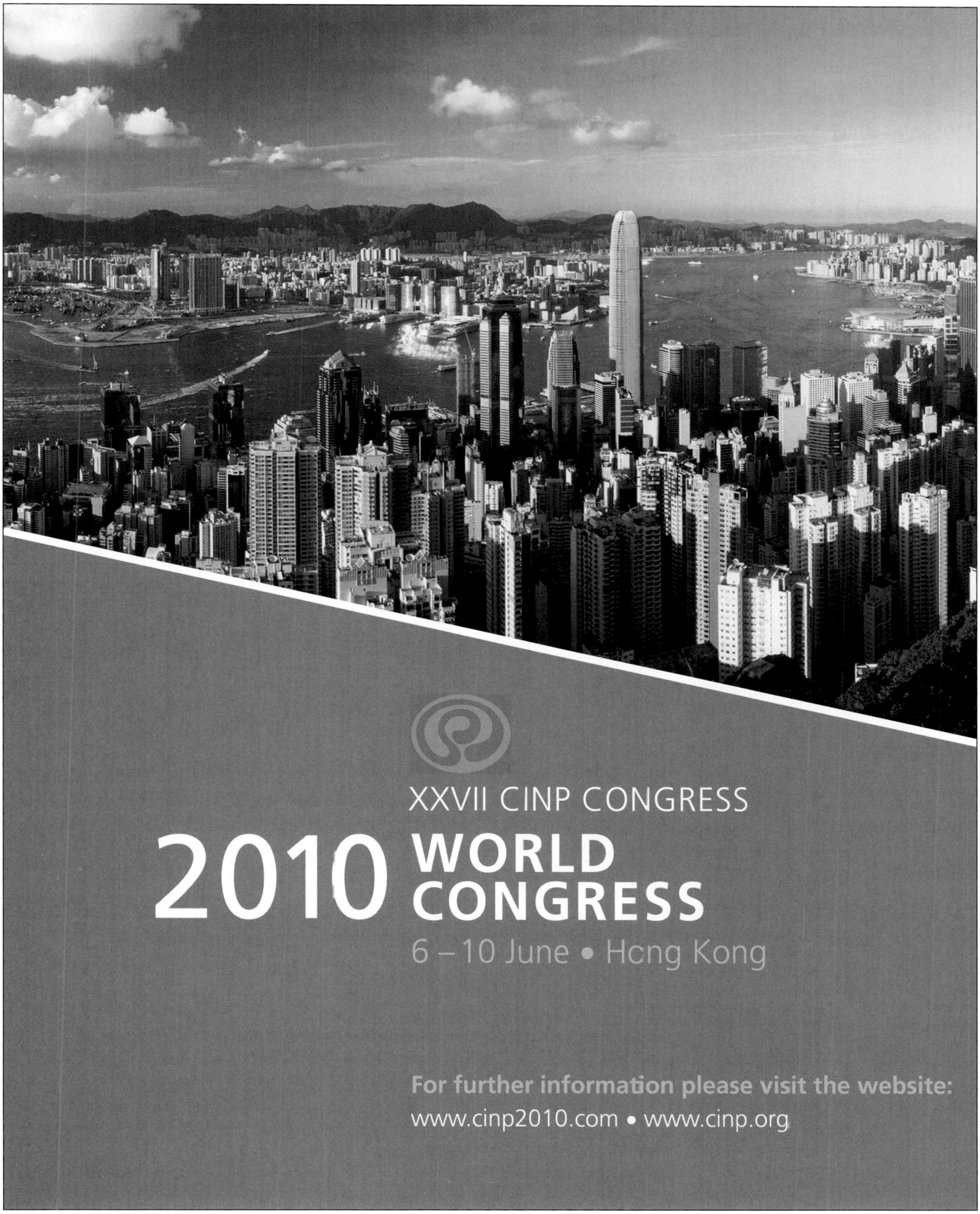
XXVII CINP CONGRESS
2010 WORLD CONGRESS
6 – 10 June • Hong Kong
For further information please visit the website:
www.cinp2010.com • www.cinp.org